Ultrasound Image Reduction Techniques: MATLAB and DSP Implementation

R. SIVAKUMAR

CONTENTS

CHAPTER NO.		TITLE	PAGE NO.
I		**INTRODUCTION**	1
	1.1	INTRODUCTION TO IMAGE PROCESSING	1
	1.2	OVERVIEW OF BIOMEDICAL IMAGE PROCESSING	2
		1.2.1 Image Enhancement	3
		1.2.2 Image Analysis	3
		1.2.3 Image Compression	4
		1.2.4 Image Synthesis	4
		1.2.5 Image Restoration	4
	1.3	IMAGE MODALITIES	5
		1.3.1 X-Ray Imaging	5
		1.3.2 Computed Tomography (CT)	6
		1.3.3 Magnetic Resonance Imaging (MRI)	7
		1.3.4 Positron Emission Tomography (PET)	7
		1.3.5 Single Photon Emission Computed Tomography (SPECT)	8
		1.3.6 Ultrasound Imaging	9
		1.3.6.1 Modes of Ultrasonography	10
	1.4	COMPARISON OF ULTRASOUND IMAGING WITH OTHER BIOMEDICAL IMAGING MODALITIES	12
	1.5	LIMITATIONS OF ULTRASOUND B-SCAN IMAGING	13
	1.6	SCOPE OF THE THESIS	14
II		**BACKGROUNG OF SPECKLE AND OVERVIEW OF DESPECKLING AND ITS PERFORMANCE ESTIMATION TECHNIQUES**	15
	2.1	BACKGROUND OF SPECKLE	15

2.2	MATHEMATICAL MOELING OF SPECKLE			16
2.3	SPECKLE PATTERN IN MEDICAL ULTRASOUND IMAGE			17
2.4	REVIEW OF LITERATURE IN SPECKLE REDUCTION TECHNIQUES			18
2.5	OVERVIEW OF DESPECKLING FILTERS			27
	2.5.1	Spatial Adaptive filters		28
		2.5.1.1	Frost filter	29
		2.5.1.2	Median filter	29
		2.5.1.3	Lee and Kuan filter	30
		2.5.1.4	Wiener filter	30
		2.5.1.5	Enhanced Frost and Enhanced Lee filter	31
		2.5.1.6	Gamma Map filter	32
		2.5.1.7	Homomorphic filter	32
	2.5.2	Wavelet Transform		33
		2.5.2.1	Continuous Wavelet Transform(CWT)	34
		2.5.2.2	Discrete Wavelet Transform(DWT)	34
		2.5.2.3	Wavelet Thresholding	35
	2.5.3	Diffusion filters		37
		2.5.3.1	Perona Malik Anisotropic Diffusion (PMAD) filter	37
		2.5.3.2	Speckle Reducing Anisotropic Diffusion(SRAD) filter	39
2.6	OVERVIEW OF IMAGE QUALITY MEASURES			41
2.7	EDGE DETECTION TECHNIQUES			44
2.8	EDGE DETECTION OPERATORS			46
	2.8.1	Sobel operator		46
	2.8.2	Robert's operator		47
	2.8.3	Prewitt's operator		48
	2.8.4	Laplacian of Gaussian operator		48
	2.8.5	Canny operator		50

III	**TOPOLOGICAL DERIVATIVE AND ITS SPECKLE NOISE REDUCTION APPLICATION IN ULTRASOUND B-SCAN IMAGES**		52
	3.1	INTRODUCTION	52
	3.2	BASIC CONCEPT OF TOPOLOGICAL DERIVATIVE	52
		3.2.1 Selection of cost function	56
	3.3	IMPLEMENTATION OF TOPOLOGICAL DERIVATIVE FOR DESPECKLING ULTRASOUND B-SCAN IMAGES	57
	3.4	ROLE OF TOPOLOGICAL DERIVATIVE IN IMAGE PROCESSING APPLICATIONS	58
IV	**EXPERIMENTAL SET-UP AND ULTROSOUND B-SCAN DATA USED FOR DEVELOPING AND TESTING SPECKLE REDUCTION ALGORITHMS**		59
	4.1	SPECIFICATION OF PCMAT SYSTEM	59
	4.2	IMAGE PROCESSING TOOLBOX IN MATLAB	60
	4.3	PROGRAMMING IN MATLAB	61
		4.3.1 Creating an M-File	61
		4.3.2 Compiling the M-File	62
	4.4	SPECIFICATION OF PCDSK SYSTEM	63
	4.5	DESCRIPTION OF TMS320C6713 DSP STARTER KIT	63
	4.6	OVERVIEW OF THE TMS320C6713 DSK	65
	4.7	MEMORY MAP	65
	4.8	CONFIGURABLE SWITCH SETTINGS	66
	4.9	POWER SUPPLY	66
	4.10	DESCRIPTION OF SOFTWARE DEVELOPMENT TOOLS	67
		4.10.1 Overview of Code Composer Studio(CCS)	67
		4.10.2 Program Development in the PCDSK System	67
	4.11	SPECIFICATION OF ULTRASOUNG B-SCAN DATA USED IN THIS STUDY	70

V	IMPLEMENTATION AND PERFORMANCE STUDY OF DESPECKLING FILTER ALGORITHMS IN THE PCMAT SYSTEM		71
	5.1	ALGORITHM INTRODUCTION	71
	5.2	TESTING DETAILS	71
	5.3	CASE STUDY	72
	5.4	DESCRIPTION OF THE DESPECKLING ALGORITHMS TESTED IN THE PCMAT SYSTEM	74
		5.4.1 Algorithm of Frost filter	76
		5.4.2 Algorithm of Median filter	76
		5.4.3 Algorithm of Lee filter	76
		5.4.4 Algorithm of Kuan filter	77
		5.4.5 Algorithm of Wiener filter	77
		5.4.6 Algorithm of Enhanced Frost filter	77
		5.4.7 Algorithm of Enhanced Lee filter	78
		5.4.8 Algorithm of Gamma Map filter	78
		5.4.9 Algorithm of Homomorphic filter	78
		5.4.10 Algorithm of Wavelet filter	79
		5.4.11 Algorithm of PMAD filter	79
		5.4.12 Algorithm of SRAD filter	79
		5.4.13 Algorithm of DTD filter	80
	5.5	DESCRIPTION OF THE EDGE DETECTION ALGORITHMS	80
		5.5.1 Algorithm of Sobel edge detection	80
		5.5.2 Algorithm of Robert's edge detection	81
		5.5.3 Algorithm of Prewitt's edge detection	81
		5.5.4 Algorithm of LoG edge detection	81
		5.5.5 Algorithm of Canny edge detection	82
	5.6	PERFORMANCE STUDY OF THE DESPECKLING FILTERS IN THE PCMAT SYSTEM	82
	5.7	DISCUSSION	93

VI	**IMPLEMENTATION AND PERFORMANCE STUDY OF DESPECKLING FILTER ALGORITHMS IN THE PCDSK SYSTEM**	116
	6.1 ALGORITHM INTRODUCTION	116
	6.2 DESCRIPTION OF DESPECKLING ALGORITHMS	116
	6.3 PERFORMANCE STUDY OF THE DESPECKLING FILTERS IN THE PCDSK SYSTEM	117
	6.4 DISCUSSION	129
VII	**CONCLUSIONS AND FUTURE SCOPE**	149

LIST OF ABBREVIATIONS

A-mode	-	Amplitude mode
AD	-	Average Difference
AIC	-	Analog Interface Chip
ANSI	-	American National Standard Institute
ARGF	-	Aggressive Region Growing Filter
ASNR	-	Average Signal to Noise Ratio
ASSF	-	Adaptive Speckle Suppression Filter
AWMF	-	Adaptive Weighted Median Filter
B-mode	-	Brightness mode
BIOS	-	Basic Input Output System
BMP	-	Bit Map Picture
CCS	-	Code Composer Studio
CNR	-	Contrast to Noise Ratio
COFF	-	Common Object File Format
CoC	-	Coefficient of Correlation
CPLD	-	Complex Programmable Logic Device
CT	-	Computed Tomography
CWT	-	Continuous Wavelet Transform
D-mode	-	Doppler mode
DCT	-	Discrete Cosine Transform
DeSpeRADO	-	Deconvolutional Speckle Reducing Anisotropic Diffusion
DRAM	-	Dynamic Random Access Memory
DSK	-	Digital Signal Processor Starter Kit
DTD	-	Discrete Topological Derivative
DWT	-	Discrete Wavelet Transform
EM	-	Electro Magnetic
EMIF	-	External Memory Interface
ENL	-	Effective Number of Looks
EPI	-	Edge Preservation Index
EVM	-	Evaluation Module
FFT	-	Fast Fourier Transform
FoM	-	Figure of Merit

FMRI	-	Functional Magnetic Resonance Imaging
GA	-	Genetic Algorithm
GAE	-	Geometric Average Error
GT	-	Gabor Transform
GUI	-	Graphical User Interface
HPI	-	Host Port Interface
HRGMF	-	Homogenous Region Growing Mean Filter
IDE	-	Integrated Development Environment
IQI	-	Image Quality Index
IRAM	-	Intelligent Random Access Memory
IV	-	Image Variance
JPEG	-	Joint Photographic Experts
JTAG	-	Joint Test Action Group
LED	-	Light Emitting Diode
LLMMSE	-	Local Linear Minimum Mean Square Errors
LMSE	-	Linear Minimum Mean Square Errors
LoG	-	Laplacian of Gaussian
LPND	-	Laplacian Pyramid Based Non linear Diffusion
LPNDSF	-	Laplacian Pyramid Based Non linear Diffusion and Shock Filter
LVQ	-	Learning Vector Quantifier
M-mode	-	Motion mode
MAP	-	Maximum A Posterior
MATLAB	-	Matrix Laboratory
McASP	-	Multichannel Audio Serial Port
MD	-	Maximum Difference
MMSE	-	Minimum Mean Squared Error
MNWD	-	Multiscale Nonlinear Wavelet Diffusion
MRI	-	Magnetic Resonance Imaging
MSE	-	Mean Square Error
MSSIM	-	Mean Structure Similarity Index Map
NAE	-	Normalized Absolute Error
NCC	-	Normalized Cross Correlation
ND	-	Nonlinear Diffusion
NMSE	-	Normalized Mean Square Error

NSD	-	Noise Standard Deviation
PC	-	Personal Computer
PCDSK	-	Personal Computer based Digital Signal Processor Starter Kit system
PCMAT	-	Personal Computer based MATLAB system
PDF	-	Probability Density Function
PDE	-	Partial Differential Equation
PET	-	Positron Emission Tomography
RGB	-	Red Green Blue
PMAD	-	Perona Malik Anisotropic Diffusion
PSNR	-	Peak Signal to Noise Ratio
RF	-	Radio Frequency
RTDX	-	Real time Data Exchange
SAR	-	Synthetic Aperture Radar
SBF	-	Squeeze Box Filter
SC	-	Structural Content
SDRAM	-	Synchronous Dynamic Random Access Memory
SI	-	Speckle Index
SND	-	Scatter Number Density
SNR	-	Signal to Noise Ratio
SNIG	-	Symmetrical Normal Inverse Gaussian
SPECT	-	Single Photon Emission Computed Tomography
SRAD	-	Speckle Reduction Anisotropic Diffusion
SSIM	-	Structure Similarity Index Map
SSRF	-	Symmetrical Speckle Reduction Filter
TDALMS	-	Two Dimensional Adaptive Least Mean Square
TI	-	Texas Instrument
US	-	Ultra Sound
USB	-	Universal Serial Bus
WT	-	Wavelet Transform
WS	-	Wavelet Series
ZAP	-	Zero adjustment procedure

LIST OF UNITS & SYMBOLS

Hz	-	Hertz
kHz	-	kilo Hertz
MHz	-	Mega Hertz
GHz	-	Giga Hertz
dB	-	Decibel
KB	-	Kilo Byte
MB	-	Mega Byte
GB	-	Giga Byte
mm	-	Millimeter
cm	-	Centimeter
FPS	-	Frames per Second
m/s	-	Meter per Second
min	-	Minute
2-D	-	Two Dimensional
3-D	-	Three Dimensional
Sec	-	Second
∇	-	Gradient operator
$\|\ \|$	-	Divergence operator
I/O	-	Input and Output
V	-	Volt
$\sim$	-	Approximately
μ	-	Mean
σ	-	Standard Deviation

FIGURE NO.	LIST OF FIGURES	PAGE NO.
Fig 1.1	Radiographic chest image	6
Fig 1.2	CT image of the Cardio vascular cavity of a cadaver	6
Fig 1.3	Axial, Coronal and Sagittal cross-section MR images of human brain	7
Fig 1.4	Sequence of axial PET images of human brain	8
Fig 1.5	SPECT image of a human brain	9
Fig 1.6	Instrumentation setup of the ultrasound imaging system	10
Fig 1.7	Typical B-Scan image setup	11
Fig 1.8	Diagrammatic representation of M-mode	11
Fig 1.9	Colour Doppler-mode image of a Fetus	12
Fig 2.1(a)	Noiseless ultrasound B-Scan image of kidney	15
Fig 2.1(b)	Noisy ultrasound B-Scan image of kidney	16
Fig 2.2	Representation of 3x3 kernel	28
Fig 2.3	Discrete wavelet transform on 2-dimensional signals	35
Fig 2.4	Hard thresholding technique	36
Fig 2.5	Representation of soft thresholding	37
Fig 2.6	Representation of edge by the change in intensity of the signal	44
Fig 2.7	First-order derivative of the original signal	45
Fig 2.8	Second-order derivative of the original signal	45
Fig 2.9	Kernels of Sobel operator	46
Fig 2.10	Kernels of Robert's operator	47
Fig 2.11	Kernels of the Prewitt's operator	48
Fig 2.12	Discrete Kernels used for approximating the Laplacian operator	49
Fig 2.13	Log kernels	49
Fig 2.14	2-D Laplacian of Gaussian (LoG) function	50
Fig 2.15	Discrete kernel for approximating the LoG with Gaussian(σ=1.4)	50
Fig 2.16	Edge orientation angle representation diagram	51
Fig 3.1	Diagrammatic representation of topological derivative	53
Fig 3.2	Pixel "s" and its neighbourhood diffusion coefficients k_s	55
Fig 4.1	PCMAT system for developing despeckling algorithms	60
Fig 4.2	View of the original and Frost filtered choroids image in the MATLAB output window after running the sample program given in Example 4.1	62
Fig 4.3	PCDSK system used for developing and testing the despeckling algorithms	63
Fig 4.4	Top view of the TMS320C6713 DSK	64
Fig 4.5	Memory map of TMS320C6713 DSK	65

Fig 4.6	Snap-shot of the contrast stretch image displayed in the PCDSK system	69
Fig 5.1	View of the ultrasound B-scan images (a) Abdomen with a calcific fibroid (IMAGE-1) (b) Kidney (IMAGE-2) (c) Lungs (IMAGE-3) (d) Heart (IMAGE-4) (e) Liver with a cyst in it (IMAGE-5) (f) Gall bladder (IMAGE-6) and (g) Pancreas-Spleen (IMAGE-7)	73
Fig 5.2	Flow chart of the speckle reduction algorithm	75
Fig 5.3	Original and despeckled images of abdomen in the PCMAT system	84
Fig 5.4	Canny edge detected images of abdomen in the PCMAT system	85
Fig 5.5	Original and despeckled images of kidney in the PCMAT system	87
Fig 5.6	Canny edge detected images of kidney in the PCMAT system	88
Fig 5.7	Original and despeckled images of liver in the PCMAT system	90
Fig 5.8	Canny edge detected images of liver in the PCMAT system	91
Fig 5.9	Histogram plot of the PSNR and Peak SNR (Canny) in the PCMAT system	98
Fig 5.10	Histogram plot of the Average Difference (AD) in the PCMAT system	99
Fig 5.11	Histogram plot of the Mean Square Error (MSE) in the PCMAT system	100
Fig 5.12	Histogram plot of the Maximum Difference (MD) in the PCMAT system	101
Fig 5.13	Histogram plot of the Normalized Absolute Error (NAE) in the PCMAT system	102
Fig 5.14	Histogram plot of the Contrast to Noise Ratio (CNR) in the PCMAT system	103
Fig 5.15	Histogram plot of the Figure of Merit (FoM) in the PCMAT system	104
Fig 5.16	Histogram plot of the Structural Content (SC) in the PCMAT system	105
Fig 5.17	Histogram plot of the Coefficient of Correlation (CoC) in the PCMAT system	106
Fig 5.18	Histogram plot of the Normalized Cross Correlation (NCC) in the PCMAT system	107
Fig 5.19	Histogram plot of the Image Quality Index (IQI) in the PCMAT system	108
Fig 5.20	Histogram plot of the Normalized Mean Square Error (NMSE) in the PCMAT system	109
Fig 5.21	Histogram plot of the Mean Structure Similarity Index Map (MSSIM) in the PCMAT system	110
Fig 5.22	Histogram plot of the Speckle Index (SI) in the PCMAT system	111
Fig 5.23	Histogram plot of the Average Signal to Noise Ratio (ASNR) in the PCMAT system	112
Fig 5.24	Histogram plot of the Image Variance (IV) in the PCMAT system	113
Fig 5.25	Histogram plot of the Noise Standard Deviation (NSD) in the PCMAT system	114

Fig 5.26	Histogram plot of the Effective Number of Looks (ENL) in the PCMAT system	115
Fig 6.1	Original and despeckled images of abdomen in the PCDSK system	119
Fig 6.2	Canny edge detected images of abdomen in the PCDSK system	120
Fig 6.3	Original and despeckled images of kidney in the PCDSK system	122
Fig 6.4	Canny edge detected images of kidney in the PCDSK system	123
Fig 6.5	Original and despeckled images of liver in the PCDSK system	125
Fig 6.6	Canny edge detected images of liver in the PCDSK system	126
Fig 6.7	Histogram plot of the PSNR and Peak SNR (Canny) in the PCDSK system	131
Fig 6.8	Histogram plot of the Average Difference (AD) in the PCDSK system	132
Fig 6.9	Histogram plot of the Mean Square Error (MSE) in the PCDSK system	133
Fig 6.10	Histogram plot of the Maximum Difference (MD) in the PCDSK system	134
Fig 6.11	Histogram plot of the Normalized Absolute Error (NAE) in the PCDSK system	135
Fig 6.12	Histogram plot of the Contrast to Noise Ratio (CNR) in the PCDSK system	136
Fig 6.13	Histogram plot of the Figure of Merit (FoM) in the PCDSK system	137
Fig 6.14	Histogram plot of the Structural Content (SC) in the PCDSK system	138
Fig 6.15	Histogram plot of the Coefficient of Correlation (CoC) in the PCDSK system	139
Fig 6.16	Histogram plot of the Normalized Cross Correlation (NCC) in the PCDSK system	140
Fig 6.17	Histogram plot of the Image Quality Index (IQI) in the PCDSK system	141
Fig 6.18	Histogram plot of the Normalized Mean Square Error (NMSE) in the PCDSK system	142
Fig 6.19	Histogram plot of the Mean Structure Similarity Index Map (MSSIM) in the PCDSK system	143
Fig 6.20	Histogram plot of the Speckle Index (SI) in the PCDSK system	144
Fig 6.21	Histogram plot of the Average Signal to Noise Ratio (ASNR) in the PCDSK system	145
Fig 6.22	Histogram plot of the Image Variance (IV) in the PCDSK system	146
Fig 6.23	Histogram plot of the Noise Standard Deviation (NSD) in the PCDSK system	147
Fig 6.24	Histogram plot of the Effective Number of Looks (ENL) in the PCDSK system	148
Fig A1	Original and despeckled images of gall bladder in the PCMAT system	155
Fig A2	Canny edge detected images of gall bladder in the PCMAT system	156

Fig A3	Original and despeckled images of heart in the PCMAT system	158
Fig A4	Canny edge detected images of heart in the PCMAT system	159
Fig A5	Original and despeckled images of lungs in the PCMAT system	161
Fig A6	Canny edge detected images of lungs in the PCMAT system	162
Fig A7	Original and despeckled images of pancreas - spleen in the PCMAT system	164
Fig A8	Canny edge detected images of pancreas - spleen in the PCMAT system	165
Fig A9	Histogram plot of the PSNR and Peak SNR (Canny) in the PCMAT system	167
Fig A10	Histogram plot of the Average Difference (AD) in the PCMAT system	168
Fig A11	Histogram plot of the Mean Square Error (MSE) in the PCMAT system	169
Fig A12	Histogram plot of the Maximum Difference (MD) in the PCMAT system	170
Fig A13	Histogram plot of the Normalized Absolute Error (NAE) in the PCMAT system	171
Fig A14	Histogram plot of the Contrast to Noise Ratio (CNR) in the PCMAT system	172
Fig A15	Histogram plot of the Figure of Merit (FoM) in the PCMAT system	173
Fig A16	Histogram plot of the Structural Content (SC) in the PCMAT system	174
Fig A17	Histogram plot of the Coefficient of Correlation (CoC) in the PCMAT system	175
Fig A18	Histogram plot of the Normalized Cross Correlation (NCC) in the PCMAT system	176
Fig A19	Histogram plot of the Image Quality Index (IQI) in the PCMAT system	177
Fig A20	Histogram plot of the Normalized Mean Square Error (NMSE) in the PCMAT system	178
Fig A21	Histogram plot of the Mean Structure Similarity Index Map (MSSIM) in the PCMAT system	179
Fig A22	Histogram plot of the Speckle Index (SI) in the PCMAT system	180
Fig A23	Histogram plot of the Average Signal to Noise Ratio (ASNR) in the PCMAT system	181
Fig A24	Histogram plot of the Image Variance (IV) in the PCMAT system	182
Fig A25	Histogram plot of the Noise Standard Deviation (NSD) in the PCMAT system	183
Fig A26	Histogram plot of the Effective Number of Looks (ENL) in the PCMAT system	184
Fig B1	Original and despeckled images of gall bladder in the PCDSK system	185
Fig B2	Canny edge detected images of gall bladder in the PCDSK system	186
Fig B3	Original and despeckled images of heart in the PCDSK system	188

Fig B4	Canny edge detected images of heart in the PCDSK system	189
Fig B5	Original and despeckled images of lungs in the PCDSK system	191
Fig B6	Canny edge detected images of lungs in the PCDSK system	192
Fig B7	Original and despeckled images of pancreas - spleen in the PCDSK system	194
Fig B8	Canny edge detected images of pancreas - spleen in the PCDSK system	195
Fig B9	Histogram plot of the PSNR and Peak SNR (Canny) in the PCDSK system	198
Fig B10	Histogram plot of the Average Difference (AD) in the PCDSK system	199
Fig B11	Histogram plot of the Mean Square Error (MSE) in the PCDSK system	200
Fig B12	Histogram plot of the Maximum Difference (MD) in the PCDSK system	201
Fig B13	Histogram plot of the Normalized Absolute Error (NAE) in the PCDSK system	202
Fig B14	Histogram plot of the Contrast to Noise Ratio (CNR) in the PCDSK system	203
Fig B15	Histogram plot of the Figure of Merit (FoM) in the PCDSK system	204
Fig B16	Histogram plot of the Structural Content (SC) in the PCDSK system	205
Fig B17	Histogram plot of the Coefficient of Correlation (CoC) in the PCDSK system	206
Fig B18	Histogram plot of the Normalized Cross Correlation (NCC) in the PCDSK system	207
Fig B19	Histogram plot of the Image Quality Index (IQI) in the PCDSK system	208
Fig B20	Histogram plot of the Normalized Mean Square Error (NMSE) in the PCDSK system	209
Fig B21	Histogram plot of the Mean Structure Similarity Index Map (MSSIM) in the PCDSK system	210
Fig B22	Histogram plot of the Speckle Index (SI) in the PCDSK system	211
Fig B23	Histogram plot of the Average Signal to Noise Ratio (ASNR) in the PCDSK system	212
Fig B24	Histogram plot of the Image Variance (IV) in the PCDSK system	213
Fig B25	Histogram plot of the Noise Standard Deviation (NSD) in the PCDSK system	214
Fig B26	Histogram plot of the Effective Number of Looks (ENL) in the PCDSK system	215

LIST OF TABLES

S.NO.	TABLES	PAGE NO.
Table 1.1	Medical image processing techniques and operations	3
Table 1.2	Comparison of Imaging Modalities	13
Table 2.1	Summarization of metrics used for estimating the performance of despeckling filters	42
Table 4.1	TMS320C6713 switch settings	66
Table 4.2	Various files generated in the CCS and their description	68
Table 4.3	Particulars of ultrasound B-scan images collected from four different sources	70
Table 5.1	Specifications of ultrasound B-Scan images	72
Table 5.2	Calculated performance metrics of the despeckling filters applied on the abdomen image in the PCMAT system	86
Table 5.3	Calculated performance metrics of the despeckling filters applied on the kidney image in the PCMAT system	89
Table 5.4	Calculated performance metrics of the despeckling filters applied on the liver image in the PCMAT system	92
Table 6.1	Calculated performance metrics of the despeckling filters applied on the abdomen image in the PCDSK system	121
Table 6.2	Calculated performance metrics of the despeckling filters applied on the kidney image in the PCDSK system	124
Table 6.3	Calculated performance metrics of the despeckling filters applied on the liver image in the PCDSK system	127
Table 6.4	Comparison of execution time of algorithms tested on the three images in the PCMAT and PCDSK systems	128
Table A1	Calculated performance metrics of the despeckling filters applied on the gall bladder image in the PCMAT system	157
Table A2	Calculated performance metrics of the despeckling filters applied on the heart image in the PCMAT system	160
Table A3	Calculated performance metrics of the despeckling filters applied on the lungs image in the PCMAT system	163
Table A4	Calculated performance metrics of the despeckling filters applied on the pancreas - spleen image in the PCMAT system	166
Table B1	Calculated performance metrics of the despeckling filters applied on the gall bladder image in the PCDSK system	187
Table B2	Calculated performance metrics of the despeckling filters applied on the heart image in the PCDSK system	190
Table B3	Calculated performance metrics of the despeckling filters applied on the lungs image in the PCDSK system	193
Table B4	Calculated performance metrics of the despeckling filters applied on the pancreas - spleen image in the PCDSK system	196
Table B5	Comparison of execution time of algorithms tested on the four images in the PCMAT and PCDSK systems	197

CHAPTER - I

INTRODUCTION

1.1 INTRODUCTION TO IMAGING

Images are the most important tool of human information transfer, since seventy percentage of human perception is through vision. However, unlike humans, who are limited to the visual band of the electromagnetic (EM) spectrum, imaging machines cover almost the entire EM spectrum, ranging from gamma to radio waves. They can operate on images generated by sources that humans are not accustomed in associating with images. These include ultrasound, electron microscopy, and computer-generated images.

An image is the optical representation of the object/specimen with the interaction of electromagnetic radiation sources like ultraviolet, visible, X-ray, infra-red, etc. The image formation can be characterized by mathematical models, which mainly depends on the radiation source, physics of interaction, image acquisition system, display specifications, etc. A simple gray level image can be described as a function $f(x, y)$ of two independent variables x and y and the amplitude of f for any coordinate (x, y) represents the intensity or gray level of an image at that point [1]. When the amplitude values of f are finite and discrete quantities, then the image is called digital image. A digital image is a 2-D discrete signal, which comprises of finite number of elements, each of which have a particular location and value called picture element/ image element/pels or pixel.

Biomedical imaging is a process of collecting information about a specific physiological structure (an organ or tissue) using a predefined characteristic property that is displayed in the form of an image. These medical images include the simplest form of chest X-ray to sophisticated images like a magnetic resonance imaging (MRI). The medical images in the form of data sets in two, three, or more dimensions convey increasingly vast and detailed information for clinical or research applications. This information has to be interpreted in a timely and accurate manner to benefit health care. The commonly used medical imaging modalities capable of producing multidimensional images for radiological applications are: X-ray, Computed Tomography (X-Ray CT), Magnetic Resonance Imaging (MRI), Positron Emission Tomography (PET), Single Photon Emission Computer Tomography (SPECT) and Ultrasound imaging. All these modern imaging methods involve sophisticated instrumentation and complex mathematical algorithms using advanced electronics and computers for data collection, image reconstruction and display.

1.2   OVERVIEW OF BIOMEDICAL IMAGE PROCESSING

Presently, all medical imaging modalities provide the image data in digital format, since image reconstruction from incomprehensible projection data, their processing, noise and distortion removal and various display methods matched to particular needs of diagnostics depend heavily on the computational aspects of medical imaging. The progress in medical imaging is significant, which depends on the advancements in information processing, in particular, the algorithm design and implementation. With the advancements in very large scale integrated circuits and software technologies, the biomedical image processing focuses on extracting clinically significant information from physiological images that can improve the performance of medical devices, which assist physicians in making more effective diagnostic decisions [2]. Over the past three decades, biomedical image processing has grown rapidly by the development of novel computational methods for diagnostic applications.

Many diagnostic medical imaging modalities are used to probe the human body both at microscopic (cell) and macroscopic (organ or system) level. The challenging task in medical image processing is the effective processing of the image to extract, quantify and interpret diagnostic/physiological information accurately in order to gain understanding and insight into the structure and function of the organs being imaged. Interpretation of the resulting images requires sophisticated image processing methods that enhance visual interpretation and image analysis methods that provide automated or semi-automated detection, measurement, and characterization [3-15]. Conversely, several mathematical transform techniques have been developed to improve the image quality, and to extract the diagnostic information of interest. The basic medical image processing techniques can be broadly classified as:

(i) enhancement
(ii) restoration
(iii) analysis
(iv) compression
(v) synthesis

Table 1.1 summarizes each technique and its related operations.

Table 1.1 Medical image processing techniques and operations

Techniques	Related operations
Enhancement	Brightness adjustment, contrast enhancement, image averaging, convolution, frequency domain filtering, edge enhancement
Restoration	Photometric correction, inverse filtering
Analysis	Segmentation, feature extraction, object classification
Compression	Lossless and lossy compression
Synthesis	Tomography, 3-D reconstruction

1.2.1 Image Enhancement

Image enhancement is a subjective phenomenon, which performs mathematical operations in spatial and frequency domains in order to enhance the interpretation or perception of image information for human understanding [3, 4, 10-16]. Several mathematical techniques viz., Fast Fourier Transform (FFT), Wavelet Transform (WT), Gabor Transform (GT), Histogram, etc are performed to modify the image brightness, contrast or the distribution of the grey levels. As a result, the pixel intensities of the enhanced image will be modified according to the transformation function applied on the input image. But, the computational cost of enhancement algorithm plays a critical role in deciding a particular algorithm for image enhancement purpose.

1.2.2 Image Analysis

Image analysis is the method of extracting information and making measurements within the image either automatically or semi-automatically. Generally, the process begins with isolating the objects of interest from the rest of the image, measuring a number of features such as size, shape and texture, and then classifying the objects into groups according to these features. For instance, in medical imaging, this permits to identify a particular lesion by comparing the features like shape and texture, which falls within or outside the tolerance value [12-16]. These analysis methods are used in classifying lesions as benign or malignant and in recognizing suspicious clusters of micro calcifications in images of particular organ.

1.2.3 Image Compression

Image Compression reduces the amount of data needed to describe an image efficiently, which would allow data storage at less cost and data transmission at high speed. For example, an image of size 512×512 pixels of 8 bit length requires about 2 MB of space, which is a comparable size of a document comprising 40 pages of text [12-15]. Thus, compression reduces the file size, so that the image can be more efficiently stored or transported electronically in a shorter time. Compression is possible because images tend to contain redundant or repetitive information. There are two main category of compression techniques viz., lossy and lossless. In medical imaging, lossless compression is mostly recommended, since it is a reversible, error-free and information preserving type. Also, the lossless compression technique exactly represents the vital image information while reconstructing the image using decompression algorithms. Smaller image files (i.e. greater compression) can be obtained with lossy compression techniques, which do not preserve all of the data of the original image, but nevertheless maintain an image of acceptable quality.

1.2.4 Image Synthesis

Image synthesis is the process of creating new images from other images or non-image data. For instance, in computed tomography, the reconstruction of axial or slice tomographic images are obtained from projection data [12-16].

1.2.5 Image Restoration

Image restoration techniques aim at reversing the degradation undergone by the image to recover the true image. The problem of image restoration has been extensively studied and several algorithms have been developed to solve this problem. Classical linear techniques restore the true image by filtering the observed image using a properly designed filter. Examples are inverse filtering, Wiener filtering, etc. [12-16].

1.3 IMAGING MODALITIES

Modern medical imaging is possibly the most progressive and also the valued diagnostic tool in human health care. Various imaging modalities such as X-ray, Computer Tomography (CT), Magnetic Resonance Imaging (MRI), Positron Emission Tomography (PET), Single Photon Emission Computer Tomography (SPECT) and ultrasound provide accurate diagnostic, anatomical as well as functional information about the particular biological system. These medical imaging modalities are briefly described in the following subsections.

1.3.1 X-Ray Imaging

X-ray is one of the most popular and oldest imaging techniques, which uses high-energy photons that penetrate through the body [16]. The absorption of X-ray by the body tissue and bone is projected on the film, which forms a two-dimensional distribution of optical density that relates to the tissue distribution inside the patient. Thus, a mapping of the three-dimensional absorption coefficient onto the two-dimensional image plane is obtained. In the case of film-based X-ray imaging, the film needs to be digitized with a film scanner to obtain a digital image. Filmless X-ray imaging uses a semiconductor detector for forming the digital image [12, 16]. Figure 1.1 shows the X-ray image of the chest.

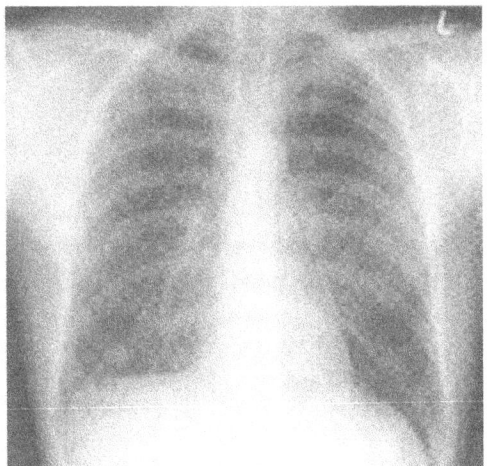

Fig 1.1 Radiographic chest image

1.3.2 Computed Tomography (CT)

In computed tomography, a number of 2D radiographs are acquired by rotating the X-ray tube around the body of the patient. The full 3D image can then be reconstructed by computer from the 2D projections using the Radon transform [17-24]. Thus, CT is essentially a 3D version of X-ray radiography, and therefore offers high contrast between bone and soft tissue and low contrast among different soft tissues. Figure 1.2 shows the cardiovascular image obtained from the CT scanner.

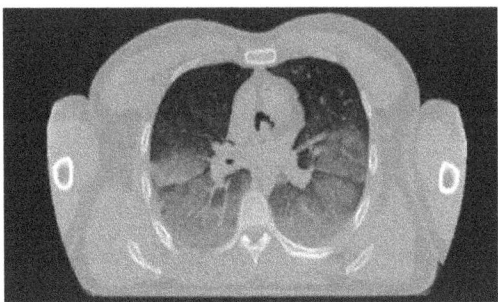

Fig 1.2 CT image of the cardiovascular cavity of a cadaver

A contrast agent (chemical solution opaque to the X-rays) is injected into the patient in order to artificially increase the contrast among the tissues of interest and so enhance image quality [17-24]. Because CT is based on multiple radiographs, the deleterious effects of ionizing radiation should be taken into account.

1.3.3 Magnetic Resonance Imaging (MRI)

Magnetic Resonance Imaging (MRI) relies on the relaxation properties of magnetically excited hydrogen nuclei of water molecules present in human body. The patient under study is kept in a magnetic field and briefly exposed to a burst of radio-frequency energy, which excites the nuclei in an elevated energy state. As the molecules return to their normal position, they release this energy into their surroundings, in a process referred to as relaxation. Different tissues relaxed at different timing, which is used to form the MRI image [17-29]. According to current medical history, MRI is considered as a harmless imaging modality, since it utilizes strong magnetic field and non-ionizing radiation in the radio frequency range [17-29]. Another advantage of MRI is that soft tissue contrast is much better than with X-rays leading to higher-quality images, especially in brain and spinal cord scans as shown in Figure 1.3. Refinements have been developed such as functional MRI (fMRI) that measures temporal variations (e.g., for detection of neural activity), and diffusion MRI that measures the diffusion of water molecules in anisotropic tissues such as white matter in the brain [27-29].

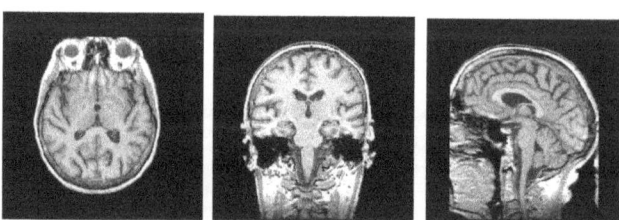

Fig 1.3 Axial, Coronal and Sagittal cross-section MR images of human brain

1.3.4 Positron Emission Tomography (PET)

In PET, radioactive isotopes are injected into the patient, which emit particles called positrons [7, 18, 19]. When the positron collides with the electron produces a pair of gamma ray photons having the same energy but moving in opposite directions. The origin of the photons can be determined from the position and delay between the photon pair on a receptor. PET is a functional imaging technique that can be used to visualize pathologies at the much finer molecular level [22-24], while MRI and CT can only detect anatomical changes. PET functional images can be obtained by employing radioisotopes that have different rates of intake for different tissues. For instance, the change of regional blood flow in various anatomical structures (as a measure of the injected positron emitter) can be visualized and relatively quantified. Since the patient has to be injected with radioactive material, PET is relatively invasive [25, 26], however, the radiation dose is similar to a CT scan. Since PET image resolution is poor that requires preprocessing to achieve the required resolution level. Figure 1.4 shows the typical PET image of the human brain.

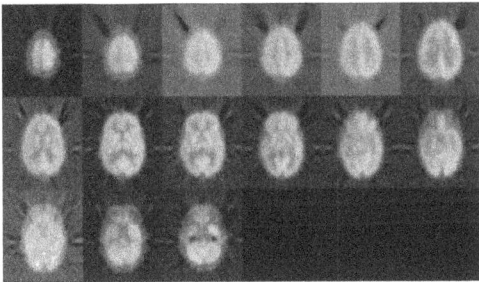

Fig 1.4 Sequence of axial PET images of human brain

1.3.5 Single Photon Emission Computed Tomography (SPECT)

The single-photon emission computed tomography (SPECT) consists of a gamma camera mounted on a gantry so that the detector can record projections from many equally spaced angular intervals around the body [12, 25]. The different acquired projections are used to reconstruct cross-sectional or 3D images by filtered back projection. Since the detected signals depend upon both the spatial distribution of the radioisotopes and the attenuation properties of the voxels, the reconstruction computations are more complicated than with X-ray CT. The main advantage of SPECT over planar imaging is the absence of super positioning of overlying and underlying signals. Figure 1.5 shows SPECT images of a human brain. From the Figure 1.5, it can be noticed that SPECT images are poor in resolution and anatomical structure as compared to CT or MR images. However, the SPECT images show radioactivity distribution in the tissue representing a specific metabolism or blood flow.

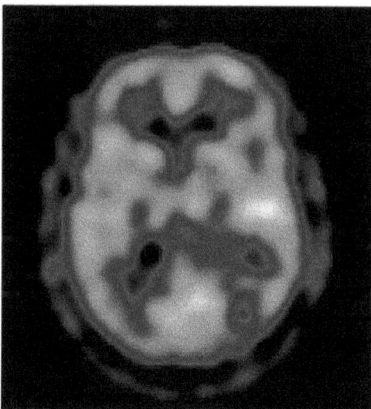

Fig 1.5 SPECT image of a human brain

1.3.6 Ultrasound Imaging

Ultrasound Imaging is a low-cost, non-invasive imaging technique widely used for diagnosis over five decades. In ultrasound imaging, the ultrasound (sound wave of frequency above 20 kHz) interacts with the different tissue structures of the body, while insonating the body at a particular anatomical position. When ultrasound passes through the different tissues, echoes are produced at the boundaries that describe or separate them. Images are then produced, which represent the acoustic reflectivity of the tissue [16]. The ultrasound imaging has been successfully used for anatomical structure identification, blood flow measurement and tissue characterization [30-38].

A typical ultrasound imaging system includes transducer (usually made up of piezoelectric material), signal processing device and display device as shown in Figure 1.6. The ultrasound transducer uses an array of piezoelectric elements that transmit ultrasound pulse into the body and receive the return echoes from the scattering structures. The frequency of the transducers employed for various diagnostic as well as therapeutic applications differs in the range of 1 to 100 MHz.

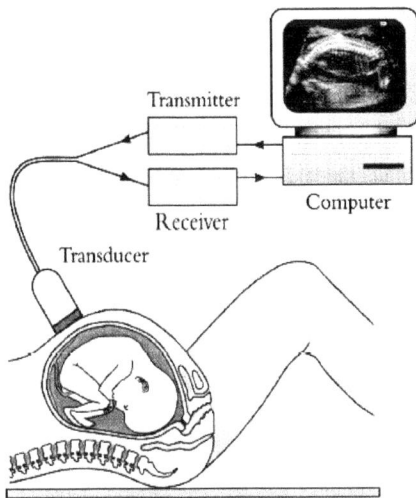

Fig 1.6 Instrumentation setup of the ultrasound imaging system

1.3.6.1 Modes of Ultrasonography

Ultrasonography can be classified into different types based on the modes of transferring the ultrasound echo signal information into a meaningful display. The important modes of ultrasound displays are described in this section.

A-mode: A single ultrasound echo measurement produces a one-dimensional map of the positions of reflecting boundaries, along the direction of the transmitted beam. This is called the A-Mode scan, or amplitude mode scans [24].

B-mode: B-mode refers to the brightness mode, in which both the X and the Y directions on the screen correspond to anatomical distances. In B-mode, each component scan line is plotted with trace brightness modulated by the variation in signal amplitude along the scan direction [24]. The principle of B-mode operation is illustrated in Figure 1.7.

M-mode: M mode refers to motion mode. The echoes are displayed as in the B-mode with momentary value of the signal modulates the brightness of the dots displayed [24]. That is, the echoes coming from moving organs are represented on the time base by moving bright dots, which leave a trace on the screen. The M-mode presentation is still fundamental in examining the function and imaging the structure of the heart. Figure 1.8 shows the diagrammatic representation of M-mode operation.

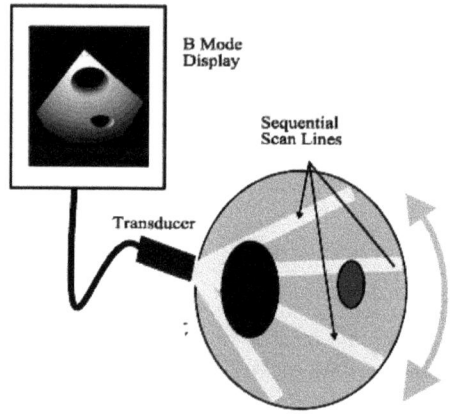

Fig 1.7 Typical B-scan image setup

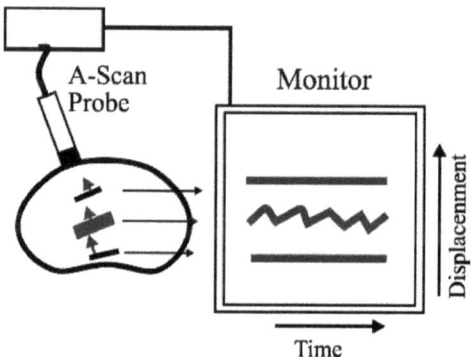

Fig 1.8 Diagrammatic representation of M-mode

D-mode: D-mode or Doppler-mode represents the shift in ultrasound frequency due to the movement of blood cell across the blood vessels or valves [24]. In the B-scan image, it is usually shown in colors viz., blue for forward and red for reverse flow with respect to the transducer. Intermediate colors for movements at lower velocities, while the echoes coming from stationary structures are presented as black-and-white. The Color Doppler image for the umbilical cord of a fetus is shown in Figure 1.9.

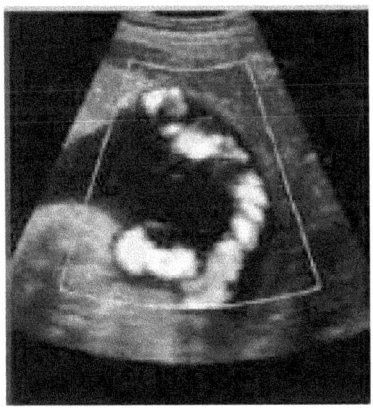

Fig 1.9 Color Doppler-mode image of a fetus

1.4 COMPARISON OF ULTRASOUND IMAGING WITH OTHER BIOMEDICAL IMAGING MODALITIES

Presently, worldwide ultrasound imaging is used as effective tool for investigating fetus status, heart conditions, tumor level etc., for routine clinical diagnosis due to its non-invasive, harmless, portable and cost-effective nature. This widespread use is evidence of the unique advantages offered by ultrasound, which complements other diagnostic imaging modalities like MRI, PET, and X-rays. Also, acoustic radiation is non-ionizing and produces few or no side effects [30]. It also has the advantage of being able to probe the mechanical properties of human tissue directly, while other techniques must infer these characteristics indirectly. The overall comparison of the medical imaging modalities are given in Table 1.2. With the widespread availability of miniature portable ultrasound systems for screening and imaging will continue to improve its usage for diagnosis.

Table 1.2 Comparison of Imaging Modalities

Specification	Common Medical Imaging Modality				
	Ultrasound	X-ray	CT	MRI	PET
Source of image	Mechanical properties	Mean tissue absorption	Tissue absorption	Biochemistry (T1 and T2)	Radio isotope Molecules
Access	Small windows	2 sides needed	Circumferential Around body	Circumferential Around body	Circumferential Around body
Spatial resolution	Frequency and axially dependent 0.3 – 3 mm	~ 1 mm	~ 1 mm	~ 1 mm	~ 5 mm
Penetration	Frequency dependent 3-25 cm	Excellent	Excellent	Excellent	Good
Safety	Very good	Ionizing radiation	Ionizing radiation	Very good	Good
Speed	100 FPS	Few min	½ min. - several min.	10 FPS	45- 60 FPS
Cost	Economic	Normal	Normal	Expensive	Very Expensive
Portability	Excellent	Good	Poor	Poor	Poor

1.5　LIMITATIONS OF ULTRASOUND B-SCAN IMAGING

Noise and artifacts can cause signal and image degradation for many medical image modalities [39]. Different image modalities exhibit distinct types of degradation. The main disadvantage of ultrasound is that it does not work well in the presence of bone or gas, and the operator needs a high level of skill in both image acquisition and interpretation to carry out the clinical evaluation.

Some of the important limitations of the ultrasound B-scan images are summarized below.

1. Spatial and geometrical information may be incorrect due to difference in speed-of-sound in different tissues, since most of the ultrasound systems are assumed speed-of-sound of human tissue as 1540 m/s [40]. Spatial compounding technique may be employed to correct this problem.

2. Lateral resolution is best at the focal length distance and widens away from this distance in a non-uniform way because of diffraction effects caused by apertures on the order of a few to tens of wavelengths [41].
3. Variation in image resolution due to depth dependence and inhomogeneous intervening tissues [42].
4. Speckle, an ultrasound textural pattern that varies with the type of biological tissues [43-45].

Several researchers have been attempting solutions for the aforementioned limitations using image processing techniques. This thesis mainly concentrated on the speckle associated with the ultrasound B-scan images and its reduction techniques in detail.

1.6 SCOPE OF THE THESIS

The primary goal of this thesis is to explore despeckling techniques and present novel technique that has better accuracy than existing methods and its testing for real-time implementation. The objectives of the research work are summarized as under.

1. To study the basic concepts of speckle, mathematical background, and constraints/limitations.
2. To explore the existing despeckling techniques and to identify the optimum technique through visual inspection and comparison of established performance metrics.
3. To explore a novel despeckling technique and comparing the results of the proposed technique with the existing/optimum techniques.
4. To implement the proposed technique in an environment suitable for studying the scope of real-time implementation.

REFERENCES

1. Gonzalez R.C., and Wood R.E., Digital Image Processing, Second Edition, Prentice Hall, 2002.
2. Haidekker M.A., Advanced Biomedical Image Analysis, John Wiley & Sons, Inc., Publication, 2011.
3. Dougherty G., Medical Image Processing Techniques and Applications, Springer 2011.
4. Exarchos T.P., Papadopoulos A., and Fotiadis D., Handbook of Research on Advanced Techniques in Diagnostic Imaging and Biomedical Applications, Medical information science reference, 2009.
5. Costaridou L., Medical Image Analysis Methods, Taylor & Francis Group, 2005.
6. Dhawan A.P., Huang H.K., and Kim D.S., Principles and Advanced Methods in Medical Imaging and Image Analysis, World Scientific Publishing Co. Pvt. Ltd, 2008.
7. Tavares J.M., and Jorge R.M., Advances in Computational Vision and Medical Image Processing, Springer, 2009.
8. González F.A., and Romero E., Biomedical Image Analysis and Machine Learning Technologies: Applications and Techniques, Medical Information Science Reference, 2010.
9. Rangayyan R.M., Biomedical Image Analysis, CRC Press LLC, 2005.
10. Acton S., and Ray N., Bio-medical Image Analysis: Segmentation, Morgan & Claypool Publisher 2009.
11. Semmlow J.L., Bio-signal and Biomedical Image Processing, Marcel Dekker, Inc. 2004.
12. Dougherty G., Digital Image Processing for Medical Applications, Cambridge University Press, 2009.
13. Jain A.K., Fundamentals of Digital Image processing, Prentice Hall, 1989.
14. Bankman N.I., Handbook of Medical Imaging Processing and Analysis, Academic Press, 2000.
15. Dhawan A.P., Medical Image Analysis, S John Wiley & Sons, Inc., Publication, 2003.
16. Base A.M., Pattern Recognition for Medical Imaging, Elsevier Academic Press, 2004.
17. Christe B.L., Introduction to Biomedical Instrumentation, Cambridge University Press, 2009.
18. Suetens P., Fundamentals of Medical Imaging, Cambridge University Press 2002.
19. Wolbarst A.B., Looking within How X-ray, CT, MRI, Ultrasound and other Medical Images are Created, and How They Help Physicians Save Lives, University of California Press, 1999.
20. Hendee W.R., and Ritenour E.R., Medical Imaging Physics, Forth Edition, A John Wiley & Sons, Inc., Publication, 2002.
21. Iniewski K., Medical Imaging, John Wiley & Sons, Inc., 2009.
22. Ogiela M.R., and Tadeusiewicz R., Modern Computational Intelligence Methods for the Interpretation of Medical Images, Springer-Verlag Berlin Heidelberg, 2008.
23. Webb S., The Physics of Medical Imaging, Taylor & Francis Group LLC, 1988.
24. Guy C., and Ffytche D., An Introduction to The Principles of Medical Imaging, Imperial College Press, 2005.

25. Angenent S., Pichon E., and Tannenbaum A., Mathematical Methods in Medical Image Processing, Bulletin (New Series) of The American Mathematical Society, Vol. 43, No.2, pp.1-32.
26. Kak A.C., and Slaney M., The Principle of Computerized Tomographic Imaging, IEEE Press, 1987.
27. Bruggen N.V., and Roberts T., Biomedical Imaging in Experimental Neuroscience, CRC Press LLC, 2003.
28. Weishaupt D., Kochli V.D., and Marincek B., How does MRI Work, Springer-Verlag Berlin Heidelberg, 2006.
29. Prasad P.V., Magnetic Resonance Imaging, Humana Press, 2006.
30. Szabo T.L., Diagnostic Ultrasound Imaging: Inside Out, Elsevier Academic Press, 2004.
31. Shiota T., 3D Echocardiography, Informa UK Ltd, 2007.
32. Brooks A., Connolly J., and Chan O., Ultrasound in Emergency Care, Blackwell Publishing Ltd, 2004.
33. Ernst A., and Kopman D.J., Ultrasound–Guided Procedures and Investigations: A Manual for the Clinician, Taylor & Francis Group, LLC2006.
34. Suri J.S., Kathuria C., Chang R.F., Molinari F., and Fenster A., Advances In Diagnostic and Therapeutic Ultrasound Imaging, Artech House, Inc., 2008.
35. Rimington H., and Chambers J.B., Echocardiography : A Practical Guide for Reporting, Second Edition, Informa Uk Ltd, 2007.
36. Ostensen H., and Tole N.M., Basic Physics of Ultrasonographic Imaging, World Health Organization, 2005.
37. Duck ., and Francis A., Ultrasound in Medicine and Medical Science Series, CRC Press, 1998.
38. Prager R.W., Ijaz. U.Z., Gee A.H., and Treece G.M., Three-Dimensional Ultrasound Imaging, Journal of Engineering in Medicine, 2010, Vol.224, No. 193, pp. 193-223.
39. Loizou C.P., and Pattichis C.S., Despeckle Filtering Algorithms and Software for Ultrasound Imaging, Morgan & Claypool, 2008.
40. Polak J.F., Doppler Sonography: An Overview in Peripheral Vascular Sonography: A practical guide, Baltimore, MD: Williams & Wilkins, 1992.
41. Cho M.H, Kang L.H, Kim J.S, and Lee S.Y, An Efficient Sound Speed Estimation Method to Enhance Image Resolution in Ultrasound Imaging, Ultrasonics, 2009, Vol.49, No.8, pp. 774-778.
42. Elatrozy T., Nicolaides A., Tegos T., Zarka A., Griffin M., and Sabetai M., The Effect of B-mode Ultrasonic Image Standardization of The Echodensity of Symptomatic and Asymptomatic Carotid Bifurcation Plaque, Int. Angiol., 1998, Vol. 17, No. 3, pp. 179–186.
43. Burckhardt C.B., Speckle in Ultrasound B-Mode Scans, IEEE Trans. on Sonics and Ultrasonics, 1978, Vol. Su-25, No. 1, pp.1-6.
44. Wagner R.F., Smith S.W., Sandrik J.M., and Lopez H., Statistics of Speckle in Ultrasound B-scans, IEEE Trans. on Sonics and Ultrasonics, 1983, Vol. 30, No.3, pp. 156–163.
45. Goodman J.W., Some Fundamental Properties of Speckle, Journal Opt. Soc. Am., 1976,Vol. 66, No. 11, pp. 1145–1149.

CHAPTER – II
BACKGROUND OF SPECKLE AND OVERVIEW OF DESPECKLING AND ITS PERFORMANCE ESTIMATION TECHNIQUES

2.1 BACKGROUND OF SPECKLE

Speckle is a random, deterministic, interference pattern in an image formed with coherent imaging modalities like ultrasound, laser and synthetic aperture radar (SAR) [1-3], which limits the visual perception and processing of structures/edges in an image. Speckle is not truly noise, since its texture often carries useful information about the image being viewed [4-6]. Speckle noise is the primary factor that has the following limitation in ultrasound imaging.

1. Contrast resolution in diagnostic ultrasound imaging limits the detectability of small low-contrast lesions and making the ultrasound images generally difficult for the non-specialist to interpret.
2. Speckle also limits the effective applications of automated computer-aided analysis such as edge detection, volume rendering, and 3D display algorithms.

As a result, speckle is most often considered as a dominant source of noise in ultrasound imaging and should be filtered out without affecting important features of the image. The effect of speckle noise on ultrasound B-scan images is clearly illustrated in Figure 2.1 (a & b).

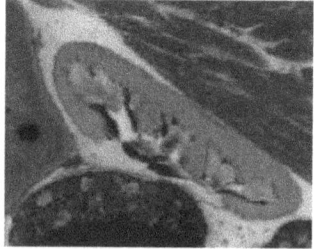

Fig 2.1(a) Noiseless ultrasound B-scan image of kidney

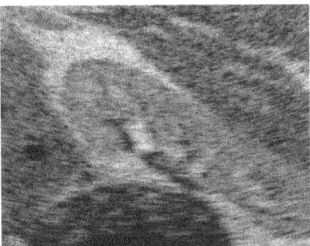

Fig 2.1(b) Noisy ultrasound B-scan image of kidney

2.2 MATHEMATICAL MODELING OF SPECKLE

Over three decades, many researchers have been proposed several models of speckle for the purpose of accurate characterization or classification of image regions and for the efficient design of despeckling filter [7-14]. The most approximated model of speckle noise in ultrasound and SAR can be described as random multiplicative noise and expressed mathematically as,

$$V_{x,y} = U_{x,y} S_{x,y} + A_{x,y} \qquad \ldots 2.1$$

where $U_{x,y}$ is the pixel without noise, $V_{x,y}$ is the noisy pixel, $S_{x,y}$ and $A_{x,y}$ represent the multiplicative and additive components of speckle noise, respectively [7-14]. Using the multiplicative model given in equation 2.1, the true intensity of the pixel $U_{x,y}$ can be calculated as a function of the intensity of the pixel $V_{x,y}$ and some local statistics calculated using the neighboring pixels.

Wagner et al., presented a stochastic first-order or second-order statistical methods for the estimation of texture or speckle within the resolution cells of the envelope-detected RF signal backscattered from near field focus zone of the transducer with high scatterer density having Rayleigh distribution with mean μ and standard deviation σ exhibited that speckle could be modeled as multiplicative noise [14]. However, speckle noise is not purely multiplicative in nature, since in homogenous regions the pixel intensity $U_{x,y}$ can be assumed as constant. Therefore, the mean is proportional to variance rather than the standard deviation.

In equation 2.1, the additive component of the speckle noise model is considerably smaller than the multiplicative component and hence $A_{x,y}$ is discarded from the model equation. Therefore, the equation 2.1 can be simplified as,

$$V_{x,y} \approx U_{x,y} S_{x,y} \quad \quad \ldots 2.2$$

This multiplicative model can be transformed into additive model using the logarithmic compression given in equation 2.3.

$$\log V_{x,y} = \log U_{x,y} + \log S_{x,y} \quad \quad \ldots 2.3$$

Equation 2.3 can be written as

$$G_{x,y} = F_{x,y} + Sl_{x,y} \quad \quad \ldots 2.4$$

where $\log V_{x,y}$ denoted as $G_{x,y}$ represents the observed pixel on the ultrasound image display after logarithmic compression and the terms $\log U_{x,y}$ and $\log S_{x,y}$ denoted as $F_{x,y}$ and $Sl_{x,y}$ represent the noise-free pixel and the noise component after logarithmic compression, respectively.

2.3 SPECKLE PATTERN IN MEDICAL ULTRASOUND IMAGE

The characteristics of speckle pattern depend on the number of scatters in a resolution cell (otherwise called as scatter number density -SND), spatial distribution and the properties of the imaging devices, which can be classified into the following three categories [15].

1. Fully formed speckle pattern due to many randomly distributed scattering within the resolution cell. e.g., Blood cells.
2. Speckle due to non-randomly distributed tissue scatters with long order. e.g., lobules in liver parenchyma.
3. Speckle due to spatially invariant coherent structure present within the random scatter region. e.g., organ surfaces and blood vessels.

2.4 REVIEW OF LITERATURE IN SPECKLE REDUCTION TECHNIQUES

Several researchers have considered the speckle in ultrasound (US) B-scan images as random noise and have obtained some agreeable measurements on image texture, whereas some other researchers have assumed the speckle as the background texture/useful signal associated with the microstructure of the tissue parenchyma used as a basis for diagnosis. This thesis mainly considered the speckle as noise and attempted to find optimum methods for removing the speckle without affecting the diagnostic information. In order to understand the depth and breadth of speckle and its reduction techniques in ultrasound B-scan images, this section presents the important research work performed over three decades.

Burckhardt made a theoretical study and experimental verification on US speckle for simple and compound scans. The author computed the speckle reduction efficiency in terms of signal-to-noise ratio (SNR) for compound scans using maximum amplitude writing and found that the reduction in speckle is almost as large as amplitude averaging. In this study, it is found that the speckle reduction depends on the number of independent amplitude values that are measured [16].

Wagner et al., analyzed the properties of the texture of B-mode phantom images near and beyond the focal zone of the transducer using the first and second order statistics. They characterized the texture/speckle using Rayleigh pdf and found that the speckle carries only the information about the transducer and its focusing pattern. They also found that the speckle cell size is inversely proportional to the pulse bandwidth in the axial direction and proportional to the transducer beam width when the speckle cell size is comparable to the resolution cell size. Finally, they predicted that the speckle cell size will be broadened when the phantom has large or cluster of particles on the scale of the resolution cell. They suggested that the outcome of their study can be used to understand clinical image texture and can be applied to clinical images of tissues having uniformly distributed scatterers [14].

Bamber et al., developed an adaptive two-dimensional filter for speckle reduction in US images based on the ratio of local variance and local mean of the image to recognize and filter fully developed speckle and retain the resolved object structures [17].

Kuan et al., addressed various adaptive speckle reduction techniques and attempted the one-point maximum a posteriori (MAP) filter and adaptive noise smoothing filter based on the local image statistics and the first-order statistics of speckle noise, respectively for despeckling US images of independent speckle samples. Further, they taken into account both the local image statistics and the correlation of speckle for speckle reduction using local linear minimum mean square error (LLMMSE) filter. They suggested that the outcome of these studies can be extended directly to process multiple frames of speckle images [18].

Donnell et al., proposed an analytical expression for the correlation between two measurements made at different spatial positions and investigated strategies for efficient incoherent averaging (compounding) for speckle reduction. They reported that the optimum aperture displacement for efficient compounding is found to be approximately one-half of the aperture length [19]. Loupes et al., presented an adaptive weighted median filter (AWMF), which combines the edge-preserving properties of the weighted median filter with the space varying properties of the local image characteristics. As a result, the AWMF reduces the speckle significantly with negligible loss to the image details, which is demonstrated in the substantial improvement in detectability of subtle grey-scale variations and small structures within the parenchyma of liver [20].

Leeman et al., proposed a two-step procedure for radio frequency A-line speckle reduction, which encompasses recognition of local occurrences of speckle effect and filling the recognized gashes through a hybrid (temporal/Fourier) method. They concluded that this procedure shows very good indication for speckle reduction without resolution loss [21]. Lopes et al., modified the most well known filters viz., Forest and Kuan by introducing two thresholds on the coefficient of variation as a function of image parameters and tested in SAR images. The authors found that the homogenous areas are adequately averaged, whereas edges and textural information are better preserved [22].

Healey et al., developed the phase acknowledging technique for the identification of large change in instantaneous frequency with respect to the carrier frequency of the image pulse for the estimation of regions of speckle corruption on the selected A-line. The authors adopted a two-stage approach called the Zero Adjustment procedure (ZAP), which describes and corrects the speckle artifact present in the amplitude and phase domain simultaneously. This method was found to be localized, robust with unchanged resolution and simple without specific statistical distribution [23]. Evans et al., introduced a non-adaptive truncated median filter of Davis for speckle reduction in ultrasound images, which achieved acceptable results with less computation complexities over the advanced adaptive filters viz., standard median, adaptive median and adaptive unsharp masking filter [24].

Steen and Olstad investigated the application of non-linear filtering technique for volume rending of medical ultrasound data, which found to increase the robustness of the gradient estimates and to smooth the homogenous regions without altering the significant monotone transitions [25]. Busse et al., explored the application of the geometric filtering method for speckle reduction in ultrasound images through effective modeling of transducer geometry, center frequency shifts and beam forming geometry for resampling of data before speckle processing, which improved the lesion detection and overall image interpretability [26]. Karaman et al., presented an adaptive speckle suppression filter (ASSF) for smoothing ultrasound B-scan images using appropriately shaped and sized local filtering kernels obtained through region growing technique employing image local statistics. The performance of the ASSF filter was compared with two other filters such as adaptive weighted median filter (AWMF) and homogenous region growing mean filter (HRGMF) on phantom and liver images [27].

Dutt and Greenleaf addressed the speckle reduction issues on log compressed ultrasound B-scan images, since the log compressed B-scan images have the advantages of reducing the dynamic range of the B-scan images for display on a monitor as well as enhancing weak back scatterers. They proposed an adaptive filter based on the K-distribution statistical model for the echo envelope to derive a parameter that was used to quantify the extent of speckle formation. This speckle quantification was used with an unsharp masking filter, which adaptively reduced the speckle and was demonstrated on images of contrast detail phantoms and on in-vivo abdominal images obtained by a clinical ultrasound system with log-compression [28]. Kofidis et al., presented a method for speckle reduction based on the combination of segmentation and optimum L-filtering and demonstrated the filter effectiveness through a comparative study with other commonly used despeckling filters. For the segmentation of homogenous regions, a modified form of the learning vector quantizer (LVQ) neural network was employed and accordingly a minimum mean-squared-error [MMSE] L-filters were designed using gray level histogram of the noisy signals and a suitable estimate of the original signals [29].

Kang et al., demonstrated a non-linear wavelet filtering method for speckle reduction in echocardiography images, which better reduced the speckle noise and less signal distortion due to its time and frequency localization capabilities. The authors also demonstrated the performance of the wavelet filter over the traditional Wiener filter [30]. Zong et al., applied shrinkage of wavelet coefficients through soft thresholding and non-linear stretching of wavelet coefficients with hard-thresholding on logarithmically transformed echocardiograms for speckle noise reduction and contrast enhancement, respectively. The authors concluded that the technique was found to be less affected by pseudo-Gibbs phenomena and the results obtained are superior both qualitatively and quantitatively than the results obtained from existing denoising techniques [31].

Hao et al., investigated the speckle reduction problem in ultrasound B-scan images using multiscale nonlinear thresholding method. In this method, the image was separated into two parts using adaptive weighted mean filter (AWMF) and the two parts are subsequently decomposed into several scales using 2D wavelet transform. The second part, which usually considered as noise was not discarded and further processed using revised Donoho's soft thresholding method. This procedure was carried out using different thresholding for different scales and finally a noise reduction factor was introduced to fit the SNR differences between the first part and second part, which resulted in more accurate signal detection at each scale. The authors performed the comparative study of the proposed method with other techniques and found that the proposed method effectively reduces the speckle noise and preserves the resolvable information in ultrasound B-scan images [32].

Abd-Elmoniem et al., developed an algorithm based on coherent anisotropy diffusion method with efficient discretization scheme for real-time visualization of ultrasound images in PC based systems. The proposed coherent anisotropic diffusion method was applied to remove the compressed speckle pattern formed by ultrasound convex B-mode sticks and showed superior results when compared with the other methods [33].

Chinrungrueng and Suvichakorn developed a 2-D weighted Savitzky-Golay filter based on the least squares fitting of a polynomial function of image intensities. The proposed method was tested on a synthetic image and an ultrasound thyroid image and its performance was compared with that of the median filter results. The results of the proposed method exhibited the same level of noise reduction and edge preservation as that of the median filter, but with far less computation time. The authors suggested that the proposed filter is suitable for filtering problems with large windows due to its complexity scales linearly with the problem size and hence the proposed filter is a promising substitute for speckle reduction in ultrasound images [34].

Achim et al., transformed the original image into a logarithmic form and then analysed the image in the multiscale wavelet domain. They modeled the wavelet sub-band decomposition of the images having non-Gaussian statistics by alpha-stable heavy-tailed distributions. The alpha-stable model was computed prior for the signal was used to design the Bayesian estimator that performs a nonlinear operation or denoising operation on the images. The authors concluded that the developed filter is more effective than the traditional thresholding method, but it is computationally expensive due to the estimation of prior distribution parameter at each scale of interest [35]. Yu and coworkers derived the speckle reducing anisotropic diffusion (SRAD) method, which exploits the instantaneous coefficient variation as a function of the local gradient magnitude and Laplacian operators. The method was tested in synthetic, real ultrasound image of carotid artery and SAR images. The results of the SRAD method were compared with three other methods viz., Lee, Frost and conventional anisotropic and exhibited that the SRAD excel over the other methods in terms of mean preservation, variance reduction and edge localization [36, 37].

Chen et al., proposed an aggressive region growing filtering (ARGF) using adaptive homogeneity threshold method based on the statistics of expected local image homogeneity for determining the appropriate shape and size of the region. This avoid premature blockage of the filtering region growth due to speckle. The filtering regions are recycled for neighboring pixels, which avoided the initialization step in homogenous regions and reduced the computation time. After determining the final filtering region, a trimmed arithmetic mean filter is employed to preserve the contrast and median filter is used to identify heterogeneous regions containing resolvable edges [38]. Huang et al., developed an adaptive symmetrical speckle-reduction filter (SSRF) based on the slop facet model to estimate the uncorrupted signal on the largest symmetrical fact centered at each target pixel, which ensured the correctness of the mean value. They adapted a two-stage approach to enhance the statistical reliability of each estimate by forming a union of a set of symmetrical despeckling windows. The algorithm was tested on synthetic as well as clinical ultrasound images and compared with three other algorithms for performance estimation, which exhibited better results than the other algorithms [39].

A novel adaptive speckle suppression and edge enhancement method based on Nakagami distribution was investigated by Shenguen and Limin. In this method, the statistics of log-compressed echo images is derived for the design of the filter and stick technique is employed to approximate certain linear features of the image locally. The stick technique estimates the most prominent linear features such as size and orientation of the stick using hypothesis test optimization and region growing method, respectively, at each point in the image, which effectively reduces the speckle and preserves edges and useful details [40]. Another method based on linear minimum mean square error (LMMSE) estimation of wavelet coefficient was proposed by Argenti and Torricelli. The estimated wavelet coefficients are rescaled using the local statistics of the degraded image, the parameters of noise model, and the wavelet filter. The output of this study revealed that the proposed method efficiently rejects speckle noise compared with the other traditional speckle reduction techniques [41].

Zhang et al., developed the two-dimensional adaptive least mean square filter (TDLMS), which track the weighted local dynamics defined to verify the local speckle formation extent. The difference between the weighted local dynamics and the ideal local dynamics decides the filter's performance in speckle reduction and details preservation [42]. Yu et al., derived a generalized SRAD partial differential equation (PDE) that seeks to minimize a cost functional of the instantaneous coefficient of variation of the image intensity function. They found that the PDE will converge to a piecewise exponential function, the derived PDE can be reformulated to process the ultrasound image. They also found that the generalized SRAD emphasized feature preservation with speckle reduction, while the conventional SRAD emphasized edge enhancement with speckle reduction [43].

A novel genetic neuro-fuzzy filter was proposed by Rafiee et al., which exploits the effectiveness of fuzzy reasoning and the ability to learn from examples. In this filter, 2-D fuzzy sets and trainable fuzzy aggregators are used. The learning method is based on real-time genetic algorithm (GA), which demonstrated an effective high-speed training of the network and satisfactory results after a few generations. The algorithm was tested in many ultrasound B-scan images and the results were validated through edge detection and comparative study with the existing techniques [44]. Yang and Fox demonstrated a compound filtering technique utilizing the advantages of the median filtering, anisotropic diffusion and image decimation and reconstruction, which accelerates the iteration process and enhances the calculation efficiency of despeckling filter. The filter was tested on artificial, speckle corrupted and medical ultrasound images and the results were compared with other traditional despeckling filter, which exhibited better results [45].

Loizou et al., carried out a comparative study of despeckling filter in carotid artery image enhancement operation. They conducted this study on ten filters, which were based on different filtering concepts such as local statistics, geometric, homomorphic, diffusion and wavelet. The performance of the filters were estimated using peak signal to noise ratio (PSNR), root mean square error (RMSE), image quality index (IQI) and geometric average error (GAE). This study suggested that the filters based on local statistics and geometric could be used as a preprocessing step for the automated segmentation of carotid plaque [46]. Acton suggested another method called deconvolutional speckle reducing anisotropic diffusion (DeSpeRADo), which enhances the edge localization ability of SRAD with reduced error interms of area estimation and improved detection of fine features [47]. Yue and coworkers proposed multiscale nonlinear wavelet diffusion (MNWD) method, which combines the sparsity and multiresolution properties of wavelet with the iterative edge preservation and enhancement feature of nonlinear diffusion. In this method, 2D dyadic wavelet transform is used for the image decomposition, speckle related components are eliminated through the iterative coarser scale diffusion and signal-related components are enhanced by the iterative compensation process. This method is validated on the synthetic and real ultrasound images and showed significant speckle reduction and edge enhancement [48, 49].

Michailovich and Tannenbaum suggested a preprocessing procedure, which modifies the speckle noise in the logarithmic image into a white Gaussian noise. This idea was tested in three different filters such as wavelet, total variation and anisotropic diffusion, which results in significant improvements in the quality of the resultant images [50]. Zhang et al., proposed Laplacian pyramid nonlinear diffusion and shock filter (LPNDSF) in which the nonlinear diffusion and shock filter are combined as single partial differential equation (PDE) in the Laplacian pyramid of an image. In this method, the nonlinear diffusion suppressed the speckle while the shock filter enhanced the edges/details [51]. Badawi and Rushdi developed a novel speckle reduction algorithm based on two local image quality parameters viz., scatterer density and texture-based contrast to weight the nonlinear diffusion process, which aimed to replace the traditional quality metrics like, SNR, PSNR, MSE and RMSE. They implemented this filter using back propagation neural network for fast parallel processing of volumetric images. The authors found that this proposed method better reduced the speckle and resolved the edges with reasonable computational speed [52].

Tay et al., presented a squeeze box filter (SBF), which considered the pixel values as stochastic process and determined the local mean and standard deviation of the pixels from an adaptively varying window for removing the outliers. This method causes aggressive smoothing in the homogeneous regions, while guaranteeing the edge preservation. The performance of this filter was studied through a comparative study with the traditional despeckling filters and found to be better than other despeckling filters [53]. Bhuiyan et al., developed a spatially adaptive wavelet method for despeckling ultrasound images by modelling the wavelet coefficients of the log-transformed reflectivity as symmetrical normal inverse Gaussian (SNIG) pdf and log-transformed speckle noise as zero-mean Gaussian pdf. Using this model, a closed form Bayesian wavelet based maximum a posteriori (MAP) denoiser was obtained. The method was experimented both in synthetic and real ultrasound images, which showed better results than the exiting methods interms of calculated SNR and visual inspection [54].

Zhang et al., demonstrated Laplacian pyramid based nonlinear diffusion (LPND) method for despeckling band-pass ultrasound images in Laplacian pyramid domain. This method estimated the nonlinear diffusion in each pyramid layer by automatically determining a gradient threshold using variation of median absolute deviation (MAD) estimator. The LPND method was tested in phantom images and compared with the SRAD and ND methods, which showed that the LPND preserved edges and small structures, where as it removed the speckle noise maximally [56]. Dantas and Costa developed a bank of wide-band two-dimensional (2-D) filters using modified Gabor functions, which split the spectrum of ultrasound image into different frequency directions. This method produces different B-mode images and each image has original information in a specific orientation. All these images were compounded, which produced images with enhanced information and reduced speckle [56].

Shankar explored a new cylindrical Bessel function based spatial filter for enhancing the contrast of speckled images. In this method, the image boundary information is determined using phase characteristics of the image. This method exhibited improvements in contrast and enhancement in boundaries of ultrasound images [57]. Vosoughi and Shamsollahi proposed a combined Wiener filter and M-band wavelet transform approach for despeckling the ultrasound images. In this approach, the image is transformed from multiplicative into additive signal using logarithmic transform. Then, two images are obtained, one using the Wiener filter and the other by subtracting the Wiener filtered image from log transformed image. Both these images are denoised using Byes Shrink despeckling filter. Finally, the summation of these two denoised images results in despeckled image. The authors validated their method both quantitatively and visual comparison [58].

Yoo et al., presented wavelet decomposition based adaptive SRAD method, which used the coarse-to-fine classification as speckle scale function. This method was validated in the simulated as well as clinical ultrasound images and compared the results with other four despeckling filters. The authors found that the proposed method performed better than the other methods [59]. Song et al., adopted a maximum a posteriori (MAP) estimator based on Rayleigh modeling for speckle reduction by manipulating the coefficients in contourlet domain. This method was tested in real ultrasound images and the results obtained were compared with other despeckling methods [60]. The outcome of the contourlet method showed effective reduction in speckle noise and preservation of the detail feature of the image.

Guo et al., illustrated several disadvantage of the spatial and wavelet filters and proposed an algorithm based on textural homogeneity histogram for speckle reduction. In this algorithm, a 2-D homogeneity histogram was built and the threshold was obtained using the maximal-entropy method. This algorithm divided the pixels into homogenous and non-homogenous groups according to the threshold. The non-homogenous pixel set is filtered using the directional average filters iteratively, which reduces the speckle noise without edge blurring. The algorithm was tested in several artificial as well clinical ultrasound images and compared with the traditional despeckling filters [61].

Khare et al., developed Daubechies complex wavelet transform based speckle reduction method, which utilizes the approximate shift invariance property and extra information in imaginary plane of the complex wavelet domain. In this method, a wavelet shrinkage factor was derived to estimate the noise-free wavelet coefficients. This method initially detected strong edges using the imaginary components of complex scaling and subsequently applied the shrinkage on magnitude of complex wavelet coefficients at the non-edge points. The shrinkage depends on the statistical parameters of complex wavelet coefficients of the noisy image. The effectiveness of this method was experimented on real ultrasound images and the results were compared with other despeckling methods [62].

Devarapu et al., investigated the application of Curvelet filter for denoising the speckle in ultrasound images. The filter was tested in various ultrasound images and the performance of the filter was estimated through calculation of performance indices such as PSNR, MSE and EPI. The results obtained from the Curvelet filter was compared with several established despeckling filters and the Curvelet filter was found to be outperformed over the other filters [63]. Huang and Yang developed a log-compressed ultrasound image model for texture identification, which results in better speckle reduction and edge preservation. The performance of the model was demonstrated through a comparative study of the proposed method with the other anisotropic diffusion methods [64]. Nedumaran et al., proposed a novel topological derivative filter for speckle reduction, which is the main research problem of this thesis and is described in Chapter III [65].

2.5 OVERVIEW OF DESPECKLING FILTERS

Over three decades, various speckle reduction filters have been proposed by biomedical researchers. The application of a particular filter depends on either local statistics for determining the noise variance within the filter or estimating the local noise variance using the effective equivalent number of looks (ENL) of the image. Several standard speckle filters such as Median, Frost, Lee, Kuan, Wiener, Wavelet, anisotropic diffusion, and speckle reduction anisotropic diffusion (SRAD) are considered as the best speckle reduction filters for the ultrasound B-scan images. All these filters have unique despeckling characteristics/approach, which performs the particular filtering operation in a moving square-window, called kernel [66, 67]. The filtering operation is performed on the basis of statistical relationship between the central pixel and its neighboring pixels as shown in Figure 2.2.

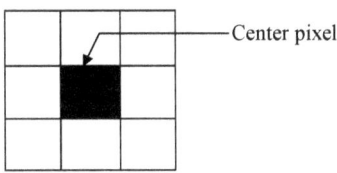

Fig 2.2 Representation of 3 x 3 kernel

The typical size of the kernel window can range from 3x3 to 33x33, but the size of the window must contain odd number of squares. If the size of the kernel is large, then it uses large pixel area for filter response calculation that possibly requires more computation time and important details will be lost due to over smoothing. On the other hand, if the kernel size is too small, speckle reduction may not be effective. In practical applications, either 3x3 or 7x7 kernel window is preferred due to better filter performance. In this research work, some of the important and novel speckle reduction filters such as spatial and frequency adaptive filters, wavelet filter, diffusion filter, and topological derivative filter have been attempted to remove the speckle noise present in ultrasound B-scan images. The basic concepts, mathematical theory and the characteristics of the afore-mentioned filters are discussed in detail in the following subsections.

2.5.1 Spatial Adaptive filters

In spatial adaptive filters, the kernel calculates the statistical information of all pixels gray values such as local mean and local variance. The calculated statistical value replaces the central pixel value of the defined kernel. Spatial filters like Frost, Median,

Lee, Kuan, Enhanced Frost, Enhanced Lee, Wiener, Gamma Map filters, and the frequency filter like Homomorphic filter are the earliest filters working directly on the intensity of the image using local statistics [68, 69]. For implementation of the spatial filters, there are three main steps involved and are given below [27].

    (i)   computation of local statistics,
    (ii)   region growing procedure and
    (iii) application of smoothening operator

The detailed description of the above-mentioned spatial adaptive filters is given in the following sub-sections.

2.5.1.1 Frost filter

Frost filter calculates the weighted sum of the pixel values within the moving kernel and replaces the particular pixel value with the calculated new value. The weighting factor decreases with distance from the particular pixel value and increases for the central pixel as the variance within the kernel increases. It is also known as adaptive and exponentially weighted averaging filter based on the coefficient of variation. The coefficient of variation is the ratio of the local standard deviation to the local mean of the degraded image [70]. This filter assumes speckle as multiplicative and stationary noise, which follows the statistics given in equation 2.5.

$$DF = \sum_{n \times n} A \delta e^{-\alpha |t|} \qquad \ldots 2.5$$

$$\text{Where } \delta = \left(\frac{4}{n \sigma'^2} \right) \left(\frac{\sigma^2}{I'^2} \right) \qquad \ldots 2.6$$

where A is the normalization constant, I'^2 is the local mean, σ is the local variance and σ'^2 is the image coefficient of variation value, $|t| = |X - X_0| + |Y - Y_0|$ and n is the moving kernel size.

2.5.1.2 Median filter

The median filter [70] is a spatial non-linear filter that calculates the median of all pixel value in the kernel and replaces the central pixel value with the calculated median. It removes pulse or spike noise in the image.

2.5.1.3 Lee and Kuan filter

The Lee [68,69] and Kuan [18] filter are based on the minimum mean square error (MMSE), which produce the speckle free image governed by the relationship given in equation 2.7 [71].

$$U(x, y) = I(x, y)W(x, y) + I'(x, y)(1 - W(x, y)) \qquad \ldots 2.7$$

where I is the mean value of the intensity in the chosen window in the raw image, I' is the mean value of the intensity after applying the despeckling filter function and $W(x,y)$ is the adaptive filter coefficient calculated using the following formula given in equations 2.8 and 2.9.

$$W(x, y) = 1 - \frac{C_B^2}{\left[C_I^2 + C_B^2\right]} \quad \text{for Lee filter} \qquad \ldots 2.8$$

$$W(x, y) = \frac{1 - C_B^2 / C_I^2}{\left[1 + C_B^2\right]} \quad \text{for Kuan filter} \qquad \ldots 2.9$$

where C_I is the coefficient of variation of the noised image and C_B is the coefficient of variation of the noise. In general, the value of W(x,y) approaches zero in uniform areas, i.e., it approaches unity at edges, which results in little modification of pixel values near edges.

2.5.1.4 Wiener filter

Wiener filter [72, 73] restores images in the presence of blur and noise. Wiener filter performs smoothing of the image based on the computation of local image variance. When the local variance of the image is large, the smoothing is little. On the other hand, if the variance is small, the smoothing will be better. This approach often produces better quality results than linear filtering, since the Wiener filtering is adaptive, more selective than a comparable linear filter. It preserves edges and other high-frequency information of the image, but requires more computation time than linear filtering.

2.5.1.5 Enhanced Frost and Enhanced Lee filter

According to Lopes et al., the ultrasound B-Scan images can be divided into the three classes based on the variation coefficients [22, 71]. The first class corresponds to the homogeneous areas in which the speckles may be eliminated simply by applying a low-pass filter. The second class corresponds to the heterogeneous areas in which the speckles are to be reduced while preserving texture. The third class includes areas containing isolated point targets, which should preserve the observed value. Based on the above considerations, the modified form of the Frost and the Lee filter functions are evaluated and are given in equations 2.10 and 2.12.

Enhanced Frost filter:

$$W(x,y) = e^{-kfunc(C_I(x',y'))|(x,y)|} \qquad \ldots 2.10$$

where $func(C_I(x',y'))$ is a hyperbolic function and it can be derived by

$$func(C_I) = \begin{cases} 0 & for\ C_I(x',y') < C_B \\ \dfrac{[C_I(x',y') - C_B]}{[C_{max} - C_I(x',y')]} & for\ C_B \leq C_I(x',y') \leq C_{max} \\ \infty & for\ C_I(x',y') > C_{max} \end{cases} \qquad \ldots 2.11$$

Enhanced Lee filter:

$$U(x,y) = \begin{cases} I'(x,y) & for\ C_I(x,y) \leq C_B \\ I(x,y)W(x,y) + I'(x,y)(1-W(x,y)) & for\ C_B < C_I(x,y) < C_{max} \\ I(x,y) & for\ C_I(x,y) \geq C_{max} \end{cases} \qquad \ldots 2.12$$

where $W(x',y') = \exp[-k(C_I(x',y') - C_B)/(C_{max} - C_I(x',y'))]$

Lopes et al., also demonstrated that these modified filters are forced to achieve average value and observed value for the homogenous and isolated point target classes, respectively without filtering in comparison with the original filters. Between these two extremes, the heterogeneous class exists, for which the modified filters have the similar forms as the original filters, but the filter responses are exaggerated due to the introduction of a hyperbolic function, which satisfied the condition that the more heterogeneous area is less smoothed [22].

2.5.1.6 Gamma Map filter

Kuan et al., [18] proposed a speckle reduction filter based on the application of maximum a posteriori (MAP) approach, which required a priori knowledge of the probability density function (PDF) of the image. Lopes et al., [23] modified the Kuan MAP filter by assuming a gamma distributed image and setting up two thresholds, since Kuan MAP filter assumed a Gaussian distribution for image reflectivity that results in negative reflectivity. The Gamma MAP filter is given by the equation 2.13.

$$U(x',y') = \begin{cases} I'(x',y') & \text{for } C_{I(x',y')} < C_B \\ \dfrac{(\alpha-L-1)I'(x',y') + \sqrt{I^2(x',y')(\alpha-L-1) + 4\alpha L I'(x',y')}}{2\alpha} & \text{for } C_B \leq C_{I(x',y')} \leq C_{\max} \\ I(x',y') & \text{for } C_{I(x',y')} > C_{\max} \end{cases} \quad ...2.13$$

where L is the Number of Looks, $C_{\max}(x',y') = \sqrt{2C_B}$ and $\alpha = \dfrac{1+C_B^2}{C_I^2(x',y') - C_B^2}$

2.5.1.7 Homomorphic filter

Homomorphic filtering performs image enhancement by applying the filter function and inverse FFT on the logarithmically compressed image [22, 46]. The filter function $H(u,v)$ may be constructed using either the band-pass or the high-boost Butter worth filter. In this study, the high-boost Butter worth technique has been employed and its mathematical formula is given in equation 2.14

$$H_{u,v} = \delta_L + \frac{\delta_H}{1+\left(\frac{D_0}{D_{u,v}}\right)^2} \qquad \text{...2.14}$$

$$D_{u,v} = \sqrt{(u-N/2)^2 2 + (v-N/2)^2} \qquad \text{...2.15}$$

where D_0 is the cut of frequency of the filter, δ_L is the low frequency gain, δ_H is the high frequency gain, u and v are the spatial coordinates of the frequency transformed image and N is the dimensions of the image in the u and v space.

2.5.2 Wavelet Transform

Wavelet theory was first proposed by Morlet and Grossman and its mathematical foundation was developed by them with Meyer [74 -77]. Later, Daubechies and Mallet developed the potential applications of wavelet in the area of digital signal processing.

In the Fourier transform, the time and frequency resolution remains constant, since the shape and length of the analysis window remains fixed. In Wavelet Transform (WT), signal decomposition is carried out on the basis functions by dilations, contractions and shift of a unique function called 'mother wavelet'. Over the years, many different wavelet basis functions have been developed by the researchers to solve many signal and image processing applications. Some of the interesting mother wavelet functions are Mexican hat, Harr, Daubechies, Coiflet, Symlet, Morlet, etc. There are different types of Wavelet transforms such as Continuous Wavelet Transform (CWT), Wavelet Series Expansion (WS) and Discrete Wavelet Transform (DWT) and the selection of the particular type depending on the domain in which it is employed and the nature of the application.

The mother wavelet function is mathematically expressed as

$$\psi(\tau,s) = \frac{1}{\sqrt{s}} \psi\left(\frac{t-\tau}{s}\right) \qquad \text{...2.16}$$

where $\psi\left(\frac{t-\tau}{s}\right)$ is the mother wavelet, the factor $\frac{1}{\sqrt{s}}$ is a normalized factor used to ensure energy across different scale, s is the scale or width of the basis function and τ is the translation in the time axis.

2.5.2.1 Continuous wavelet transform (CWT)

Continuous wavelet transform of $f(t)$, with respect to the wavelet $\psi(t)$ is defined as,

$$CWT(\tau,s) = \frac{1}{\sqrt{s}} \int_{-\infty}^{\infty} f(t)\psi\left(\frac{t-\tau}{s}\right)dt \qquad \ldots 2.17$$

where τ is the translation coefficient and s is the scaling coefficient. Continuous wavelet transform analyzes the signal through the continuous shifts of a scalable function over a time plane. This technique results in redundancy and it is numerically impossible to analysis at infinite number of wavelet sets.

2.5.2.2 Discrete wavelet transform (DWT)

Discrete Wavelet Transform (DWT) approach scales and translates the mother wavelets in discrete steps, which reduces the redundancy problem in CWT. The DWT is mathematically expressed as,

$$DWT(\tau_0, s_0) = \frac{1}{\sqrt{s_0^j}} \int_{-\infty}^{\infty} f(t)\psi\left(\frac{t - k\tau_0 s_0^j}{s_0^j}\right)dt \qquad \ldots 2.18$$

where s_o^j is the scaling factor, τ_0 is the translating factor, k and j are just integers.

In the case of images (2-D signals), the discrete wavelet transform decompose the image into various sub-bands and is given in Figure 2.3.

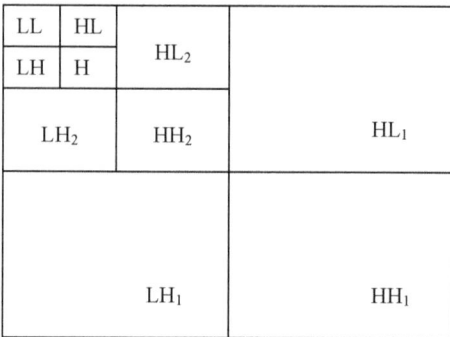

Fig 2.3 Discrete wavelet transform on 2-dimensional signals

In the Figure 2.5, the sub-bands HH_k, HL_k, LH_k, $k = 1, 2,..., j$ are called the details, where k is the scale and j denotes the largest or coarsest scale in decomposition. Here, LL_k is the low-resolution component. To remove the unwanted wavelet coefficient or noise in the detail components of the sub-bands, thresholding is applied. To construct the denoised images from the modified coefficients, inverse discrete wavelet transform is applied.

2.5.2.3 Wavelet Thresholding

Wavelet thresholding is the decomposition technique that converts the signal or image into wavelet coefficients by comparing the detail coefficients with the given threshold and set to zero if its magnitude is less than the threshold, otherwise, it is retained or modified according to the threshold rule [78, 79]. This technique is used to distinguish the noise from the significant information found in signals and images. The selection of the threshold values in image denoising plays a very important role in the removal of noise, since too much denoising smoothed the images and reducing the sharpness of the image.

Several methods have been found in the literature for wavelet thresholding and some of the important thresholding methods for image denoising include VisuShrink, SureShrink and BayesShrink [78 - 81]. Also, there are two types of thresholding strategies available viz., hard-thresholding and soft-thresholding. The hard-thresholding can be mathematically defines as [79],

$$T_H = \begin{cases} x \ for \ |x| \geq t \\ 0 \ in \ all \ other \ regions \end{cases} \quad ...2.19$$

where t is the threshold value. A plot of the hard-thresholding is shown in Figure 2.4

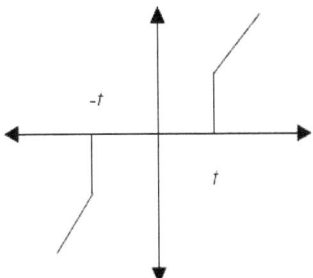

Fig 2.4 Hard thresholding technique

From the plot shown in Figure 2.4, it is found that all coefficients whose magnitude value greater than the selected threshold value t keeps the present value and those with magnitudes smaller than t are set to zero. Soft thresholding is the process by which the coefficients with greater than the threshold are shrunk towards zero after comparing to the threshold value. It is diagrammatically represented in Figure 2.5 and its mathematical definition is given in equation 2.20 [79].

$$T_H = \begin{cases} sign(x)(|x|-t) \ for \ |x| > t \\ 0 \ in \ all \ other \ regions \end{cases} \quad ...2.20$$

From the Figure 2.5, it can be seen that the soft thresholding is much better than the hard thresholding, since soft thresholding has smooth transition from the threshold region to the zero region that produces smooth images whereas in hard thresholding the transition is abrupt, which results in discontinuous or artifacts in the recovered images. Besides, soft-thresholding has smaller minimum mean squared error than the hard-thresholding.

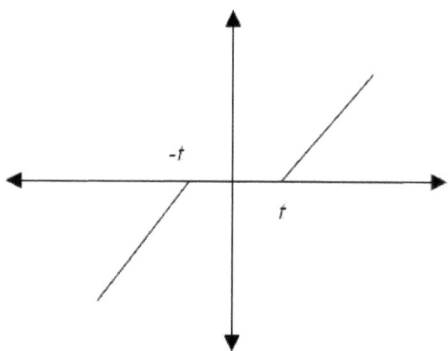

Fig 2.5 Representation of soft thresholding

2.5.3 Diffusion filters

Diffusion filters may be applied directly on the image for removing the speckle noise by solving partial differential equation. An anisotropic diffusion filter performs contrast enhancement and noise reduction without requiring the power spectrum information of the image [82]. In this research work, two diffusion filters have been attempted and their descriptions are given in the following sub-sections.

2.5.3.1 Perona Malik Anisotropic Diffusion (PMAD) filter

Perona Malik Anisotropic Diffusion filter (PMAD) is based on three criteria viz., causality, immediate localization and piecewise smoothing. Causality criteria guarantee that no spurious detail should be generated while passing from the finer to coarser scales. Immediate localization ascertains the sharpness of the region boundaries and coincidence with the semantically meaningful boundaries at each resolution. The piecewise smoothing guarantees intra-region smoothing over inter-region smoothing at all scales.

Based on the above criteria, Perona and Malik proposed a diffusion method based on the nonlinear PDE to avoid the blurring and localization problems of linear diffusion filtering [82 - 85]. The PMAD filter mathematical expression is given in equation 2.21.

$$T_H = \begin{cases} \dfrac{\partial I}{\partial t} = div\left[c|\nabla I|.\nabla I\right] \\ I(t=0) = I_0 \end{cases} \qquad \ldots 2.21$$

where ∇ is the gradient operator, div the divergence operator, $|\ |$ denotes the magnitude, c(x) the diffusion coefficient, and I_0 the initial image. They suggested two diffusion coefficients

$$C(x) = \frac{1}{1+(x/k)^2} \qquad \ldots 2.22$$

$$C(x) = \exp[-(x/k)^2] \qquad \ldots 2.23$$

where k is an edge magnitude parameter.

In this method, the gradient magnitude is utilized to detect the image edge/boundary as a step discontinuity in intensity. In the above equation, if $|\nabla I| \gg k$, then $c|\nabla I| \to 0$, and we have an all-pass filter; if $|\nabla I| \ll k$, then $c|\nabla I| \to 1$, and isotropic diffusion (Gaussian filtering) is achieved.

The discrete form of the equation 2.21 is expressed by,

$$I_s^{t+\Delta t} = I_s^t + \frac{\Delta t}{|\bar{\eta}_s|} \sum_{p \in \bar{\eta}_s} C(\nabla I_{s,p}^t) \nabla I_{s,p}^t \qquad \ldots 2.24$$

where I_s^t is the discretely sampled image, s denotes the pixel position in a discrete two-dimensional (2-D) grid, and Δt is the time step size, $\bar{\eta}_s$ represents the spatial neighborhood of pixel s, $|\bar{\eta}_s|$ is the number of pixels in the window (usually four, except at the image boundaries), and $\Delta I_{s,p}^t = I_p^t - I_s^t$, $\forall p \in \bar{\eta}_s$.

The advantages of anisotropic diffusion include intra-region smoothing and edge preservation and perform well for images corrupted by additive noise. In cases where images contain speckle, anisotropic diffusion will actually enhance the speckle, instead of eliminating the noise [36].

2.5.3.2 Speckle Reducing Anisotropic Diffusion (SRAD) filter

SRAD is an adaptive filter using soft-threshold technique to modify the quality of image in homogenous regions, small features and regions near edges. It inhibits diffusion across edges and allows diffusion on either side of the edge, which results in both preservation and enhancement of the edges. Yu and Acton suggested a PDE-based SRAD approach, which allows the generation of an image scale space without bias due to filter window size and shape [36]. For a given intensity image $I_0(x,y)$ having finite power and non-zero values in the image domain Ω, the output image $I(x,y; t)$ is estimated according to the PDE relationship given in equation 2.25.

$$\begin{cases} \partial I(x,y;t)/\partial t = div[c(q)\nabla I(x,y;t)] \\ I(x,y;0) = I_0(x,y), \left(\dfrac{\partial I(x,y;t)}{\partial \vec{n}}\right)_{d\Omega=0} \end{cases} \quad \ldots 2.25$$

where $d\Omega$ represents the envelop of Ω, $\vec{n}$ is the outer normal to the $d\Omega$ and

$$C(q) = \dfrac{1}{1+[q^2(x,y;t)-q_0^2(t)]/[q_0^2(t)(1+q_0^2(t))]} \quad \ldots 2.26$$

or

$$C(q) = \exp\{-[q^2(x,y;t)-q_0^2(t)]/[q_0^2(t)(1+q_0^2(t))]\} \quad \ldots 2.27$$

where $q(x,y; t)$ is the instantaneous coefficient of variation and $q_0(t)$ is the speckle scale function.

The value of $q(x,y; t)$ can be determined using equation 2.28.

$$q(x,y;t) = \sqrt{\dfrac{(1/2)(|\nabla I|/I)^2 - (1/4)^2(\nabla^2 I/I)^2}{[1+(1/4)(\nabla^2 I/I)]^2}} \quad \ldots 2.28$$

The instantaneous coefficient of variation produces high values at the high contrast regions and edges whereas it gives low values at homogenous regions. Therefore, using the equations (2.26) and (2.27), the amount of smoothing can be effectively controlled.

By assuming that the diffusion should be isotropic in a uniform area, the function for $q_0(t)$ can be derived using the equation 2.29.

$$I_{i,j}^{t+\nabla t} = I_{i,j}^t + \frac{\Delta t}{4}(I_{i+1,j}^t + I_{i-1,j}^t + I_{i,j+1}^t + I_{i,j-1}^t + 4I_{i,j}^t) \qquad \ldots 2.29$$

For a given $\sigma(t)$ and the standard deviation of $I_{i,j}^t$ in a homogenous region, the standard deviation of $I_{i,j}^{t+\Delta t}$ in the region can be calculated by assuming that the pixel in this region are statistically independent to each other and identically distributed. From the statistical formula for variance of a sum of random variables and from the equation (2.29) we can calculate the standard deviation using equation 2.30.

$$\sigma(t+\Delta t) = \sqrt{(1-\Delta t)^2 \sigma^2(t) + (\Delta t/4)^2 4\sigma^2(t)} \qquad \ldots 2.30$$

But, the local mean remains the same before and after the iteration, hence $q_0(t+\Delta t)$ becomes,

$$q_0(t+\Delta t) = q_0(t)\sqrt{(1-\Delta t)^2 + (\Delta t)^2 + (\Delta t)^2/4} \qquad \ldots 2.31$$

For $\Delta t \ll 1$, $(\Delta t)^2$ term can be neglected in equation (2.31), and we have,

$$\sqrt{1-2\Delta t} \approx 1-\Delta t \qquad \ldots 2.32$$

Expanding the above equation (2.31) using Taylor series expansion and neglecting higher order terms we have,

$$q_0(t+\Delta t) - q_0(t) + q_0(t)\Delta t \approx 0 \qquad \ldots 2.33$$

Dividing the above equation by Δt on both sides and taking the limit as $\Delta t \to 0$, we have

$$\dot{q}_0(t) + q_0(t) \approx 0 \qquad \ldots 2.34$$

Where $\dot{q}_0(t)$ is the first derivative of $q_0(t)$ with respect to t. Solving equation (2.34) gives,

$$q_0(t) \approx q_0 \exp[-t] \qquad \ldots 2.35$$

From equation 2.35, it is clear that the speckle will be reduced exponentially through the diffusion process. This result can be achieved from equation (2.30), only when the values of $I_{i,j}^t$, in the homogenous region are truly independent. But, in practical situation the iteration of diffusion should be smaller than the value predicted by equation 2.35. To control the exponential decay rate, a constant ($\rho<1$) is introduced in equation 2.35 resulting in equation 2.36.

$$q_0(t) \approx q_0 \exp[-\rho t] \qquad \ldots 2.36$$

For a given values of q_0 and ρ, any speckled image can be denoised using equation 2.36 without choosing the homogenous regions. Another way of finding q_0 from intensity and mean variance over a homogenous area at t can be performed using equation 2.37.

$$q_0(t) = \frac{\sqrt{\operatorname{var}[z(t)]}}{z(t)'} \qquad \ldots 2.37$$

where $\operatorname{var}[z(t)]$ and $z(t)'$ are the intensity variance and mean, respectively over a homogenous area at t.

2.6 OVERVIEW OF IMAGE QUALITY MEASURES

The quality of the images, in particular medical images, must be guaranteed in order to perform clinical tasks such as lesion identification and classification efficiently and to measure the ability of the image processing technique to improve the quality of the particular imaging modality. Most of the recent studies pointed out that the performance of the equipment in producing the image is assessed by the expert's opinion, which differs due to intraobserver and interobserver variability. Image degradation is the most important aspect of image quality, a few studies have been attempted to perform physical measurements of degradation. In the case of ultrasound B-scan image, the quality of the image is important when evaluating the performance of the particular speckle suppression technique. To quantify the performance of the despeckling filters, several well-established performance metrics were found in the literature [86 – 97]. In this research work, we have chosen the following nineteen quality measures viz., Average Difference (AD), Mean-Square-Error (MSE), Peak Signal to Noise Ratio (PSNR), Maximum Difference (MD), Normalized Absolute Error (NAE), Structural Content (SC), Coefficient of Correlation (CoC), Normalized Cross Correlation (NCC), Image Quality Index (IQI), Speckle Index (SI), Average Signal to Noise Ration (ASNR), Image Variance (IV), Noise Standard Deviation (NSD), Equivalent Number of Looks (ENL), Mean Structure Similarity Index Map (MISSIM), Normalized Mean Square Error (NMSE), Contrast to Noise Ratio (CNR), Geometric Average Error (GAE), and Figure of Merit (FoM) for estimating the performance of the proposed despeckling filter and execution time. In addition to this, five edge detection methods were attempted in this study in order to represent the performance of the despeckling filters graphically for visual inspection and peak SNR calculation. The definition, mathematical expression, range and the physical interpretation of the afore-mentioned quality metrics are summarized in Table 2.1.

Table 2.1 Summarization of metrics used for estimating the performance of despeckling filters

Performance Metrics	Mathematical Expression	Definition	Range of value for better Performance (Min/Max/Close to Unity)
Average Difference (AD)	$AD = \dfrac{1}{MN} \sum_{j=1}^{M} \sum_{k=1}^{N} \left| X_{j,k} - X'_{j,k} \right|$	Mean difference of the two (Original and denoised) images divided by the size of the image	AD is maximum for dissimilar images and minimum for similar images. The range of AD is from 0 to 255.
Mean Square Error (MSE)	$MSE = \dfrac{1}{MN} \sum_{j=1}^{M} \sum_{k=1}^{N} (X_{j,k} - X'_{j,k})^2$	The average of the square of the difference between original and the denoised image divided by the size of the image (the error). Represents the average difference between images.	Higher and lower MSE values indicate larger and smaller differences between the original and denoised images, respectively. MSE will be equal to zero for identical images. For completely dissimilar images, the MSE value becomes 255.
Peak Signal to Noise Ratio (PSNR)	$PSNR = 10 \log_{10} \dfrac{(2^n - 1)^n}{MSE} = 10 \log_{10} \left(\dfrac{255^2}{MSE} \right)$	Measure of the performance of the speckle noise removal. It is a ratio between the maximum possible power of the signal and the noise content.	Typical value is between 30 and 50 dB. Higher PSNR values show better image quality. For identical images, the MSE become zero and the PSNR is undefined.
Maximum Difference (MD)	$MD = Max\left(\left| X_{j,k} - X'_{j,k} \right| \right)$	Maximum error difference between the original and denoised images.	MD gives the maximum difference values in the pixel level.
Normalized Absolute Error (NAE)	$NAE = \dfrac{\sum_{j=1}^{M} \sum_{K=1}^{N} \left| X_{j,k} - X'_{j,k} \right|}{\sum_{j=1}^{M} \sum_{K=1}^{N} X_{j,k}}$	Normalized absolute error is the measure of error prediction accuracy of the image	Its value ranges between 0 and 1. Lower value indicates that the error between the original and denoised images is smaller.
Structural Content (SC)	$SC = \dfrac{\sum_{j=1}^{M} \sum_{K=1}^{N} X_{j,k}^2}{\sum_{j=1}^{M} \sum_{K=1}^{N} (X'_{j,k})^2}$	Measure of similarity between original and denoised images.	For identical images it should be one.
Coefficient of Correlation (CoC)	$CoC = \dfrac{\sum_{j=1}^{M} \sum_{K=1}^{N} (X'_{j,k} - \bar{X}'_{j,k})(X_{j,k} - \bar{X}_{j,k})}{\sqrt{\sum_{j=1}^{M} \sum_{K=1}^{N} (X'_{j,k} - \bar{X}'_{j,k})^2 \sum_{j=1}^{M} \sum_{K=1}^{N} (X_{j,k} - \bar{X}_{j,k})^2}}$	Measure of edge preservation in the denoised image.	Its value is 1 and 0 for identical and completely uncorrelated images, respectively. Its value becomes –1 if they are completely anti-correlated.
Normalized Cross Correlation (NCC)	$NCC = \dfrac{\sum_{j=1}^{M} \sum_{K=1}^{N} (X_{j,k})(X'_{j,k})}{\sum_{j=1}^{M} \sum_{K=1}^{N} X_{j,k}^2}$	It is a correlation based image quality measure.	Its value becomes unity for identical images.
Image Quality Index (IQI)	$IQI = \dfrac{4\sigma_{xx'} \overline{XX'}}{\left[\sigma_x^2 + \sigma_{x'}^2 \right] \left[\bar{X}^2 + (\bar{X}')^2 \right]}$	Degree of distortion in terms of loss of correlation, mean distortion and variance distortion.	Its dynamic range is between -1 and 1. For identical images the value of image quality index is unity.

Metric	Formula	Description	Remarks
Speckle Index (SI)	$SI = \dfrac{1}{MN} \sum_{j=1}^{M} \sum_{K=1}^{N} \dfrac{\sigma(X)}{\mu(X)}$	Measure of speckle removal in terms of average contrast of the image	If SI is low then the image quality is improved.
Average Signal to Noise Ratio (ASNR)	$ASNR = \dfrac{1}{SI}$	Measures average deviation of the speckle with respect to the mean value of the image.	Less for noisy images and increases with the degree of denoising.
Image Variance (IV)	$\sigma^2 = \dfrac{1}{MN} \sum_{j=1}^{M} \sum_{k=1}^{N} (X_{j,k} - \bar{X}_{j,k})^2$	Determines the contents of the speckle in the image.	A lower value gives smoother image as more speckles is reduced.
Noise Standard Deviation (NSD)	$NSD = \dfrac{SORT((\sum_{j=1}^{M}\sum_{k=1}^{N}(X_{j,k}-NMV)^2)}{MN}$ where $NMV = \dfrac{\sum_{j=1}^{M}\sum_{k=1}^{N} X_{j,k}}{MN}$	Determines the quantity of the speckle in the image	NSD value will be less for the images with minimum quantity of the speckle.
Effective Number of Looks (ENL)	$ENL = \dfrac{[NMV]^2}{[NSD]^2}$	Measure of speckle level in ultrasound image over a uniform image region.	A large value of ENL reflects the better quantitative performance of the filter. The value also depends on the size of the testing region.
Mean Structure Similarity Index Map (MSSIM) Structure similarity index map (SSIM)	$MSSIM = \dfrac{1}{MN} \sum_{j=1}^{M}\sum_{K=1}^{N} SSIM[(X_{j,k}),(X'_{j,k})]$ where $SSIM(X,X') = \dfrac{(2\mu_X \mu_{X'}+C_1)(2\sigma_{XX'}+C_2)}{(\mu_X^2+\mu_{X'}^2+C_1)(\sigma_X^2+\sigma_{X'}^2+C_2)}$	MSSIM and SSIM are used to compare luminance, contrast and structure of two different images. It can be treated as a similarity measure of two different images	The MSSIM value should be closer to unity for optimal measure of similarity.
Normalized Mean Square Error (NMSE)	$NMSE = \dfrac{\sum_{j=1}^{M}\sum_{k=1}^{N}(X_{j,k}-X'_{j,k})}{\sum_{j=1}^{M}\sum_{k=1}^{N} X_{j,k}^2}$	Measure the variation of the mean square error.	The measured value of NMSE value is small for similar images and is zero for identical images
Contrast to Noise Ratio (CNR)	$CNR = \dfrac{|\mu' - \mu''|}{\sqrt{\sigma_1^2 + \sigma_2^2}}$	Measure the contrast ratio of the image with respect to the background	The CNR provides a quantitative measure of the detect ability of low contrast lesions with respect to high contrast lesion or from the background media.
Geometric Average Error (GAE)	$GAE = \left(\prod_{j=1}^{M}\prod_{k=1}^{N} \sqrt{X_{j,k}-X'_{j,k}} \right)^{\frac{1}{MN}}$	Measure the information between the original and the despeckled images.	The value of GAE is approaching zero if there is a very good transformation (small differences) between the original and despeckled images; otherwise, the value of GAE is high.
Figure of Merit (FoM)	$FoM = \dfrac{1}{\max(N_e, N_i)} \sum_{j=1}^{N} \dfrac{1}{1+d_j^2 \alpha}$	Measure the performance of edge preservation of the image	The value of FoM ranges between 0 and 1, and is unity for the ideal edge detection.

2.7 EDGE DETECTION TECHNIQUES

Edge detection is the most common approach for identifying and locating sharp discontinuities that characterize the boundaries in an image using first and second order derivatives. Usually, the edge detection process significantly reduces the amount of data and filters out information of an image. There are several edge detection methods found in the literature and can be broadly classified in two categories, namely gradient and Laplacian [98-109]. In the gradient method, the edges are detected by finding the maximum and minimum in the first-order derivative of the image. In the Laplacian method, the edges are identified by searching the zero crossing in the second-order derivative of the image. There are several edge detection operators available including Sobel, Robert's, Prewitt's, Laplacian of Gaussian (LoG) and Canny. In the classical methods, the image is convolved with the operator and identified the edges where large gradient is found in the image, whereas returned with zero for uniform regions. Each operator is designed to be sensitive to certain types of edges and the selection of a particular operator depends on edge orientation, noise environment and edge structure. The geometry of the operator determines a characteristic direction in which it is most sensitive to edges and can be optimized to look for horizontal, vertical, or diagonal edges [98-100].

The edge detection using first-order and second-order derivatives can be demonstrated by an example. A signal with an edge is illustrated as the jump in the intensity of the signal as shown in Figure 2.6.

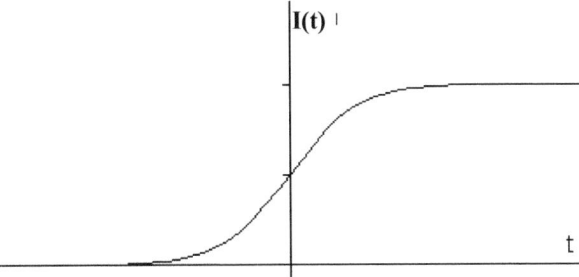

Fig 2.6 Representation of edge by the change in intensity of the signal

The first-order derivative (gradient) of the signal is shown in Figure 2.7.

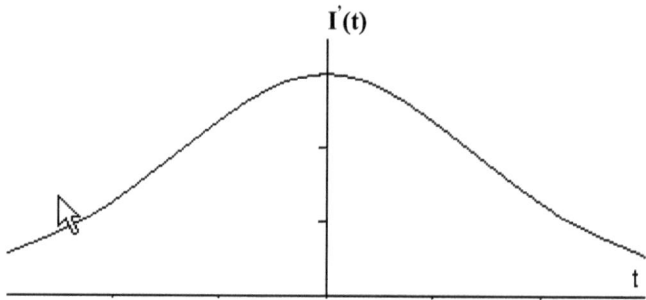

Fig 2.7 First-order derivative of the original signal (shown in Fig 2.6)

The second-derivative of the signal is shown in Figure 2.8.

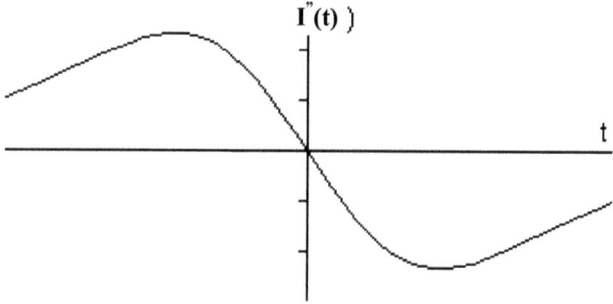

Fig 2.8 Second-order derivative of the original signal (shown in Fig 2.6)

From the Figure 2.7, it is found that the maximum gradient is located at the centre of the original signal, which forms the characteristic of the gradient filters like Sobel [98-100]. The second derivative shows a zero value where a maximum value is found for the first derivative, which forms the foundation for the Laplacian filters. As a result, either the maximum of the first derivative or zeros of the second derivatives can be used as deciding parameter for edge detection. But, in the case of the first derivative, a threshold value is set for the identification of edges. By comparing the gradient with the threshold value, the pixel values higher than the threshold are identified as edges.

2.8 EDGE DETECTION OPERATORS

2.8.1 Sobel operator

Sobel operator consists of a pair of 3×3 convolution kernels as shown in Figure 2.9. In this one kernel is obtained by rotating the other kernel by 90°.

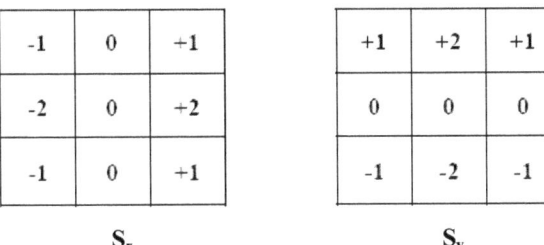

S_x S_y

Fig 2.9 Kernels of Sobel operator

These kernels are designed to respond maximally to edges of the two perpendicular directions relative to the pixel grid [98, 99, 101- 104]. The kernels are applied to the input image separately, which produced separate gradient components in each orientation denoted as S_x and S_y as shown in Figure 2.9. To calculate the absolute gradient magnitude at each point, the values of S_x and S_y are combined together using equation 2.37.

$$|S| = \sqrt{S_x^2 + S_y^2} \quad \ldots 2.37$$

The approximate magnitude can be computed using the equation 2.38, which computes the value much faster.

$$|S| = |S_x| + |S_y| \quad \ldots 2.38$$

The angle of orientation of the edge can be computed using equation 2.39, which gives the spatial gradient of the edge.

$$\theta = \arctan\left[\frac{S_y}{S_x}\right] \quad \ldots 2.39$$

2.8.2 Robert's operator

The Robert's operator consists of a pair of 2x2 convolution kernel as shown in Figure 2.10. In this operator, one kernel can be obtained by simply rotating the other kernel by 90° and the output pixel value is the estimated absolute magnitude of the spatial gradient of the corresponding input pixel.

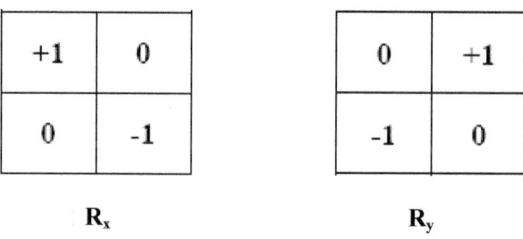

Fig 2.10 Kernels of the Robert's operator

These kernels are designed to respond maximally to edges running at 45° to the two perpendicular directions relative to the pixel grid. Similar to the Sobel kernels, the two kernels are applied separately to the input image in order to obtain the output gradient components separately. Then, these two components are combined together according to the equation 2.40, to obtain the absolute gradient magnitude at each point [98, 99,101,104,105].

The gradient magnitude is given by:

$$|R| = \sqrt{R_x^2 + R_y^2} \quad \ldots 2.40$$

For faster computation of the gradient magnitude, equation 2.41 is used

$$|R| = |R_x| + |R_y| \quad \ldots 2.41$$

The spatial gradient can be calculated using the equation 2.42.

$$\theta = \arctan\left[\frac{R_y}{R_x}\right] - \frac{3\pi}{4} \quad \ldots 2.42$$

2.8.3 Prewitt's operator

The Prewitt's operator is similar to the Sobel operator, but the kernels are designed to give spectral response very fast in the x, y directions. The kernels are shown in Figure 2.11. It is suitable for well-contrasted noiseless images [98, 99, 101, 102, 106].

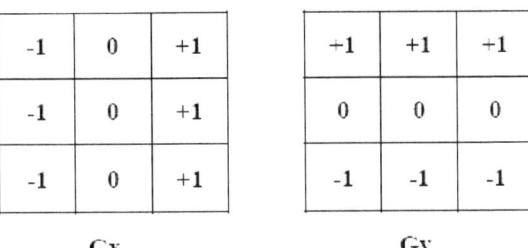

Fig 2.11 Kernels of the Prewitt's operator

2.8.4 Laplacian of Gaussian operator

Laplacian of a Gaussian (LoG) is a two-dimensional isotropic measure, which calculates the second spatial derivative of an image. It operates on single gray level image and produces another gray level image. Also, it detects rapid intensity variation regions and hence, it is more often used for edge detection [98, 99, 103, 104, 107].

For given pixel intensity values of $J(x,y)$, the Laplacian operator $L(x,y)$ of an image can be calculated using the equation 2.43

$$L(x,y) = \frac{\partial^2 J}{\partial x^2} + \frac{\partial^2 J}{\partial y^2} \qquad \ldots 2.43$$

Usually the images are acquired and processed in the digital domain; therefore, the edges are estimated using discrete convolution kernels, which can approximate the second derivatives of the Laplacian. Three common kernels are used for discrete convolution and are shown in Figure 2.12.

0	+1	0
+1	-4	+1
0	+1	0

+1	+1	+1
+1	-8	+1
+1	+1	+1

-1	+2	-1
+2	-4	+2
-1	+2	-1

Fig 2.12 Discrete kernels used for approximating the Laplacian operator

These three kernels are sensitive to noise, since they approximate the second derivative measurements. This can be rectified by applying the Gaussian smoothing before the application of the Laplacian operator. Also, Gaussian smoothing reduces the high frequency component before differentiation. Since the convolution operation obeys the associative property, therefore, the Gaussian smoothing operator can be convolved with the Laplacian operator and the resulting hybrid operator can be convolved with the image to achieve the expected result. This combined operation has the following advantages:

1. Requires fewer arithmetic operations, since both the Gaussian and the Laplacian kernels are usually much smaller than the image.
2. The LoG kernel can be pre-calculated in advance so that only one convolution needs to be performed at the run-time of the algorithm.

The two-dimensional LoG function centered on zero with Gaussian standard deviation σ can be written as,

$$LoG(x, y) = -\frac{1}{\pi\sigma^4}\left[1 - \frac{x^2 + y^2}{2\sigma^2}\right]e^{-\frac{x^2+y^2}{2\sigma^2}} \qquad \text{...2.44}$$

For example, a two-dimensional Laplacian of Gaussian function and its simulated graph are shown in the Figure 2.13 and 2.14, respectively. The LoG is approximated by the discrete kernel for a Gaussian (σ = 1.4) is shown in Figure 2.15.

0	1	0
1	-4	1
0	1	0

Fig 2.13 LoG kernel

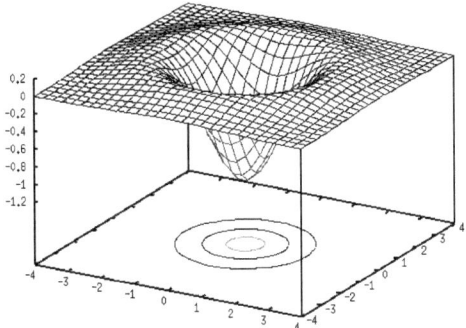

Fig 2.14 2-D Laplacian of Gaussian (LoG) function (Note: *x* and *y* axes are marked in terms of standard deviations (σ))

0	+1	+1	+2	+2	+2	+1	+1	0
+1	+2	+4	+5	+5	+5	+4	+2	+1
+1	+4	+5	+3	0	+3	+5	+4	+1
+2	+5	+3	-12	-24	-12	+3	+5	+2
+2	+5	0	-24	-40	-24	0	+5	+2
+2	+5	+3	-12	-24	-12	+3	+5	+2
+1	+4	+5	+3	0	+3	+5	+4	+1
+1	+2	+4	+5	+5	+5	+4	+2	+1
0	+1	+1	+2	+2	+2	+1	+1	0

Fig 2.15 Discrete kernel for approximating the LoG with Gaussian (σ = 1.4)

From the Figure 2.14, it is shown that the Gaussian is increasingly narrow and the LoG kernel becomes the same as the simple Laplacian kernel as shown in Figure 2.13. This is due to smoothing with a very narrow Gaussian (σ < 0.5 pixels) on a discrete grid, which has no effect on the Laplacian kernel. Therefore, the simple Laplacian can be treated as limiting case of the Log for narrow Gaussian on discrete grid.

2.8.5 Canny operator

The Canny edge detection operator is widely considered to be the standard and optimum edge detection algorithm in the image-processing domain [100,103,104,107-109]. This method is formulated on the basis of the following criteria.

1. Low error rate – No edge should be missed and false edge should not be identified.
2. Edge points be well localized – The distance between the actual edge and the edge found out by the operator should be minimum.
3. One response to single edge – To avoid multiple responses to a single edge.

Based on the above three criteria, Canny formulated the edge detection operator, which follows the following six steps.

Step1: Smoothing using Gaussian Kernel, which removes the blurring and noise effects
Step2: Finding the gradients using Sobel operator, which detects the edges based on the gradient value
Step3: Computing the edge direction in the image using the gradient values calculated in the x, y direction
Step4: Relating the edge direction to a direction traced in the image using edge orientation angle representation diagram shown in Figure 2.16
Step5: Applying non-maximum suppression to trace along the edge in the edge direction to found out the pixel values that is not considered as edge
Step6: Applying Hysteresis to eliminate streaking effect

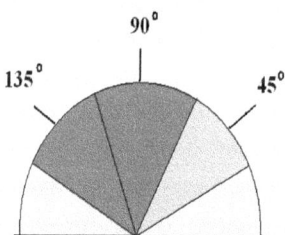

Fig 2.16 Edge orientation angle representation diagram

[Note: The orientation angle can be identified using the angle representation diagram shown in Figure 2.16. In this Figure, if the edge direction falls in the **yellow range** (0 to 22.5 & 157.5 to 180 degrees), then it is assigned as 0 degrees or in the **green range** (22.5 to 67.5 degrees), then it is set to 45 degrees or in the **blue range** (67.5 to 112.5 degrees), then it is assigned as 90 degrees or in the **red range** (112.5 to 157.5 degrees), it is assigned as 135 degrees.]

REFERENCES

1. Goodman J.W., Some Fundamental Properties of Speckle, Journal Opt. Soc. Am.,1976,Vol. 66, No. 11, pp. 1145–1149.
2. Prager R.W., Gee A.H., Treece G.M., and Berman L., Speckle Detection in Ultrasound Images Using First Order Statistics, GUED/F-INFENG/TR *415*, University of Cambridge, Dept. of Engineering, July 2002,pp. 1–17.
3. Sirohi, R. S., Speckle Metrology Optical Engineering, Marcel Dekker, Inc., 1993.
4. Anderson M.E., and Trahey G.E., A seminar on k-space Applied to Medical Ultrasound. [Online]. Available:http://dukemil.egr.duke.edu/Ultrasound/k-space/, April 2000.
5. Rabal H.J., and Braga A.R., Dynamic Laser Speckle and Applications, Taylor & Francis Group, CRC Press, 2009.
6. Achim A., Panagiotis E., Tsakalides, and Bezerianos A., SAR Image Denoising via Bayesian Wavelet Shrinkage Based on Heavy-Tailed Modeling, IEEE Trans. on Geoscience and Remote Sensing, 2003, Vol. 41, No. 8, pp. 1773-1784.
7. Sudha S., Suresh G.R., and Sukanesh R., Speckle Noise Reduction in Ultrasound Images Using Context-Based Adaptive Wavelet Thresholding, IETE Journal of Research, 2009,Vol.55, No.3, pp.135-143.
8. Huang M., Huang Y., and Wang M., Speckle Reduction of Ultrasound Image Based on Contourlet Transform, Int. Computer Symposium, Dec. 2004, Taipei, Taiwan, pp.178-182.
9. Saad S.A., Speckle Reduction of Ultrasound Images Using Wavelets Analysis, IMIBE 2006, pp.51-54.
10. Shi Z., And Fung B.K., A Comparison of Digital Speckle Filters, 0-7803-1497-2194, Canadian Crown, 1994, pp. 2129-2133.
11. Maini R., and Aggarwal H., A Novel Technique for Speckle Noise Reduction on Medical Images, International Journal of Applied Engineering Research, 2010, Vol. 5 No.1, Pp. 1–8.
12. Kuan D.T., Sawchuk A.A., Strand T.C., And Chavel P., Adaptive Noise Smoothing Filter for Images with Signal-Dependent Noise, IEEE Trans. on Pattern Analysis and Machine Intelligence, 1985, Vol. Pami-7, No. 2, pp. 165-177.
13. Fernández A.S., Ferrero S.V.G., Fernández M.M., and López C.A., Automatic Noise Estimation in Images Using Local Statistics. Additive and Multiplicative Cases, Image And Vision Computing 27, 2009, pp.756–770.
14. Wagner R.F., Smith S.W., Sandrik J.M., and Lopez H., Statistics of speckle in ultrasound B-scans, IEEE Trans. On Sonics and Ultrasonics, May 1983, Vol. 30, No.3, pp. 156–163.
15. Abd-Elmoniem K.Z., Kadah Y.M., and Youssef A.M., Real Time Adaptive Ultrasound Speckle Reduction and Coherence Enhancement, IEEE, 07803-6297-7.2000, pp.172-175.
16. Burckhardt C. B., Speckle in Ultrasound B-Mode Scans, IEEE Trans. on Sonics and Ultrasonics, 1978, Vol.25, No.1 pp. 1 – 6.
17. Bamber J.C., and Daft C., Adaptive Filtering for Reducing of Speckle Noise in Ultrasonic Pulse Echo Images, Ultrasonics, 1986, Pp. 41-44.
18. Kuan D.T., Sawchuk A., Strand T.C., and Chavel P., Adaptive Restoration of Images with Speckle, IEEE Trans. on Acoustics Speech and Signal Processing, 1987, Vol. Assp-35, No.3, pp. 373-383.

19. Donnell O.M., and Silverstein D.S., Optimum Displacement for Compound Image Generation in Medical Ultrasound, IEEE Trans. on Ultrasonics, Ferroelectrics, and Frequency Control, 1988, Vol.35, No.4, pp. 470-476.
20. Loupes T., Mcdicken W.N., and Allan P.L., An Adaptive Weighted Median Filter for Speckle Suppression in Medical Ultrasonic Images, IEEE Trans. on Circuits And Systems, 1989, Vol. 36, No. 1, pp.129-135.
21. Leeman S., Gatenby J.C., Forsberg F., and Hoddinott J.C., Speckle Reduction in Two Easy Steps, IEEE Ultrasonic Symposium, 1989, pp.927-930.
22. Lopes A., Touzi R., and Nezry E., Adaptive Speckle Filters and Scene Heterogeneity, IEEE Trans. on Geoscience and Remote Sensing,1990, Vol. 28, No. 6, pp. 992-1000.
23. Healey A.J., Forsberg F., and Leeman S., Processing Techniques for Speckle Reduction in Medical Ultrasound Images, IEEE Colloquium on Image Processing in Medicine, 1991, pp. 6/1-6/4.
24. Evans A.N., and Nixon M.S., Speckle Filtering in Ultrasound Images for Feature Extraction IEEE Acoustic Sensing and Imaging, 1993, Conference Publication No. 369, pp. 44-49.
25. Steen E., and Olstad B., Volume Rendering in Medical Ultrasound Imaging based on Nonlinear Filtering, IEEE winter workshop on Nonlinear Digital Signal Processing, 1993, pp. 6.1- 6.6.
26. Busse L.J., Crimmins T.R., and Fienup J.R., A Model Based Approach to Improve the Performance of the Geometric Filtering Speckle Reduction Algorithm, IEEE Ultrasonics Symposium, 1995, pp.1353-1356.
27. Karaman M., Kutay M.A., and Bozdagi G., An Adaptive Speckle Suppression Filter for Medical Ultrasonic Imaging, IEEE Trans. on Medical Imaging, 1995, Vol. 14, No. 2, pp. 283-292.
28. Dutt V. and Greenleaf J.F., Adaptive Speckle Reduction Filter for Log Compressed B-Scan Images, IEEE Trans. on Medical Imaging, 1996, Vol. 15, No. 6, pp. 802-813.
29. Kofidis E., Theodoridi S., Kotropoulosc C., and Pitas I., Nonlinear Adaptive Filters for Speckle Suppression in Ultrasonic Images, Elsevier Signal Processing, 1996, Vol. 52, pp.357-372.
30. Kang C.S., Lee M.S., and Hong H.S., Noise Reduction of Echocardiographic Images Using Wavelet Filtering, International Conference on signal Processing Proceedings, 1998, pp.267-270.
31. Zong X., Laine F.A., and Geiser A.E., Speckle Reduction and Contrast Enhancementof Echocardiograms via Multiscale Nonlinear Processing, IEEE Trans. on Medical Imaging, 1998, Vol. 17, No. 4, pp.532-540.
32. Hao X., Gao S., and Gao X., A Novel Multiscale Nonlinear Thresholding Method for Ultrasonic Speckle Suppressing, IEEE Trans. on Medical Imaging, 1999, Vol. 18, No. 9, pp.787-794.
33. Abd-Elmonieum Z.K., Youssef M.A., and Kadah M.Y., Real-Time Speckle Reduction and Coherence Enhancement in Ultrasound Imaging via Nonlinear Anisotropic Diffusion IEEE Trans. on Biomedical Engineering, 2002, Vol. 49, No. 9, pp.997-1014.
34. Chinrungrueng C., and Suvichakorn A., Fast Edge-Preserving Noise Reduction for Ultrasound Images, IEEE Trans. on Nuclear Science, 2001, Vol. 48, No. 3,pp. 849-854.
35. Achim A., Bezerianos A., and Tsakalides P., Novel Bayesian Multiscale Method for Speckle Removal in Medical Ultrasound Images, IEEE Trans. on Medical Imaging, 2001, Vol. 20, No. 8, pp. 772-783.

36. Yu Y., and Acton S.T., Speckle Reducing Anisotropic Diffusion, IEEE Trans. on Image Processing, 2002, Vol.11, No.11, pp.1260- 1270.
37. Yu Y., Molloy J.A., and Acton S.T., Three-Dimensional Speckle Reducing Anisotropic Diffusion, IEEE Conference Record of the 37th Asilomar Conference on Signals, Systems and Computers, 2003, Vol.2, pp. 1987- 1991.
38. Chen Y., Yin R., Flynn P., and Broschat S.D., Aggressive Region Growing for Speckle Reduction in Ultrasound Images, Elsevier, Pattern Recognition Letters, 2002, Vol. 24, pp.677–691.
39. Huang C.H., Chen Y.J., Wang D.S, and Chen M.C., Adaptive Ultrasonic Speckle Reduction Based on the Slope-Facet Model, Elseiver, Ultrasound in Medicine and Biology, 2003 Vol. 29, No. 8, Pp. 1161–1175.
40. Shengwen G., and Limin L., An Adaptive Speckle Suppression and Edge Enhancement Technique, Journal of Electronics, 2003, Vol.20, No.5, pp. 353-361.
41. Argenti F., and Torricelli G., Speckle Suppression in Ultrasonic Images Based on Undecimated Wavelets, EURASIP Journal on Applied Signal Processing, 2003, pp. 470–478.
42. Zhang L.C., Wong E.M.C., Koh L.M., and Ng L.S., An Adaptive Filter for Speckle Reduction in Medical Ultrasound Image Processing, 8th IEEE International Conference on Control, Automation, Robotics and Vision, 07803-8653, 2004, pp.654-658.
43. Yu Y., Molloy J.A., and Acton S.T., Generalized Speckle Reducing Anisotropic Diffusion for Ultrasound Imagery, 17th IEEE Symposium on Computer-Based Medical Systems, 2004, pp. 279- 284.
44. Rafiee A., Moradi H.M., and Farzaneh R.M., Novel Genetic-Neuro-Fuzzy Filter for Speckle Reduction from Sonography Images, Journal of Digital Imaging, 2004 Vol.17, No.4, pp.292-300.
45. Yang Z., and Fox D.M., Speckle Reduction and Structure Enhancement by Multichannel Median Boosted Anisotropic Diffusion, EURASIP Journal on Applied Signal Processing, 2004, Vol.16, pp. 2492–2502.
46. Loizou C.P., Pattichis C.S., Christodoulou I.C., Istepanian H.S.R., Pantziaris M., and Nicolaides A., Comparative Evaluation of Despeckle Filtering in Ultrasound Imaging of the Carotid Artery, IEEE Trans. on Ultrasonics, Ferroelectrics, and Frequency Control, 2005, Vol. 52, No. 10, pp.1653-1669.
47. Acton S.T., De-convolution speckle reducing anisotropic diffusion, IEEE International Conference on Image Processing, 2005, Vol.1, pp. I- 4.
48. Yue Y., Croitoru M.M., Bidani A., Zwischenberger B.J., and Clark W.J., Ultrasound Speckle Suppression and Edge Enhancement Using Multiscale Nonlinear Wavelet Diffusion, IEEE 27th Annual International Conference of the Engineering in Medicine and Biology Society, 2005, pp. 6429-6432.
49. Yue Y., Croitoru M.M., Bidan A., Zwischenberger B.J., and Clark W.J., Nonlinear Multiscale Wavelet Diffusion for Speckle Suppression and Edge Enhancement in Ultrasound Images, IEEE Trans. on Medical Imaging, 2006, Vol.25, No. 3, pp. 297-311.
50. Michailovich V.O., and Tannenbaum A., Despeckling of Medical Ultrasound Images, IEEE Trans. on Ultrasonics, Ferroelectrics, and Frequency Control, 2006, Vol. 53, No. 1 pp.64-78.
51. Zhang F., Yoo M.Y., Zhang L., Koh M.L., and Kim Y., Multiscale Nonlinear Diffusion and Shock Filter for Ultrasound Image Enhancement, IEEE Computer Society Conference on Computer Vision and Pattern Recognition, 2006, Vol. 2, pp. 1972- 1977.

52. Badawi M.A., and Rushdi A.M., Speckle Reduction in Medical Ultrasound: A Novel Scatterer Density Weighted Nonlinear Diffusion Algorithm Implemented as a Neural-Network Filter, IEEE 28th Annual International Conference on Engineering in Medicine and Biology, 2006, pp. 2776-2782.
53. Tay C.P, Acton S.T., and Hossack A.J., Ultrasound Despeckling Using an Adaptive Window Stochastic Approach, IEEE International Conference on Image Processing, 2006, pp. 2549-2552.
54. Bhuiyan M.I.H., Ahmad M.O., and Swamy M.N.S., Wavelet-Based Despeckling of Medical Ultrasound Images with The Symmetric Normal Inverse Gaussian Prior, IEEE International Conference on Acoustics, Speech and Signal Processing 2007, 4244-0728, pp.721-724.
55. Zhang F., Yoo M.Y., Koh M.L., and Kim Y., Nonlinear Diffusion in Laplacian Pyramid Domain for Ultrasonic Speckle Reduction, IEEE Trans. on Medical Imaging, 2007, Vol.26, No.2, pp.200-211.
56. Dantas G.R., and Costa T.E, Ultrasound Speckle Reduction Using Modified Gabor Filters, IEEE Trans. on Ultrasonics, Ferroelectrics and Frequency Control, 2007, Vol.54, No. 3, pp. 530-538.
57. Shankar P.M., Contrast Enhancement and Phase-sensitive Boundary Detection in Ultrasonic Speckle Using Bessel Spatial Filters, IET Image Processing, 2008, Vol. 3, No. 2, pp. 41–51.
58. Vosoughi A., and Shamsollahi B.M., Speckle Noise Reduction of Ultrasound Images Using M-band Wavelet Transform and Wiener Filter in a Homomorphic Framework, International Conference on Bio Medical Engineering and Informatics, Indexed in IEEE Computer Society, 2008, 978-0-7695, pp.510-515.
59. Yoo B., Park H., Ryu J., Hwang K., and Nishimura T., Wavelet Decomposition Based Speckle Reduction Method for Ultrasound Images by Using Speckle Reducing Anisotropic Diffusion, Proceedings of the World Congress on Engineering and Computer Science, 2008, 978-988-98671-0-2.
60. Song X.Y., Zhang S., Song K.O., Yang W., and Chen Y.Z., Speckle Suppression for Medical Ultrasound Images Based on Modeling Speckle with Rayleigh Distribution in Contourlet Domain, Proceedings of the 2008 International Conference on Wavelet Analysis and Pattern Recognition, Hong Kong, 30-31 Aug. 2008, pp.194-199.
61. Guo Y., Cheng H.D., Tian J., And Zhang Y., A Novel Approach To Speckle Reduction In Ultrasound Imaging, Elsevier, Ultrasound in Med. & Biol.,2009, Vol. 35, No. 4, pp. 628–640.
62. Khare A., Khare M., Jeong Y., Kim H., and Jeon M., Despeckling of Medical Ultrasound Images Using Daubechies Complex Wavelet Transform, Elsevier, Signal Processing, 2009, pp.1-12.
63. Devarapu K.V., Murala S., and Kumar V., Denoising of Ultrasound Images Using Curvelet Transform, Proceedings of the International Conference on Computer and Automation Engineering (ICCAE2010), Singapore, 26-28 Feb. 2010, pp.447-451.
64. Huang J., and Yang X., A PDE based Method for Speckle Reduction of Log-compressed Ultrasound Image, International Journal of Image, Graphics and Signal Processing, 2011,Vol.3, pp.17-24.
65. Nedumaran D., Sivakumar R., Sekar V., and Gayathri M.K., Speckle Noise Reduction In Ultrasound Biomedical B-Scan Images Using Discrete Topological Derivative, Elsevier, Ultrasound in Med. & Biol., 2012, Vol. 38, No. 2, pp. 276–286.

66. Solbo S., and Eltoft T., Homomorphic Wavelet-Based Statistical Despeckling of SAR Images, IEEE Trans. on Geoscience and Remote Sensing, 2004, Vol. 42, No. 4, pp. 711-721.
67. Mastriani M., and Giraldez E.A., Enhanced Directional Smoothing Algorithm for Edge-Preserving Smoothing of Synthetic-Aperture Radar Images, Measurement in Biomedicine, 2004, Vol. 4, No. 3, pp. 1-11.
68. Lee J.S., Digital Image Enhancement and Noise Filtering by Use of Local Statistics, IEEE Trans. on Pattern Analysis and Machine Intelligence, 1980, Vol. PAMI-2, No. 2, pp.165-168.
69. Lee J.S., Refined Filtering of Image Noise Using Local Statistics, Computer Vision, Graphics, and Image Processing, 1981, Vol.15, No. 2, pp.380-389.
70. Maini R., and Aggarwal H., Performance Evaluation of Various Speckle Noise Reduction Filters on Medical Images, International Journal of Recent Trends in Engineering, 2009, Vol.2, No. 4, pp.22-25.
71. Souag N., Speckle Reduction in Echocardiographic Images, 14th European Signal Processing Conference (EUSIPCO 2006) Proceeding, Florence, Italy, Sept pp.4-8.
72. Jain A.K., Fundamentals of Digital Image Processing, First Edition, Prentice-Hall, Inc, 1989.
73. Gonzalez R.C., and Woods R.E., Digital Image Processing, Third Edition, Pearson Education, 2008.
74. Graps A., An Introduction to Wavelets, IEEE Computational Science and Engineering, 1995, Vol. 2, No. 2. pp. 1-18.
75. Jansen M., and Oonincx P., Second Generation Wavelets and Applications, 2005, Springer-Verlag London Limited.
76. Michel M., Misiti Y., Oppenheim G., and Jean-Michel Poggi., Wavelets and their Applications, 2007, ISTE Publication.
77. Polikar R., Fundamental Concepts and an Overview of the Wavelet theory, Second edition, 1998, Rowan University.
78. Donoho D.L., and Johnstone M.I., Adapting to Unknown Smoothness via Wavelet Shrinkage, Journal of American Statistical Association, 1995, Vol.90, No.432, pp.1200-1224.
79. Donoho D.L., De-Noising by Soft-Thresholding, IEEE Trans. on Information Theory, 1995, Vol. 41, No. 3, pp. 613- 627.
80. Antoniadis A., and Bigot J., Wavelet Estimators in Non-parametric Regression: A Comparative Simulation Study, Journal of Statistical Software, 2001, Vol. 6, No.6, pp.1-83.
81. Grace C.S., Yu B., and Vetterli M., Adaptive Wavelet Thresholding for Image Denoising and Compression, IEEE Trans. on Image Processing, 2000, Vol. 9, No. 9, pp. 1532-1546.
82. Perona P., and Malik J., Scale-Space and Edge Detection Using Anisotropic Diffusion, IEEE Trans. on Pattern Analysis and Machine Intelligence, 1990, Vol. 12, No. 7, pp. 629-639.
83. Acton S.T., Multigrid Anisotropic Diffusion, IEEE Trans. on Image Processing, 1998, Vol.7, No. 3, pp.280-291.
84. Weickert J., Anisotropic Diffusion in Image Processing, Stuttgart Publishers, 1998, pp.26-27.
85. Yu Z., and Bajaj C., Anisotropic Vector Diffusion in Image Processing, IEEE Explorer, International Conference on Image Processing (ICIP 2002), pp.828-831.

86. Eskicioglu M.A., and Fisher S.P., Image Quality Measures and their Performance, IEEE Trans. on Communications, 1995, Vol.43, No.12, pp.2959-2965.
87. Grgic S., Grgic M., and Mrak M., Reliability of Objective Picture Quality Measures, Journal of Electrical Engineering, 2004, Vol.55, No.1-2, pp.3-10.
88. Gupta K.K., and Gupta R., Despeckle and Geographical Feature Extraction in SAR Images by Wavelet Transform, Elsevier, ISPRS Journal of Photogrammetry & Remote Sensing, 2007, Vol. 62, No.2, pp.473–484.
89. Avcibas I., Sankur B., and Sayood K., Statistical Evaluation of Image Quality Measures, Journal of Electronic Imaging, 2002,Vol.11, No.2, pp.206–223.
90. Neto A.M., Rittner L., Leite N., Zampieri D.E., Lotufo R., and Mendeleck A., Pearson's Correlation Coefficient for Discarding Redundant Information in Real Time Autonomous Navigation System, 16th IEEE International Conference on Control Applications, Part of IEEE Multi-conference on Systems and Control, 2007, pp.426-631.
91. Gupta S., Kaur L., Chauhan R.C., and Saxena S.C., A Versatile Technique for Visual Enhancement of Medical Ultrasound images, Elsevier, Digital Signal Processing, 2007, Vol.17, No.3, pp.542–560.
92. Wang Z., and Bovik A., A universal image quality index, IEEE Signal Processing Letters, 2002, Vol. 9, No.3, pp.81-84.
93. Srivastava R., Gupta J.R.P., and Parthasarthy H., Comparison of PDE based and Other Techniques for Speckle Reduction from Digitally Reconstructed Holographic Images, Elsevier, Optics and Lasers in Engineering, 2010, Vol.48, No.5, pp.626–635.
94. Nasri M., and Nezamabadi H., Image denoising in the wavelet domain using a new adaptive Thresholding function, Elsevier, Neurocomputing, 2009, Vol.72, No.6, pp.1012–1025.
95. Wang Z., Bovik C.A., Sheikh R.H., and Simoncelli P.E., Image Quality assessment: from Error visibility to structural similarity, IEEE Trans. on Image Processing, 2004, Vol.13, No.4, pp.600-612.
96. Thitaikumar A., Krouskop T.A., and Ophir J., Signal-to-noise ratio, Contrast-to-Noise Ratio and their Trade-offs with Resolution in Axial-shear Strain Elastography, Physics in Medicine and Biology, 2007, Vol.52, No.1, pp.13-28.
97. Zhang Y., Cheng H.D., Tian J., Huang J., and Tang X., Fractional Sub Pixel Diffusion and Fuzzy Logic Approach for Ultrasound Speckle Reduction, Elsevier, Pattern Recognition, 2010, Vol.43, No.8, pp. 2962-2970.
98. Maini R., and Aggarwal H., Study and Comparison of Various Image Edge Detection Techniques, International Journal of Image Processing, 2009, Vol.3, No.1, pp.1-12.
99. Tuneja M., and Sandu P.S., Performance Evaluation of Edge Detection Techniques for Images in Spatial Domain, International Journal of Computer Theory and Engineering, 2009, Vol.1, No.5, pp.614-621.
100. Shriram K.V., Dharmendra T., Sivaraman R., and Karthick S., Automotive Image Processing Techniques Using Canny Edge Detection, International Journal of Engineering Science and Technology, 2010, Vol.2, No.7, pp2632-2643.
101. Senthilkumaran V., and Rajesh R, Edge Detection Techniques for Image Segmentation: A Survey of Soft Computing Approaches, International Journal of Recent Trends in Engineering, 2009, Vol.1, No.2, pp.250-254.
102. Sobel I., On Calibrating Computer Controlled Cameras for Perceiving 3-D Scenes, Session 24, Perception for Robots, pp.646-657.

103. Yadav R., Tyagi R., and Malviya L.D., Low Magnitude Edge Detection Algorithm, International Journal of Computer Applications, 2011, Vol.23, No.2, pp.16-19.
104. Lakshmi S., and Sankaranarayanan V., A Study of Edge Detection Techniques for Segmentation Computing Approaches, International Journal of Computer Applications, Special Issues, CASCT 2010, pp.35-41.
105. Maini R., and Aggarwal H., Analyzing Robert's Edge Detector for Digital Images Corrupted with Noise, International Journal of Computer and Network Security, 2010, Vol.2, No.1, pp.35-40.
106. Singh S.K., and Kathane A., Various Methods for Edge Detection in Digital Image Processing, International Journal of Computer Science and Technology, 2011, Vol.2, No.2, pp.188-190.
107. Kumar T., and Sahoo G., A Novel Method of Edge Detection Using Cellular Automate, International Journal of Computer Applications, 2010, Vol.9, No.4, pp.38-44.
108. Canny J., A Computer Approach to Edge Detection, IEEE Trans. on Pattern Analysis and Machine Intelligence, 1986, Vol.8, No.6, pp.679-698.
109. Nadernejad E., and Sharifzadeh S., Edge Detection Techniques Evaluations and Comparisons, Applied Mathematical Sciences, 2008, Vol.2, No.31, pp.1507-1520.

CHAPTER – III

TOPOLOGICAL DERIVATIVE AND ITS SPECKLE NOISE REDUCTION APPLICATION IN ULTRASOUND B-SCAN IMAGES

3.1 INTRODUCTION

Topological derivative is a structural mechanics concept initially conceived to deal with topology optimization problems and, later on, it has been successfully adapted to solve inverse problems, material properties characterization and image processing problems [1-4]. Many researchers adapted this technique for solving the image processing problems, especially image segmentation and image restoration [5-22]. The major advantage of topological derivative is that it reduces noise to maximum extent while preserving the image details. Unlike standard filters, this method does not blur the edges and hence the image features are retained and only noise is reduced. An image can be viewed as a piecewise smooth function and edges can be considered as a set of singularities. The topological derivative allows quantifying the sensitivity of a problem when the domain under consideration is perturbed by changing its topology, for example by the introduction of an arbitrary shaped hole, an inclusion or a source term.

3.2 BASIC CONCEPTS OF TOPOLOGICAL DERIVATIVE

Topological derivative quantifies the sensitivity of a problem when the domain is perturbed by changing its topology (by the introduction of heterogeneity such as hole, inclusion, source term, etc) [21-27]. For example, a domain Ω under consideration is perturbed by the introduction of small holes (topology changes) in Ω as shown in Figure 3.1 [21, 22]. In the Figure 3.1, Ω is the domain under perturbation, Υ_ε is the crack of length ε centered at the pixel n, $\psi(\Omega)$ is the cost function assigned before perturbation and $\Psi_\varepsilon(\Omega_\varepsilon)$ or $\Psi_\varepsilon(\Omega \setminus \Upsilon_\varepsilon)$ is the cost function after perturbation.

Considering Ω as a bounded open set in $\mathbb{R}^N$ (N =2, 3) and Υ_ε as a crack of length ε centered at point $\hat{x} \in \Omega$ (Figure 3.1), the cost function becomes,

$$\Psi_\varepsilon(\Omega_\varepsilon) = \Psi(\Omega) + f(\varepsilon) D_T(\hat{x}) + 0 f((\varepsilon)) \qquad \ldots 3.1$$

where $f(\varepsilon)$ is the known positive function going to zero with ε and $D_T(\hat{x})$ is the topological derivative at point $\hat{x}$. Since $f(\varepsilon)$ is positive, by introducing a perturbation at any point $\hat{x}$ where D_T is negative, the cost function ψ will be decreased.

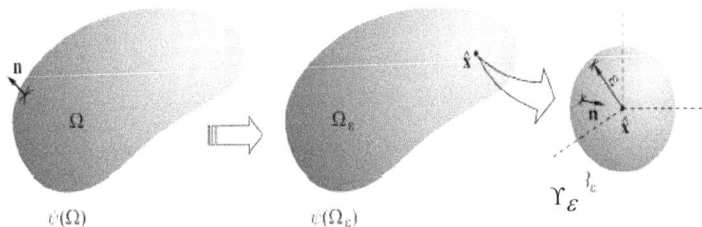

Fig 3.1 Diagrammatic representation of topological derivative

Thus, D_T can be taken as an indicator function defining the best places where the perturbations could be introduced in order to reduce the value of the cost function. Cost function quantifies the degree of similarity between two images, which simply adjust the parameters of the appropriate transformation model until the cost function reaches a local optimum [28]. With the limiting value ($\varepsilon \to 0$), Equation (3.1) can be modified by dividing with $f(\varepsilon)$, and is given in the equation 3.2.

$$D_T \tilde{x} = \lim_{\varepsilon \to 0} \frac{\Psi_\varepsilon(\Omega \setminus \Upsilon_\varepsilon) - \Psi(\Omega)}{f(\varepsilon)} \qquad \ldots 3.2$$

$$\Psi_\varepsilon(\Omega \setminus \Upsilon_\varepsilon) = \Psi(\Omega) + f(\varepsilon) D_T(\tilde{x}) + \ldots \qquad \ldots 3.3$$

where $f(\varepsilon)$ is a positive function that decreases monotonically so that $f(\varepsilon) \to 0$ with $\varepsilon \to 0^+$. The topological derivative (D_T) given by equation (3.2) has been recognized as a powerful tool to solve topology optimization problem. In this research work, the discrete version of the topological derivative is used as an indicator function to find an optimal topology of the B-scan image in the presence of diffusion, which will preserve edges and valuable diagnostic information and reduce the speckle noise present in the ultrasound B-scan images. Larrabide et al., [23] proposed a computationally efficient Discrete Topological Derivative (DTD) concept, which used the cost functional (for the discrete approach) represented by the equation 3.4.

$$\Psi(u_i^s) = \sum_s \sum_{p \in n^s} k^{s,p} \hat{\Delta} u_i^{s,p} . \hat{\Delta} u_i^{s,p} \qquad ...3.4$$

where $k^{s,p}$ is the diffusion of pixel s with neighbors p and $n^s = \{w,e,n,s\}$ denotes the neighbors of the pixel s, and u_i^s is the intensity of the image pixel. Also, $\hat{\Delta}u_i^{s,p}$ is defined by the equation 3.5.

$$\hat{\Delta}u_i^{s,p} = u_i^p - u_i^s \qquad ...3.5$$

and u_i^s is explicitly computed using the expression 3.6.

$$u_i^s(k^s) = u_{i-1}^s + \Delta t \sum_{p \in n^s} k^{s,p} \hat{\Delta} u_{i-1}^{s,p} \qquad ...3.6$$

where i ≥1 represents the iteration number, $k^s = \{k^{s,w}, k^{s,e}, k^{s,n}, k^{s,s}\}$ denotes the set of diffusion coefficient associated with the pixel s and Δt is the artificial time step size. Here, we assume that $k^{s,p}=0$, is the pixel at which the perturbation is introduced for the pixel s with the neighbor p. Since u_i^s is the explicit function of the set k^s, the best configuration of k^s can be found out by computing u_i^s, which preserve the image details and remove the noise. The exact total variation of the cost functional for a given perturbation in $k^{s,p}$ can be calculated using the expression 3.7

$$\Psi(u_i^s(k_\varepsilon^s)) = \Psi(u_i^s(k^s)) + D_T(s, k_\varepsilon^s) \qquad ...3.7$$

where $D_T(s, k_\varepsilon^S)$ represents the total variation of the cost functional due to perturbation on the diffusivity coefficient at pixel s characterized by the set k_ε^S. In our case, we assume that $k_\varepsilon^S \in \{0, k_0\}$, and then the set of all possible configuration of k^s can be defined as shown in equation 3.8.

$$C(s) := \begin{cases} k^s = (k^{s,w}, k^{s,e}, k^{s,n}, k^{s,s}); k^{s,p} \in \{0, k_0\}, \\ p = \{w, e, n, s\} \end{cases} \quad \ldots 3.8$$

There are sixteen different combinations for k^s (since each neighbor has $k^{s,p}=0$ or $k^{s,p}=k_0$, so that $2^4=16$ combinations are available). The cost functional having the value zero has been discarded and in the remaining 15 possible combinations, C_σ denotes the non-perturbed combination corresponding to the isotropic case defined by the combination $k_{iso}^S = (k_0, k_0, k_0, k_0)$, which is the subset of C. Hence, the cost function C contains the remaining 14 combinations. Pixel "s" and its neighborhood, and their corresponding diffusion coefficient k_s are illustrated in Figure 3.2.

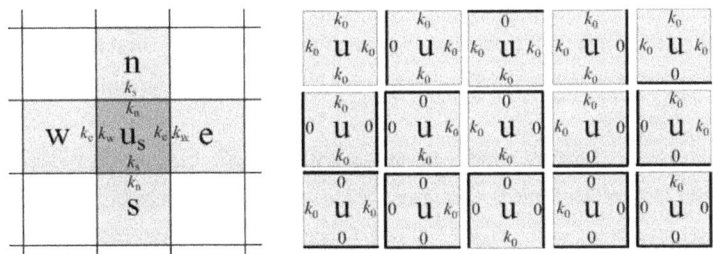

Fig 3.2 Pixel "s" and its neighborhood diffusion coefficients k_s

To compute the value of D_T of a specific pixel, perturbation is introduced in the form of changing a particular pixel s (denoted by the set k_{iso}^S) by $k_\varepsilon^S \in C_\sigma$. The cost function $\Psi_\varepsilon(_\varepsilon u_i^S)$ becomes,

$$\Psi_\varepsilon(_\varepsilon u_i^S) = \Psi(u_i^S) - \sum_{p \in n^S} k^{S,P} \hat{\Delta} u_i^{S,P} \cdot \hat{\Delta} u_i^{S,P} + \sum_{p \in n^S} k_\varepsilon^{S,P} \hat{\Delta}_\varepsilon u_i^{S,P} \cdot \hat{\Delta}_\varepsilon u_i^{S,P} \quad \ldots 3.9$$

If $_\varepsilon u_i^S = u_i^S(k_\varepsilon^S)$ and $u_i^S = u_i^S(k_{iso}^S)$, then using equation 3.6, the value $\hat{\Delta}_\varepsilon u_i^{S,P} = u_i^P - _\varepsilon u_i^S$ can be obtained. From equation 3.7 and 3.9, the total variation of the cost functional ψ due to the perturbation k_ε^S can be written as,

$$D_T(s, k_\varepsilon^S) = \sum_{p \in n^S} k_\varepsilon^{S,P} \hat{\Delta}_\varepsilon u_i^{S,P} \cdot \hat{\Delta}_\varepsilon u_i^{S,P} - \sum_{p \in n^S} k^{S,P} \hat{\Delta} u_i^{S,P} \cdot \hat{\Delta} u_i^{S,P}$$
$$\ldots 3.10$$

In this research work, the discrete topological derivative algorithm for despeckling the ultrasound B-scan image has been formulated using the concept detailed above.

3.2.1 Selection of cost function

Choosing the correct cost function depends on particular image problem. In this work, the cost function proposed by Larrabide et al., was chosen for the speckle noise reduction problem in ultrasound B-scan images [22, 23, 28]. In the case of B-scan ultrasound images, it is a difficult task to differentiate the soft images from speckle noise. For this, we introduced diffusion to the B-scan image to preserve the important information of the soft tissues and edges from the speckle noise. The diffusion coefficient k is allowed to assume values of 0 and 1 only, and we stopped the diffusion (setting k = 0), where there is a chance to lose image features. This ($k = 0$) can be seen as the introduction of a crack, which will stop the diffusivity effect and preserve edges and soft tissue information in the B-scan image. These singularities can only occur along the edge pixel boundaries when neighboring pixels having $k = 0$ along the edge share, hence no diffusion occurs between them. Thus, the cost functional quantifies the values of the diffusion coefficient k and the gradient corresponding to a given image, when the DTD results in minimized cost function.

DTD is computed according to the energy norm function of a B-scan image with the introduction of cracks. The DTD is used as seed for a path parameter to find the best pixels using method of diffusion. Also, the diffusion coefficients are calculated in 16 different possibilities. This robust algorithm has two parameters for controlling the percentage of pixels to put crack and find the tolerance value to stop the iteration. Even though DTD guaranteed optimum despeckling, still it requires the intervention of the user to identify the cost function for the sensitivity of desired image quality.

3.3 IMPLEMENTATION OF TOPOLOGICAL DERIVATIVE FOR DESPECKLING ULTRASOUND B-SCAN IMAGES

The topological derivative algorithm has been modified for the ultrasound B-scan image speckle reduction. For implementing the topological algorithm on the ultrasound B-scan image, the image was divided into 5x5 blocks and then the topological algorithm was applied on the ultrasound B-scan images. Topological derivative calculation requires large memory space and long computational time due to its huge quantity of data and computational complexity. After the calculation of topological derivative, the denoised block images are combined together to form the overall denoised image. This methodology reduces the memory space requirements as well as the computational time, since the calculation of DTD is performed in a 5x5 blocks that requires very small memory space and reduced computations.

The main idea behind DTD algorithm is to compute the topological derivative for an appropriate cost functional introduced as perturbation in a pixel in order to identify its diffusion with the neighboring pixels. Here, the topological derivative is used as an indicator function to find the best pixels to introduce the perturbation that will remove noise and preserve the relevant image characteristics. The DTD algorithm takes the raw ultrasound B-scan image as an input. To apply the cost function to a single pixel, the input image is enlarged to a single pixel level. Now, the cost function is applied to the single pixel identified for perturbation. The diffusion coefficient of the cost function applied is calculated for the 16 different possibilities (assuming that there are four neighboring pixels surrounding the perturbed pixel). At this stage, the topological derivative is initialized as indicator function to compute the total variation in the cost function. Then, the cost function of the first iteration is calculated and compared with the tolerance value (the tolerance value will be fixed a value greater than zero). If the cost function is less than the tolerance value, the iteration is stopped, otherwise it will continue for determining the new value of cost function by applying another value of the diffusion coefficient. If the iteration is stopped, the gradient for the new image and old image is calculated for sensitivity analysis. Then, the topological derivative value is used for reshaping the despeckled image. This procedure is repeated for all the pixels in the image.

3.4 ROLE OF TOPOLOGICAL DERIVATIVE IN IMAGE PROCESSING APPLICATIONS

Topological derivative is a well established technique for solving the topology optimization and inverse problem as well as material property characterization. The inherent potential of this technique motivated interdisciplinary applications to several other fields of science and technology. One such potential application is the image processing, since image processing is the integral part of almost all fields in science, technology and engineering. Some of the important topology based images processing applications found in the literature are presented below.

Kong and Rosenfield summarized several applications of topology in digital image processing operations such as digitization, connected component labeling and counting, boundary extraction, contour filling, and thinning [5]. Caselles and Monasse described the topographic description as a local and contrast invariant description of images and its various applications in efficient shape description, image comparison, image registration and extraction of image features like edges, corners, etc., [6]. Sekar and Nedumaran applied discrete topological derivatives for the restoration of high quality fingerprint images [16]. Larrabide et al., proposed algorithm using topological sensitivity analysis and anisotropic diffusion method for image segmentation and image restoration applications and demonstrated the performance of the algorithm over the existing methods [22, 23]. Krishnaveni and Radha applied topological derivative for the segmentation of images for sign language recognition system [26]. Belaid et al., employed topological gradient as a tool to detect the edges of medical images for image restoration application [27].

In this thesis, the application of topological derivative for speckle noise reduction in ultrasound B-scan images was attempted and its performance was studied and compared with other established despeckling methods [29].

REFERENCES

1. Cea J., Garreau S., Guillaume P., and Masmoud M., The Shape and Topological Optimizations Connection, Elsevier, Computer Methods in Applied Mechanics and Engineering, 1999, Vol.188, No.2, pp.713-726.
2. Sokolowski J., Zochowski A., On the Topological Derivative in Shape Optimization, SIAM Journal of Control Optimization, 1999, Vol. 37, No. 4, pp.1251–1272.
3. Eschenauer H.A., Kobelev V.V., and Schumacher A., Bubble Method for Topology and Shape Optimization of Structures, Springer, Structural and Multidisciplinary Optimization, 1994, Vol.8, No.1, pp.42–51.
4. Novotny A.A., Feijoo R.A, Taroco E.A., and Padra C., Topological Sensitivity Analysis, Journal of Computer Methods in Applied Mechanics and Engineering, 2003, Vol.192, No.7, pp.803–829.
5. Kong T.Y., and Rosenfeld A., Topological Algorithms for Digital Image Processing, Elsevier Science, Netherland, 1996.
6. Caselles V., and Monasse P., Geometric Description of Images as Topographic Maps, Springer Heidelberg Dordrecht, London, 2010.
7. Stancl D.L., and Stancl M.L., Real Analysis with Point-Set Topology, Marcel Dekker, New york, 1987.
8. Eshrig H., Topology and Geometry for Physics, Springer-Verlag, Berlin Heidelberg, New york, 2011.
9. Guzina B.B., and Bonnet M., Topological Derivative for the Inverse Scattering of Elastic Waves, Journal of Mech. Appl. Math, 2004, Vol. 57, No. 2, pp.161–179.
10. Novotny A.A., Feij´oo R.A., Padra C., and Taroco E., Topological Derivative for Linear Elastic Plate Bending Problems, Elsevier, Control and Cybernetics, 2005, Vol. 34, No.1, pp. 339-361.
11. Novotny A.A, Feij´oo R.A, Taroco E., and Padra C., Topological Sensitivity Analysis for Three Dimensional Linear Elasticity Problem, Elsevier, Computer Methods in Applied Mechanics and Engineering, 2007, Vol.196, No.41-44, pp. 4354-4364.
12. Giusti S.M., Novotny A.A., Neto E.A., and Feij´oo R.A., Topological Derivative in Multi-scale Heat Conduction Models, Proceedings of the European Congress on Computational Methods in Applied Sciences and Engineering (ECCOMAS 2008) Venice June 30 –July 5, 2008.
13. Cardone G., Nazarov S.A, and Sokolowski J., Topological Derivatives in Piezoelectricity, Hall Version, 2008, Vol.1, No.1, pp.1-37.
14. Grzanek M., Nowakowski A., and Sokolowski J., Topological Derivatives of Eigen Values and Neural Networks in Identification of Imperfections, Journal of Physics: Conference Series, 2008, Vol.135, No.012046, pp. 1- 8.
15. Amstutz S., Giusti S.M., Novotny A.A., and Neto E.A., Topological Derivative for Multi-scale Linear Elasticity Models Applied to The Synthesis of Microstructures, International Journal for Numerical Methods in Engineering, 2009, Vol.9, No.18, pp. 1 – 37.
16. Sekar V., and Nedumaran D., Restoration of Fingerprint Images Using Discrete Version of the Topological Derivative, Proceedings of the third UK Sim European Symposium on Computer Modeling and Simulation (EMS2009), Athens 25-27 Nov.2009, pp. 225-230.

17. Iguernane M., Nazarov S.A., Roche J.R., Sokolowski J., and Szulc K., Topological Derivatives for Semi Linear Elliptic Equations, Int. J. Appl. Math. Comput. Sci., 2009, Vol. 19, No. 2, 191–205.
18. Takezawa A., Nishiwaki S., and Kitamura M., Shape and Topology Optimization Based on the Phase Field Method and Sensitivity Analysis, Journal of Computational Physics, 2010, Vol.229, No.7, pp.2697-2718.
19. Bertsch C., Cisilino A.P., and Calvo N., Topology Optimization of Three-Dimensional Load-Bearing Structures Using Boundary Elements, Journal of Advances in Engineering Software, 2010, Vol.41, No.5, pp. 694-704.
20. Canelas A., Novotny A.A., and Roche R.J., A New Method for Inverse Electromagnetic Casting Problems Based on The Topological Derivative, Journal of Computational Physics, 2011, Vol.230, No.9, pp. 3570-3588.
21. Yoon G.H., Topological Layout Design of Electro-Fluid-Thermal-Compliant Actuator, Journal of Computer Methods in Applied Mechanics and Engineering, 2012, Vol. 209-212, No.14, pp.28-44.
22. Larrabide I., Feijóo R.A., Novotny A.A., and Taroco E.A., A Medical Image Enhancement Algorithm Based on Topological Derivative and Anisotropic Diffusion, Proceedings of the XXVI Iberian Latin-American Congress on Computational Methods in Engineering (CILAMCE –2005), Brazil, 19-21 Oct.2005, pp. 1 – 14.
23. Larrabide I., Feijóo R.A., Novotny A.A., and Taroco E.A., Topological Derivative: A tool for Image Processing. Elsevier, Computers and Structures 2008, Vol.86, No.14, pp.1386-1403.
24. Auroux D., Masmoudi M., and Belaid L., Image Restoration and Classification by Topological Asymptotic Expansion, Variational Formulations in Mechanics: Theory and Applications - CIMNE, Spain 2007, pp. 1 - 20.
25. Novotny A.A., Feijoo R.A., Taroco E.A., and Padra C., Topological Sensitivity Analysis for Three Dimensional Linear Elasticity Problem, 6th World Congress on Structural and Multidisciplinary Optimization, Brazil, 30 May-03 June2005, pp.1-10.
26. Krishnaveni M., and Radha V., A Topological Derivative Based Image Segmentation for Sign Language Recognition System Using Isotropic Filter, International Journal of Computer Science and Information Security, 2009, Vol.6, No.3, pp. 41-45.
27. Belaid L.J., Jaoua M., Masmoudi M., and Siala L., Image Restoration and Edge Detection by Topological Asymptotic Expansion, C. R. Acad. Sci. Paris, Ser. I, 2006, Vol. 342, No.5, pp.313–318.
28. Bankman I.N., Handbook of Medical Imaging Processing and Analysis, Academic Press, 2000.
29. Nedumaran D., Sivakumar R., Sekar V., and Gayathri M.K., Speckle Noise Reduction in Ultrasound Biomedical B-Scan Images Using Discrete Topological Derivative, Elsevier, Ultrasound in Med. & Biol., 2012, Vol. 38, No. 2, pp. 276–286.

CHAPTER – IV

EXPERIMENTAL SET-UP AND ULTRASOUND B-SCAN DATA USED FOR DEVELOPING AND TESTING SPECKLE REDUCTION ALGORITHMS

In this research work, the despeckling algorithms were developed and tested using two different experimental set up viz.,
1. Personal Computer (PC) Based MATLAB (PCMAT) system
2. Personal Computer (PC) Based TMS320C6713 DSK (PCDSK) system

The specification of both the systems and their functions are described in the following sections.

4.1 SPECIFICATION OF PCMAT SYSTEM

The PCMAT system was intended to develop despeckling algorithm in off-line, which comprises of Intel Pentium 4 processor with a clock speed of 3 GHz and 2 GB memory. The despeckling algorithm were developed using high performance technical computing language MATLAB (Version: MATLAB 7.1), which integrates computation, visualization and programming of the problems and solutions in matrix notation very easily and rapidly [1]. In addition to this, MATLAB has built-in toolboxes for data acquisition, modeling, simulation, prototyping, data analysis, exploration, visualization, scientific and engineering graphics, and application development including the graphical user interface (GUI). Toolboxes are comprehensive collections of MATLAB functions (M-files) that extend the MATLAB environment to solve particular classes of problems. There are special toolboxes available in the MATLAB for imaging, signal processing, neural network, fuzzy logic toolbox and wavelet. For DSP programming in MATLAB environment, an integrated platform called SimuLink [1-5] is available for model-based design and simulation of dynamic systems. The developed PCMAT system used for developing the despeckling algorithm is shown in Figure 4.1.

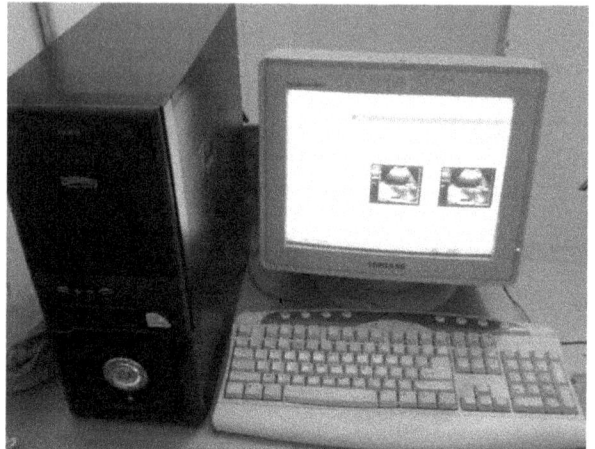

Fig 4.1 PCMAT system for developing despeckling algorithms

4.2 IMAGE PROCESSING TOOLBOX IN MATLAB

MATLAB has in-built image-processing toolbox that extends the MATLAB computing environment to offer functions and interactive tools for enhancing and analyzing images in various fields viz., aerospace/defense, astronomy, remote sensing, medical and scientific imaging, and materials science [6]. This toolbox supports a wide range of image processing operations, including

- Neighborhood and block operation
- 2-D filters, linear filters, and novel filter design
- Image analysis including pixel and region
- Binary and grayscale morphology
- Spatial transformation
- Image registration, segmentation, and deblurring
- FFT, DCT, and radon transform
- Region-of-interest processing
- Multidimensional image processing

In this work, all the despeckling filters were developed by applying the 2-D adaptive noise removal filtering, analysis and enhancement function available in the MATLAB 7.1.

4.3 PROGRAMMING IN MATLAB

MATLAB is a high-level language that includes data structures, functions, control flow statements, input/output, and object-oriented capabilities. The important steps involved in the program development of despeckling filters are presented in the following sub-sections.

4.3.1 Creating an M-File

M-files are programs written on a sequence with .m extension (For example filename.m) using text editor window available in the MATLAB [1]. This file extension (.m) creates the respective file as MATLAB M-file, which simply executes a series of MATLAB statements, or functions that accepts arguments and produces output.

The following two types of M-files are used in the MATLAB environment namely.

1. Script M-Files - It operates on data in the workspace and does not accept input arguments or return output arguments. It is used to perform a task many times automatically.
2. Function M-Files - It accepts input arguments and returns output arguments using the internal variables. It is used for developing specific applications.

In this work, we mostly used the functions available in MATLAB for our program development. The algorithms were developed using only two or three lines of code, which would require many hundreds of lines of code while using other programming languages. A sample M-file developed for speckle reduction using Frost filter is given in Example 4.1.

```
%% Read the image and perform filtering
im1 = rgb2gray(imread ('choroids_leme .bmp'));
filt1 = frost(im1);
image = double(im1);
filtered_image = double(filt1);
fprintf(f1, '\n \t abd_frost filter');
%% Show the original and filtered.
figure('Position',[30,90,900,300])
subplot(1,3,1)
imshow(im1);
title('Original Image');

subplot(1,3,2)
imshow(filt1);
title('Filtered image (Frost filter)');
```

Example 4.1 Sample program for speckle reduction using Frost filter

4.3.2 Compiling the M-File

For compiling the M-File, the editor window is opened and executed using "Run" option (in the editor window). If the program has any error, it will be displayed in the command window; otherwise, the command window will show the history of execution as per program sequence. The sample Frost filter program given in Example 4.1 was complied and tested on the ultrasound B-scan images of choroids. The Frost filtered image output obtained from the sample program and the original image are displayed in the MATLAB output window as shown in Figure 4.2.

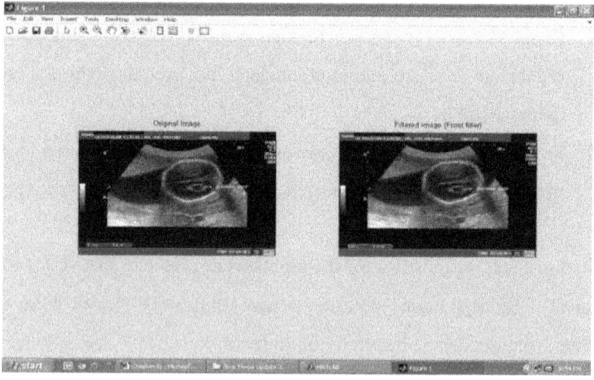

Fig 4.2 View of the original and Frost filtered choroids image in the MATLAB output window after running the sample program given in Example 4.1

4.4 SPECIFICATION OF PCDSK SYSTEM

The PCDSK system comprises of a Texas Instruments DSP TMS320C6713 digital signal processor starter kit (DSK) interfaced with the personal computer (PC) through universal serial bus (USB). The PC has Intel Pentium 4 processor with a clock speed of 3 GHz and 2 GB memory. The algorithms were developed using Code Composer Studio (CCS Version: 3.1), an integrated develop environment (IDE) for communicating with the TMS320C6713 DSK to access its various functionalities and for developing and testing the algorithms. Figure 4.3 shows the PCDSK system used for developing and testing the proposed despeckling algorithms in this work.

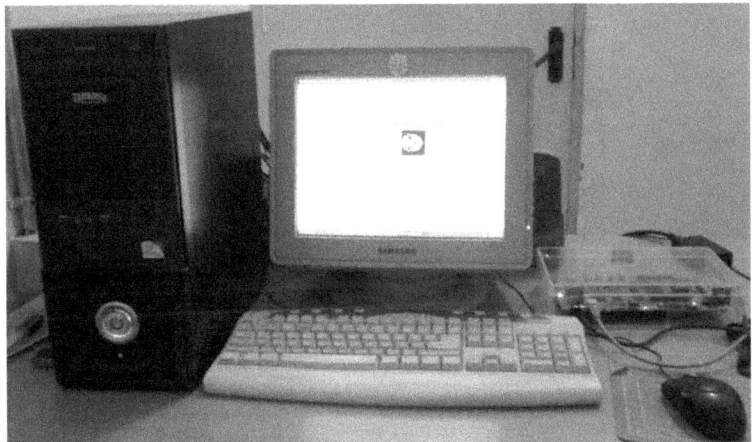

Fig 4.3 PCDSK system used for developing and testing the despeckling algorithms

4.5 DESCRIPTION OF TMS320C6713 DSP STARTER KIT

The TMS320CC6713 DSK is a low-cost standalone development platform that enables the users to evaluate and develop applications for the TI C6713 DSP. The DSK also serves as a hardware reference design for the TMS320C6713 DSP [7-9]. Figure 4.4 shows the top-view of the TMS320C6713 DSP Starter Kit (DSK), which consists of a floating-point digital signal processor (TMS320C6713).

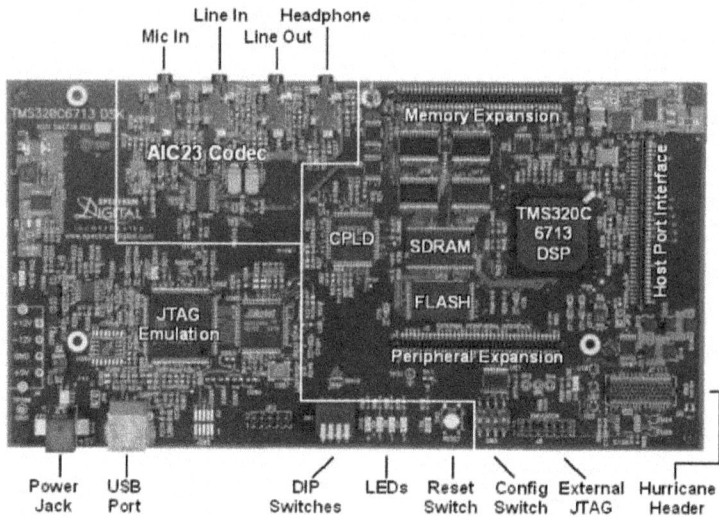

Fig 4.4 Top view of the TMS320C6713 DSK

The board can be easily interfaced with the personal computer through the universal serial bus (USB). The DSK comprises of the following on-board devices that suit a wide variety of application environments.

- A Texas Instruments' TMS320C6713 DSP operating at 225 MHz.
- An AIC23 stereo codec.
- 8 Mbytes of synchronous DRAM.
- 512 KB of non-volatile Flash memory.
- Software board configuration through registers implemented in CPLD
- Configurable boot options.
- Standard expansion connectors for daughter card use.
- JTAG emulation through on-board JTAG emulator with USB host interface or external emulator.
- Single voltage power supply (+5V)

In this work, this DSK board was used to perform the various despeckling filter operations on ultrasound B-scan images.

4.6 OVERVIEW OF THE TMS320C6713 DSK

The 6713 DSP on the DSK is interfaced with the on-board peripherals through a 32-bit wide External Memory Interface (EMIF). The SDRAM, Flash and CPLD (complex programmable logic device) are all connected to the same EMIF bus. The CPLD has a register based user interface that allows the user to configure the board by reading and writing to its registers. It also provides four LED signals, which could help the programmers by indicating the status of the hardware during debugging. A reset button is provided on the board to allow the user to reset the board whenever necessary. A 5 V external power supply is used to power the board. On-board switching voltage regulators provide the +1.26 V DSP core voltage and +3.3 V I/O supplies. The board is held in reset until these supplies are within operating specifications. Code Composer communicates with the DSK through an embedded joint test action group (JTAG) emulator with a USB host interface. The DSK can also be used with an external emulator through the external JTAG connector [7].

4.7 MEMORY MAP

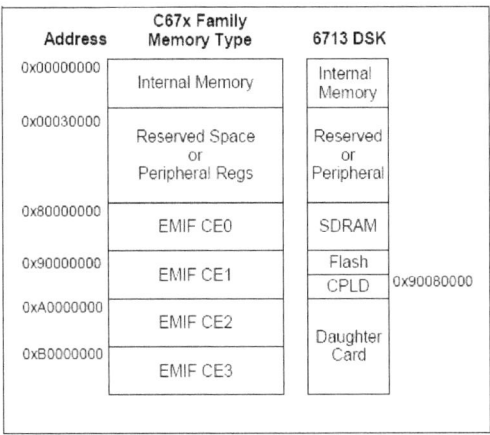

Fig. 4.5 Memory map of TMS320C6713 DSK

The C67xx family of DSPs has a large byte addressable address space, in which the program code and data can be placed anywhere in the unified address space. The addresses are always 32-bits wide. Figure 4.5 shows the memory map of the address space of a generic and specific 6713 processor. By default, the internal memory sits at the beginning of the address space. Portions of the internal memory can be reconfigured in software as L2 cache rather than fixed RAM.

4.8 CONFIGURABLE SWITCH SETTINGS

The DSK has four configuration switches that allow users to control the operational state of the DSP when it is released from reset. The configuration switch 1 controls the endianness of the DSP, while switches 2 and 3 configure the boot mode, when the DSP starts executing. Configuration switch 4 controls the on-chip multiplexing of host port interface (HPI) and multichannel audio serial port (McASP) signals brought out to the HPI expansion connector. By default all switches are off, which corresponds to EMIF boot (out of 8-bit Flash) in little endian mode and HPI signals available on the HPI expansion connector. The complete TMS320C6713 DSK switch settings are summarized in the Table 4.1

Table 4.1 TMS320C6713 switch settings

Switch 1	Switch 2	Switch 3	Switch 4	Configuration of Description
OFF				Little endian (default)
ON				Big endian
	OFF	OFF		EMIF Boot from 8-bit Flash (default)
	OFF	ON		HPI/Emulation boot
	ON	OFF		32-bit EMIF boot
	ON	ON		16-bit EMIF boot
			OFF	HPI enabled on HPI pins (default)
			ON	McASP1 enabled on HPI pins

4.9 POWER SUPPLY

The DSK operates on a single +5 V external power supply, which is internally, converted into +1.26 V and +3.3V using separate voltage regulators in the DSK [7]. The DSP core is energized with the +1.26 V supply whereas the I/O buffers are powered with the +3.3V supply. There is a provision in the DSK to power the daughter card with +12V and -12V using the external power connector (J6).

4.10 DESCRIPTION OF SOFTWARE DEVELOPMENT TOOLS

Texas Instruments provided the necessary software development tools for the TMS320C6713 DSK called Code Composer Studio (CCS) and its features are discussed in this section.

4.10.1 Overview of Code Composer Studio (CCS)

Code Composer Studio (CCS) is an integrated development environment (IDE) to develop programs for the TMS320C6000 processors [10-12], which includes C/C++ compiler, assembler, linker, debugger and other utilities. It supports real-time processing such as analysis, scheduling, and data exchange with DSP/BIOS. The C/C++ compiler of the CCS supports the American National Standards Institute (ANSI) C programs and converts into an efficient and compact C6000 assembly language source code using sophisticated optimization procedures. The assembler creates a machine-language object file from an assembly source code. The linker produces an executable file by combining object files and object libraries. The executable file can be uploaded on the DSK and executed on the DSP. The debugger has an ability to show data graphically so that a user can find and fix errors quickly and efficiently. DSP/BIOS has scalable real-time kernels, which can be designed for real-time applications such as scheduling, synchronization and host-to-target communication. It allows analysis of an application program in real time without stopping the digital signal processor. CCS keeps all information of an application in a project file (with extension .pjt). When C is used to develop a project, the following files need to be prepared by the programmer viz., C source code file(s) (with extension .c); and a linker command file (with extension .cmd).

4.10.2 Program Development in the PCDSK System

All the application programs are developed in the CCS environment as project file (.pjt). In the project file, all the related files such as source file, command file, header file, library files, etc., must be included before building the project [13-17]. The various files appended and generated while compiling the project files have specific functions and are summarized in Table 4.2.

Table 4.2 Various files generated in the CCS and their description

File Name	Description
Project file (filename.pjt)	Project file and folder will be generated, while creating a project, which consists of all source and support files related with the project.
filename.h	Header of the image filter function included in the image library (img62x.lib)
Filename.c	Source C program for the despeckling filter
filename.lib	Library file, such as the run-time support library file rts6700.lib
filename.cmd	Linker command file that maps sections to memory
filename.out	Executable file created by the linker called as Common Object File Format (COFF), which should be uploaded in the DSP and execute as the application program in the DSK

In addition, we have used the following support files developed by Chassaing [13] and Qureshi [14] in our despeckling application programs viz.

1. Header file (C6xdskinit.h) - For initializing the DSK [13]
2. Command file (C6713.cmd) - For internal memory (IRAM) mapping [13]
3. Driver library (drv6x.lib) - For enabling imaging processing library [14]
4. Peripheral support library (dev6x.lib) – For initializing the peripherals [14].

Using the above-mentioned programming concepts, an application program was developed [14] in the PCDSK system for contrast stretch and is given in the Example 4.2. To test the program, the image was resized (128x128 or 256x256) and converted in to a data file (.dat), since the DSK supports .dat format of specific sizes only. The data file (.dat file) was injected into the application program using in_img and the processed image was saved in the out_img option. The input and output images were viewed in the graph property dialog window. In the PCDSK system, the contrast stretch program (Example 4.2) was executed and tested on the ultrasound B-scan images and the results are shown in Figure 4.6

```
#include <board.h> /* EVM library */
#include <limits.h>
#include <stdio.h>
#define _TI_ENHANCED_MATH_H 1
#include <math.h>
/* image dimensions */
#define X_SIZE 128
#define Y_SIZE 128
#define N_PIXELS X_SIZE*Y_SIZE
```

```c
unsigned char in_img[N_PIXELS];
/* Input & output buffer both will not fit in   internal chip RAM, this pragma places the
   output buffer in off-chip RAM */
#pragma DATA_SECTION (out_img, "SBSRAM");
unsigned char out_img[N_PIXELS]; /* scratch buffer needed by IMGLIB */
void compute_range(unsigned char *pin, int N, float percentile1, float percentile2,
           unsigned char *pbin1, unsigned char *pbin2)
{       unsigned short cumsum = 0, /* running tally of the cumulative sum */
                T1 = round((float)N * percentile1), /* threshold for 1st bin */
                T2 = round((float)N * percentile2); /* threshold for 2nd bin */
        int ii, jj;
        /* buffers must be initialized to zero */
        memset(t_hist, 0, sizeof(unsigned short)*1024);
        memset(hist, 0, sizeof(unsigned short)*256);
}       void contrast_stretch(unsigned char *pin,
        unsigned char *pout,
{       unsigned char a, b; /* lower & upper bounds for scaling function */
        float scale, pixel;
        int ii; /* estimate dynamic range of the input */
        compute_range(pin, N, .05, 0.95, &a, &b);
                /* apply linear scaling function to input pixels, taking care to handle overflow & underflow */
        scale = 255.0/(float)(b-a);
        for (ii=0; ii<N_PIXELS; ++ii) {
                pixel = round( (float)(pin[ii] - a) * scale ); /* clamp to 8 bit range */
                pout[ii] = (pixel<0.f) ? 0 : ((pixel>255.0) ? 255 : pixel);
        }
} int main(void)
{       evm_init(); /* initialize the board */
        contrast_stretch(in_img, out_img, N_PIXELS);
        printf("contrast stretch completed");
}
```

Example 4.2 Contrast Stretch program tested in the PCDSK system

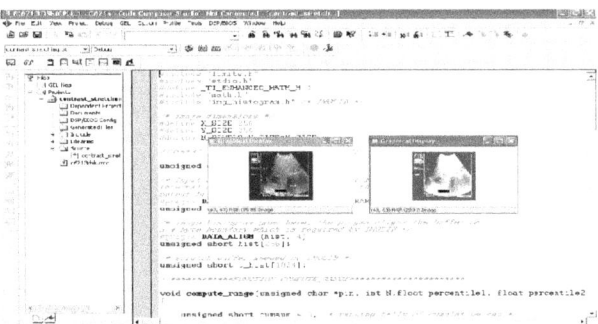

Fig 4.6 Snap-shot of the contrast stretch image displayed in the PCDSK system

4.11. SPECIFICATION OF ULTRASOUND B-SCAN DATA USED IN THIS STUDY

The algorithm was tested on more than 200 ultrasound B-scan images of various organs obtained from four different sources in both the PCMAT and PCDSK systems. The details of the organization, specifications of the ultrasound B-scan machine (model, make), image size and image format are summarized in Table 4.3.

Table 4.3 Particulars of ultrasound B-scan images collected from four different sources

S. No.	Firm	Make	Model	Image Size	Image Format
1	M/s. Sri Ramachandra Medical College and Hospital	GE	Vivid 7 Dimension '05	640x480	JPEG
2	M/s. Mithil Scan Center	MINDRAY	DC6	640x480	BMP
3	M/s. Saravana Scan Center	SIEMENS	G40	1024x768	JPEG
4	Open web database source (http://www.ultrasound-images.com/)	PROVIDIAN		300x225	JPEG

REFERENCES

1. www.mathworks.com
2. Davis T.A., and Sigmon K., MATLAB® Primer, Seventh Edition, Chapman & Hall CRC, 2005.
3. Sayood K., Learning Programming Using MATLAB, Morgan & Claypool Publishers, 2007.
4. MATLAB The Language of Technical Computing, MathWorks Inc., 2004.
5. Gonzalez R.C., Woods E.R., and Eddins S.L., Digital Image Processing Using MATLAB, Pearson Education, 2004.
6. Raeve W.D., Implementation of Biomedical Image Processing Algorithms, GVA-ELAI-UPM, 2003.
7. TMS320C6713 DSK, Technical Reference, DSP Development Systems, Spectrum Digital Corporation, 2003.
   http://c6000.spectrumdigital.com/dsk6713/V2/docs/dsk6713_TechRef.pdf
8. Tan E.J., and Heinzelman W.B., DSP architectures: past, present and futures, ACM SIGARCH Computer Architecture News 2003, Vol. 31, No. 3, pp. 6-19.
9. TMS320C6000 Technical Brief, Literature Number: SPRU197D, February 1999.
10. Code Composer Studio Getting Started Guide, Literature Number: SPRU509H, Texas Instruments, Dallas, TX, October 2006.
11. Code Composer Studio Users Guide, Literature No: SPRU328A, Texas Instruments, Dallas, TX, August 1999.
12. TMS320C6000 Programmer's Guide, Literature No: SPRU198D, Texas Instruments, Dallas, TX, March 2000.
13. Chassaing R., Digital Signal Processing and Applications with the C6713 and C6416, Wiley Inter Science, New Jersey, USA, 2005.
14. Qureshi S., Embedded Image Processing on the TMS320C6000 DSP, Labcyte Inc., Palo Alto, CA, USA, 2005.
15. Chassaing R., DSP Applications Using C and the TMS320C6x DSK, John Wiley & Sons, Inc., USA, 2002.
16. Kehtarnavaz N., Real Time Digital Signal Processing Based on the TMS320C6000, Elsevier, Newnes, USA, 2005.
17. Tretter S.A., Communication System Design Using DSP Algorithms with Laboratory Experiments for the TMS320C6713 DSK, Springer, New York, USA, 2008.

CHAPTER-V

IMPLEMENTATION AND PERFORMANCE STUDY OF DESPECKLING FILTER ALGORITHMS IN THE PCMAT SYSTEM

5.1 ALGORITHM INTRODUCTION

In the PCMAT system, all despeckling algorithms were developed in the MATLAB 7.1 (MathWorks, Natick, MA, USA). The algorithm comprised of the programs for eight despeckling spatial filters viz. Frost, Median, Lee, Kuan, Wiener, enhanced Frost, enhanced Lee, Gamma map, one frequency filter viz., Homomorphic, (mentioned in Chapter II, Section 2.5.1) two diffusion filters viz., PMAD and SRAD [1] (mentioned in Chapter II, Section 2.5.3), one multi-resolution wavelet filter [2-5] (mentioned in Chapter II, Section 2.5.2) and discrete topological derivative (DTD) filter [6] (discussed in Chapter III). In addition to this, programs for twenty performance metrics (discussed in Chapter II, Section 2.6) are incorporated. Further, the program for five edge detection methods such as Sobel, Robert's, Prewitt's, Laplacian of Gaussian (LoG) and the Canny edge detection with Peak SNR calculation (given in Chapter II, Section 2.8) are included for comparing the performance of the despeckling filters. Of the five edge detection methods, Canny edge detection performed well over the other methods due to its minimized false and missing actual edge detection as well as minimized multiple response to an actual edge [7-10]. As a result, the Canny edge detection and its Peak SNR values are given in this chapter for comparison of the performance of the despeckling filters.

5.2 TESTING DETAILS

All the algorithms were tested on more than 200 ultrasound B-scan images of various organs like abdomen, kidney, liver, gall bladder, heart, lungs and pancreas-spleen, etc, obtained from four different sources (mentioned in Chapter-IV, Section 4.11). The results obtained were compared for grading the performance of the despeckling filters using the following methods.

1. Visual inspection of the raw and filtered images by trained sonologist/radiologist.
2. Comparison of calculated performance metrics
3. Comparison of the Canny edge detected raw and despeckled images with the calculated peak SNR value.

5.3 CASE STUDY

In this research work, over 200 ultrasound B-scan images of various human organs have been tested in the developed algorithms. But, due to the limitation in maximum number of pages prescribed for thesis submission, seven example ultrasound B-scan images are presented here based on the sonologist/radiologist suggestion, since these images contains hypo and hyper ecogenic regions, which is mostly degraded by the speckle noise. The details of the seven images used for presentation in this thesis are given in Table 5.1. The B-scan view of the raw images taken for this study is given in Figure 5.1 (a-g). In this Chapter, three example images for abdomen, kidney and liver, ultrasound B-scan images tested in the PCMAT system are presented. The remaining four ultrasound B-scan images tested in the PCMAT system are given in the Appendix-A.

Table 5.1 Specifications of Ultrasound B-scan Images

Sample name	Content of the Image	Size (in pixels)	Format
IMAGE - 1	Abdomen calcific fibroid	290x350	BMP/JPEG
IMAGE - 2	Kidney	290x350	BMP/JPEG
IMAGE - 3	Lungs	290x350	BMP/JPEG
IMAGE - 4	Heart	290x350	BMP/JPEG
IMAGE - 5	Liver cyst	290x350	BMP/JPEG
IMAGE - 6	Gall Bladder	290x350	BMP/JPEG
IMAGE - 7	Pancreas-Spleen	290x350	BMP/JPEG

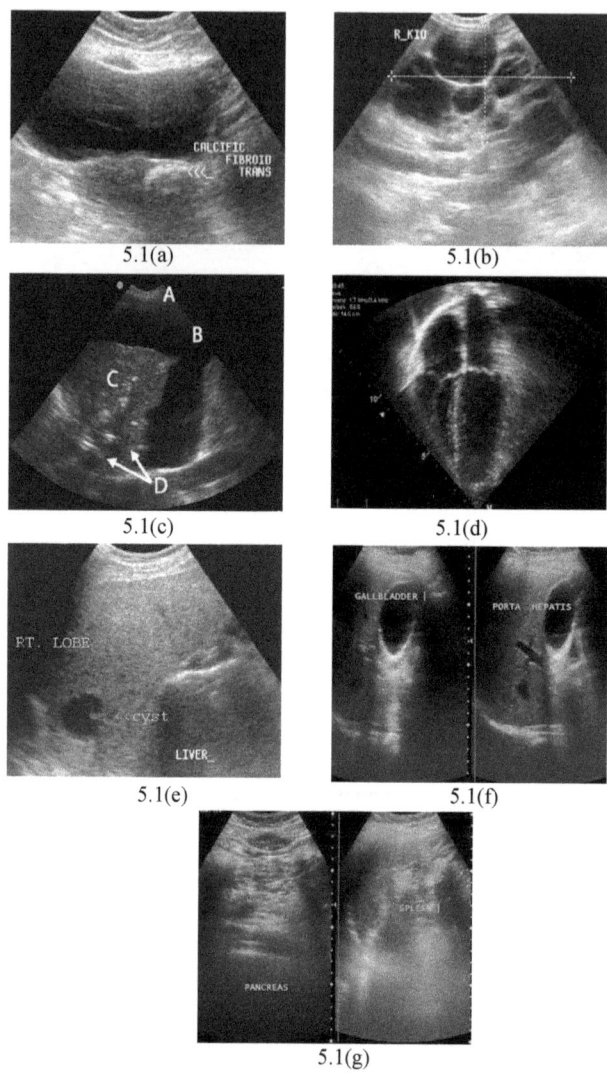

Fig 5.1 View of the ultrasound B-scan images (a) Abdomen with a calcific fibroid (IMAGE-1) (b) Kidney (IMAGE-2) (c) Lungs (IMAGE-3) (d) Heart (IMAGE-4) (e) Liver with a cyst in it (IMAGE-5) (f) Gall bladder (IMAGE-6) and (g) Pancreas – Spleen (IMAGE-7)

5.4 DESCRIPTION OF THE DESPECKLING ALGORITHMS TESTED IN THE PCMAT SYSTEM

The complete flowchart of all the despeckling algorithms used in this study and tested in the PCMAT system is given in Figure 5.2. The program execution comprises of the following steps in a sequence and is summarized below.

Step 1   In the initial step, the raw/original ultrasound B-scan image is taken for applying the despeckling filters as per the format detailed in Table 5.1

Step 2   Then, conversion of the existing RGB image into gray scale image is performed for clearly viewing the image details

Step 3   At this step, DTD filter function selection is checked, since DTD filter involved different processing steps than the others. If DTD is chosen, then resize the input image into 5x5 blocks. For the calculation of DTD, the cost function is applied to one of the pixels of the chosen 5x5 block and calculated the DTD values using threshold values (described in Chapter-III, section 3.3). This procedure should be repeated for all other pixels of the chosen 5x5 block

Step 4   Add all the DTD values of the chosen 5x5 block for creating the despeckled image. Repeat the steps 3 and 4 for other 5x5 blocks of the raw image. If all the 5x5 blocks of the image are DTD filtered, then the DTD filtered image is displayed in a window

Step 5   If DTD is not chosen at Step 3, then the spatial, frequency, wavelet, and diffusion filter functions are called in a sequence. Each filter function (Described in the following sub-sections) is applied separately in a sequence and calculated the despeckled images. Then, the raw and the despeckled images are displayed in a window. Using the raw and despeckled image data, the nineteen performance metrics mentioned in Chapter-II, Section 2.6 are calculated, displayed and stored in a file for future use

Step 6   Step 5 is repeated for all the seven spatial filters, one wavelet filter and two diffusion filters using the filter equations mentioned in Chapter-II, Section 2.5

Step 7   Using the raw and the despeckled image data obtained in Step 5, the algorithm for the five edge detection techniques mentioned in Chapter-II, Section 2.7 are called in a sequence. In the edge detection stage, one of the five edge detection operator (mentioned in Chapter-II, Section 2.8) is applied to the raw and despeckled images, which detected the respective edge values. Using the edge values of the raw and despeckled images, the peak SNR value is calculated. Finally, the edge detected images for the raw and the despeckled filters are displayed in a window. The calculated peak SNR is displayed on the command window. This process is repeated for all the five edge detection methods.

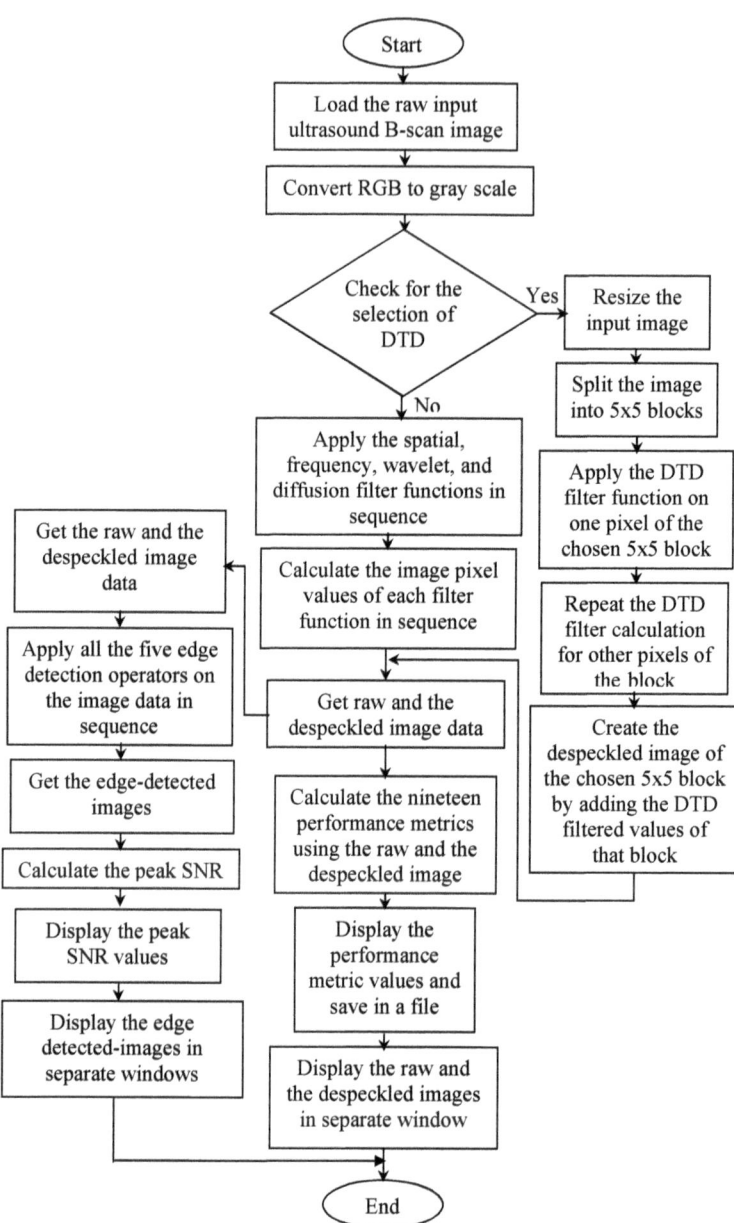

Fig 5.2 Flow chart of the speckle reduction algorithm

In the following sub-sections, all the techniques given in the overall flowchart (Figure 5.2) is described in detail. In all these filter operations, the first two steps (Step 1 & 2) are common and hence both the steps are left in the following discussion.

5.4.1 Algorithm of Frost filter

Step 1   The raw gray scale image data in the BMP/JPEG format is converted into double precision format in order to get linear scaling for both the X and Y coordinates.

Step 2   Then, the Frost filter function expressed in Chapter-II, Section 2.5.1.1 is applied on the chosen cell of the image. This filter calculated the weighted sum of the cell values in the filter function. The calculated value is substituted in the center pixel of the cell.

Step 3   The procedure mentioned in Step 2 is repeated for the whole image and finally raw and Frost filtered images are displayed.

5.4.2 Algorithm of Median filter

Step 1   The raw gray scale image data in the BMP/JPEG format is converted into double precision format in order to get linear scaling for both the X and Y coordinates.

Step 2   Then, the Median filter function given in Chapter-II, Section 2.5.1.2 is applied on the chosen window of the image. It calculates the median value and the calculated median value are substituted in the central pixel.

Step 3   Step 2 is repeated for the whole image and finally the raw and median filtered images are displayed.

5.4.3 Algorithm of Lee filer

Step 1   The raw gray scale image data in the BMP/JPEG format is converted into double precision format in order to get linear scaling for both the X and Y coordinates.

Step 2   Lee filter function given in Chapter-II, Section 2.5.1.3 is applied on the image data. It calculates the coefficient of variation of despeckled image and raw image using the standard deviation and mean of the respective images for the chosen window. Then, the calculated coefficients are substituted in the weighting function given in equation 2.8.

Step 3   Step 2 is repeated for the remaining windows in the image. Then, the raw and the Lee filtered images are displayed.

5.4.4 Algorithm of Kuan filter

Step 1 The raw gray scale image data in the BMP/JPEG format is converted into double precision format in order to get linear scaling for both the X and Y coordinates.

Step 2 Kuan filter function given in Chapter-II, Section 2.5.1.3 is applied on the image data. It calculates the coefficient of variation of despeckled image and raw image using the standard deviation and mean of the respective images for the chosen window. Then, the calculated coefficients are substituted in the weighting function given in equation 2.9.

Step 3 Step 2 is repeated for the remaining windows in the image. Then, the raw and the Kuan filtered images are displayed.

5.4.5 Algorithm of Wiener filter

Step 1 The raw gray scale image data in the BMP/JPEG format is converted into double precision format in order to get linear scaling for both the X and Y coordinates.

Step 2 Wiener filter function given in Chapter-II, Section 2.5.1.4 is implemented in the chosen window of the image, which calculates the power spectra of the chosen window for the original and the noisy image using the periodogram estimation. From the power spectra the despeckled image is obtained through inverse filtering and noise smoothing.

Step 3 Step 2 is repeated for the entire image. Then, the raw and Wiener filtered images are displayed.

5.4.6 Algorithm of Enhanced Frost filter

Step 1 The raw gray scale image data in the BMP/JPEG format is converted into double precision format in order to get linear scaling for both the X and Y coordinates.

Step 2 The enhanced Frost filter function given in equation 2.10 is applied on the chosen window of the image, which calculates the coefficients using the noise variance, mean, and standard deviation of the image. Then, the calculated values are substituted in weighting function given in equation 2.11.

Step 3 Step 2 is repeated for the remaining windows of the image. Then, the raw and enhanced Frost filtered images are displayed.

5.4.7 Algorithm of Enhanced Lee filter

Step 1   The raw gray scale image data in the BMP/JPEG format is converted into double precision format in order to get linear scaling for both the X and Y coordinates.

Step 2   The enhanced Lee filter function given in equation 2.10 is applied on the chosen window of the image, which calculates the noise variation coefficients using the variance, mean, and standard deviation of the image. Then, the calculated values are substituted in weighting function given in equation 2.12.

Step 3   Step 2 is repeated for the remaining windows of the image. Then, the raw and enhanced Lee filtered images are displayed.

5.4.8 Algorithm of Gamma Map filter

Step 1   The raw gray scale image data in the BMP/JPEG format is converted into double precision format in order to get linear scaling for both the X and Y coordinates.

Step 2   Apply the Gamma map filter function given in equation 2.13 on the chosen window of the raw image. This is performed by calculating the mean, standard deviation, variance of the noise in the image.

Step 3   Step 2 is repeated for the other windows of the image. Then, the raw and Gamma map filtered images are displayed.

5.4.9 Algorithm of Homomorphic filter

Step 1   The raw gray scale image data in the BMP/JPEG format is converted into double precision format in order to get linear scaling for both the X and Y coordinates.

Step 2   2D-FFT with Butterworth high boost filter given in equation 2.14 is applied to the chosen window of the raw image, which suppresses the low frequency components in the image. Then, logarithmic operator is applied to the Fourier transformed image that performs logarithmic compression on the image. The compressed image is subjected to inverse FFT to obtain the despeckled image in the space domain.

Step 3   Step 2 is repeated for the other windows of the image to obtain the whole despeckled image. Finally, the raw and Homomorphic filtered images are displayed.

5.4.10 Algorithm of Wavelet filter

Step 1   The raw gray scale image data in the BMP/JPEG format is converted into double precision format in order to get linear scaling for both the X and Y coordinates.

Step 2   The wavelet function (db1 to 4) is applied on the selected window, which decomposes the image into sub bands. For each sub band, the noise variance, standard deviation and scale parameters are calculated. Then, soft thresholding is applied to the sub bands such as LHi, HLi and HHi to remove the magnitude of the wavelet coefficients that are below the threshold value and retain/modify the coefficients that are above the threshold value. The LLi sub band is subjected to Wiener filter, which remove the noise present in that level. Then, all the sub band values are used to reconstruct the denoised image.

Step 3   Step 2 is repeated for all the other windows of the image. Finally, the raw and wavelet filtered images are displayed.

5.4.11 Algorithm of PMAD filter

Step 1   The raw gray scale image data in the BMP/JPEG format is converted into double precision format in order to get linear scaling for both the X and Y coordinates.

Step 2   The PMAD filter function given in equation 2.21 is applied on the chosen window of the raw image, which calculates the diffusion coefficients using the gradient magnitude of the chosen image. This procedure finds out the edges/boundaries in the image.

Step 3   Step 2 is repeated for the remaining windows of the image. Then, the raw and PMAD filtered images are displayed.

5.4.12 Algorithm of SRAD filter

Step 1   The raw gray scale image data in the BMP/JPEG format is converted into double precision format in order to get linear scaling for both the X and Y coordinates.

Step 2   The SRAD filter function given in equation 2.25 on the selected window of the raw image, which calculates the speckle scaling function and instantaneous coefficient of variation of the image. The instantaneous coefficient of variation values are substituted in equation 2.26 or 2.27, which results in smoothing of high contrast and homogenous regions.

Step 3   Step 2 is repeated for the remaining windows of the image. Then, the raw and SRAD filtered images are displayed.

5.4.13 Algorithm of DTD filter

Step 1   The raw gray scale image data in the BMP/JPEG format is converted into double precision format in order to get linear scaling for both the X and Y coordinates.

Step 2   The ultrasound image is enlarged to one pixel level and the perturbation is applied to the enlarged single pixel in the form of a cost function given in equation 3.9, which calculates the diffusion co-efficient of the cost function to the neighboring pixels. Now, the discrete topological derivative (DTD) given in equation 3.10 is initialized, which is a measure of the total variation in the cost function for the applied perturbation. Then, the cost function of the first iteration is calculated and compared with the tolerance value (the tolerance value will be fixed a value greater than zero). If the cost function is less than the tolerance value, the iteration is stopped, otherwise it will continue for determining the new value of cost function by applying another value of the diffusion coefficient. If the iteration is stopped, the gradient for the new and old image is calculated for sensitivity analysis. Then, the topological derivative value is used for reshaping the despeckled image.

Step 3   The procedure mentioned in Step 2 is repeated for all the pixels in the image. Finally the raw and DTD filtered images are displayed.

5.5 DESCRIPTION OF THE EDGE DETECTION ALGORITHMS

5.5.1 Algorithm of Sobel edge detection

Step 1   The raw/despeckled image data is taken for applying the Sobel edge detection operator.

Step 2   The Sobel kernels S_x, S_y described in Chapter II, Section 2.8.1 is applied to the image, which calculate the edges in the two perpendicular (x, y) directions of the selected 3x3 window. The gradient and the orientation of the edges are determined using the calculated kernels S_x, S_y in equations 2.37 and 2.39.

Step 3   The step 2 is repeated for the remaining 3x3 windows of the image. Then, the Sobel edge detected image of the raw/despeckled image is displayed.

5.5.2 Algorithm of Robert's edge detection

Step 1   The raw/despeckled image data is taken for applying the Robert's edge detection operator.

Step 2   The Robert's kernels R_x, R_y described in Chapter II, Section 2.8.2 is applied to the image, which calculate the edges in the two perpendicular x, y directions of the selected 2x2 window. The gradient and the orientation of the edges are determined using the calculated kernels R_x, R_y in equations 2.40 and 2.42.

Step 3   The step 2 is repeated for the remaining 2x2 windows of the image. Then, the Robert's edge detected image of the raw/despeckled image is displayed.

5.5.3 Algorithm of Prewitt's edge detection

Step 1   The raw/despeckled image data is taken for applying the Prewitt's edge detection operator.

Step 2   The Prewitt's kernels G_x, G_y described in Chapter II, Section 2.8.3 is applied to the image, which calculate the edges in the two perpendicular (x, y) directions of the selected 3x3 window. The gradient and its orientation of the edges are determined by substituting the calculated kernels G_x, G_y in equations 2.37 and 2.39 in place of S_x, S_y.

Step 3   The step 2 is repeated for the remaining 3x3 windows of the image. Then, the Prewitt's edge detected image of the raw/despeckled image is displayed.

5.5.4 Algorithm of LoG edge detection

Step 1   The raw/despeckled image data is taken for applying the LoG edge detection operator.

Step 2   The three kernels of the Laplacian operator mentioned in Chapter-II, Section 2.8.4 are convolved with the Gaussian smoothing operator given in equation 2.44, which generated a hybrid operator that is convolved with the chosen 3x3 image window. This operation detects the edges and removes the high frequency noise.

Step 3   Step 2 is repeated for the remaining 3x3 windows of the image. Finally, the LoG edge detected image of the raw/despeckled image is displayed.

5.5.5 Algorithm of Canny edge detection

Step 1   The raw/despeckled image data is taken for applying the Sobel edge detection operator.

Step 2   Gaussian kernel mentioned in Chapter-II, Section 2.8.5 is applied to the selected pixel window for removing the blurring and noise effects. Then, the Sobel operator algorithm given in section 5.5.1 is applied to detect the edges and the orientation based on the calculated gradient values. Next, non-maximum suppression operator is applied to trace along the edge to found out the false edges. Then, hysteresis is applied to remove the streaking effect.

Step 3   Step 2 is repeated on the other windows of the image. Then, the Canny edge detected image of the raw/despeckled image is displayed.

5.6 PERFORMANCE STUDY OF THE DESPECKLING FILTERS IN THE PCMAT SYSTEM

The speckle reduction algorithms were tested on over 200 ultrasound B-scan images of various organs collected from four sources (Given in Chapter-IV, Section 4.11, Table 4.3). In this chapter, the results of the three important case studies (abdomen, kidney and liver) suggested by the sonologist/radiologist are presented here in the following format for easy comparison of the results obtained.

1. A collection of the raw image with the thirteen despeckled images of the three case studies is given for visual inspection of the performance of the speckle reduction filter and the assessing the ability of the filters in retaining the information/details by the sonologist or radiologist.

2. Five Edge detection methods were tested on all the images, but Canny edge detection was proved to be the better method for detecting both strong and weak edges of medical images according to the references given [6-10]. As a result, a collection of Canny edge detected images of thirteen despeckled filters are given for the three case studies for estimating the performance of the despeckling filters.

3. A collection of nineteen performance metrics calculated for the thirteen despeckling filters with the time for execution of the respective filter algorithm are tabulated for comparison of the performance of the filters. In addition, the peak SNR value calculated for the Canny edge detected image of

each despeckling filter is given in the table for comparing the despeckling filter efficiency in identifying the edges.

In the case study 1, the raw/original ultrasound B-scan image of abdomen with calcified fibroid is taken. The raw image with the thirteen despeckling filters output images of the abdomen are given in Figure 5.3. The Canny edge detected images of the thirteen filters are given in Figure 5.4. The calculated nineteen performance metrics, execution time and the calculated peak SNR values of the Canny edge detected images of the thirteen despeckling filters for the abdomen image are summarized in Table 5. 2.

In case study 2, the raw/original ultrasound B-scan image of kidney is used. The raw image with the thirteen despeckling filters output images of the kidney are given in Figure 5.5. The Canny edge detected images of the thirteen despeckling filters are given in Figure 5.6. The calculated nineteen performance metrics, execution time and the calculated peak SNR values of the Canny edge detected images of the thirteen despeckling filters for the kidney image are summarized in Table 5.3.

Likewise, in case study 3, the raw/original ultrasound B-scan image of liver is used. The raw image with the thirteen despeckling filters output images of the liver are given in Figure 5.7. The Canny edge detected images of the thirteen despeckling filters are given in Figure 5.8. The calculated nineteen performance metrics, execution time and the calculated peak SNR values of the Canny edge detected images of the thirteen despeckling filters for the liver image are summarized in Table 5.4.

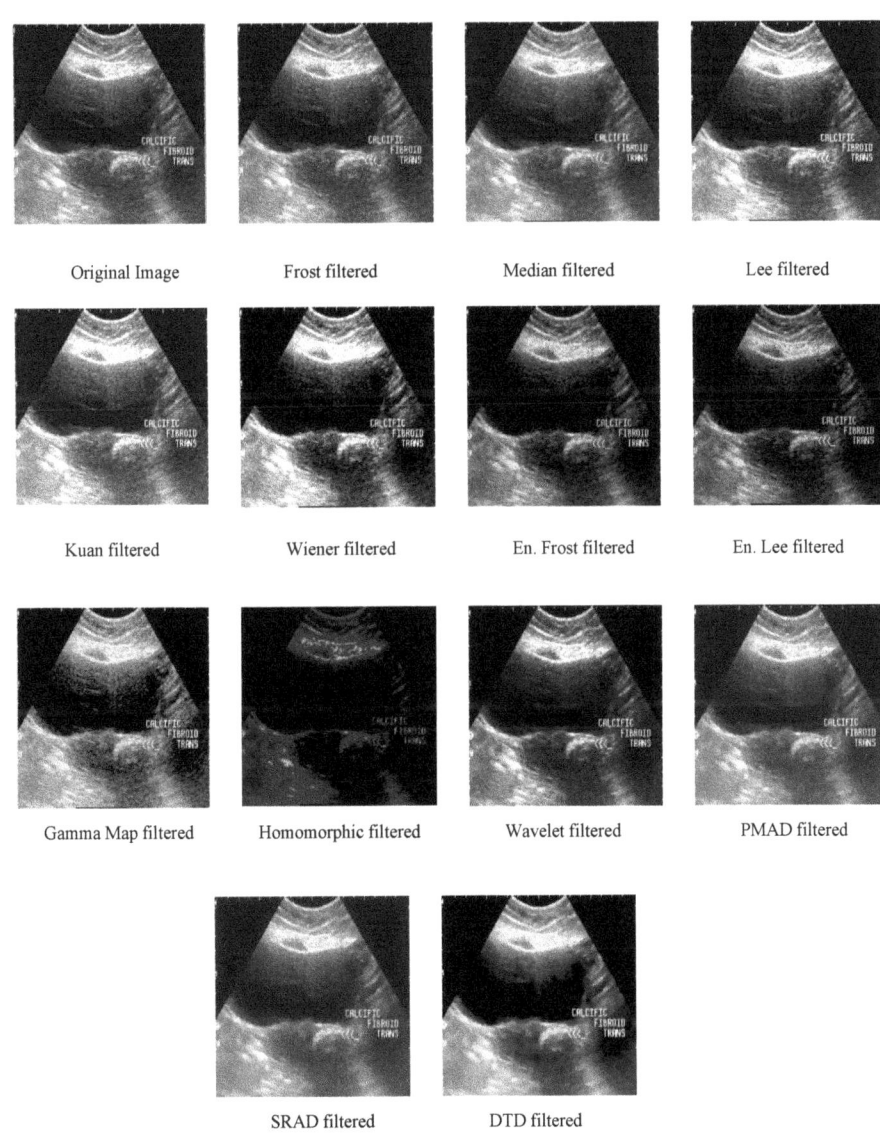

Fig 5.3 Original and despeckled images of abdomen in the PCMAT system

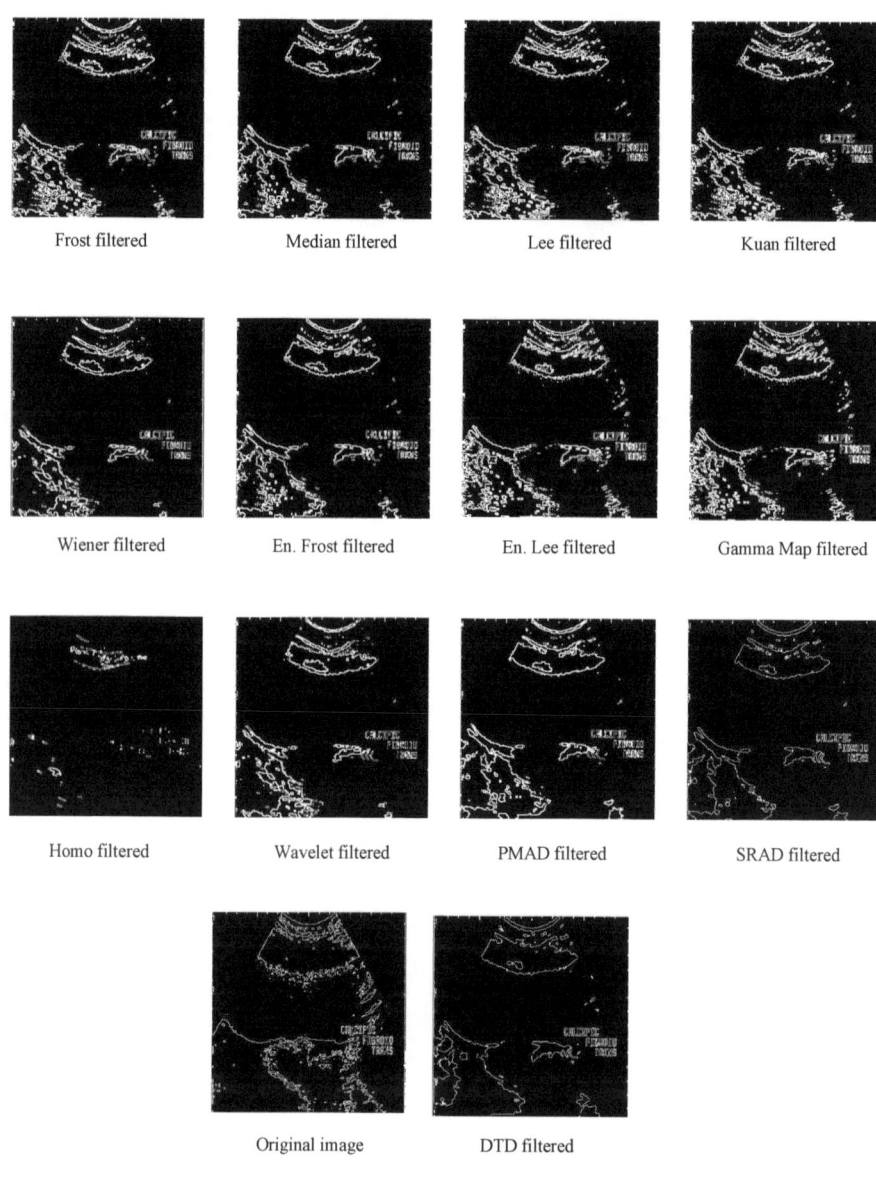

Fig 5.4 Canny edge detected images of abdomen in the PCMAT system

Table 5.2 Calculated performance metrics of the despeckling filters applied on the abdomen image in the PCMAT system

Group	Metrics	Frost	Median	Lee	Kuan	Homo morphic	Wiener	En. Frost	En Lee	GAM	Wavelet	PMAD	SRAD	DTD
Quality metrics	PSNR in dB	30.43	29.95	27.92	27.49	8.28	33.61	22.87	21.25	25.123	20.39	26.42	27.26	36.52
	PSNR (Canny) in dB	16.54	16.78	15.23	17.14	6.48	21.47	17.25	18.46	17.58	23.45	18.42	22.05	25.21
	AD	0.15	0.27	0.18	0.48	77.07	0.02	12.87	15.67	9.82	17.28	24.67	0.05	0.30
	MSE	112.81	118.75	138.25	134.45	9648.96	98.31	170.74	168.55	152.84	194.21	125.25	147.22	78.43
	MD	122	157	158	181	253.19	35	93	107	67	114	157	245	146
	NAE	0.052	0.04	0.06	0.06	0.98	0.04	0.16	0.19	0.124	0.21	0.31	0.12	0.09
	CNR	1.48	2.83	4.05	5.64	2.07	2.94	1.613	1.92	1.20	2.02	2.81	8.36	4.21
	FoM	0.52	0.51	0.48	0.46	0.11	0.55	0.48	0.47	0.51	0.54	0.37	0.49	0.56
Similarity metrics	SC	1.01	1.01	1.02	1.02	4023.05	1.07	0.77	0.73	0.82	0.71	0.62	1.04	1.02
	CoC	0.99	0.99	0.98	0.98	0.93	0.99	0.98	0.97	0.98	0.97	0.94	0.96	0.98
	NCC	0.99	0.99	0.98	0.98	0.02	0.98	0.96	0.98	0.98	0.94	0.91	0.97	0.99
	IQI	0.97	0.97	0.96	0.97	0.00	0.97	0.97	0.97	0.97	0.96	0.92	0.97	0.98
	GAE	0.00	0.00	0.00	0.00	0.00	0.00	0.00	0.00	0.00	0.00	0.00	0.00	0.00
	NMSE	1.89	6.93	8.14	2.75	0.96	7.62	0.026	0.03	0.015	0.04	0.09	5.58	1.48
	MSSIM	0.91	0.93	0.88	0.88	0.059	0.98	0.78	0.72	0.85	0.68	0.56	0.61	0.71
	SI	0.12	0.14	0.13	0.13	0.10	0.21	0.15	0.16	0.21	0.17	0.15	0.21	0.26
Speckle metrics	ASNR	1.34	1.33	1.43	1.33	1.02	1.32	1.39	1.45	1.37	1.41	1.43	1.39	1.36
	IV	0.092	0.089	0.094	0.086	118.46	0.068	0.12	0.14	0.13	0.17	-0.098	0.22	0.21
	NSD	6.29	6.24	4.79	6.21	2.47	6.27	8.52	9.01	7.94	9.34	1.08	6.28	6.32
	ENL	2.15	2.12	2.23	2.03	2.04	1.48	1.44	1.59	1.35	1.26	2.14	2.38	2.15
	Execution time in sec	18.16	4.28	22.36	25.38	4.58	4.18	18.14	24.48	19.18	2.49	8.26	6.98	37.46

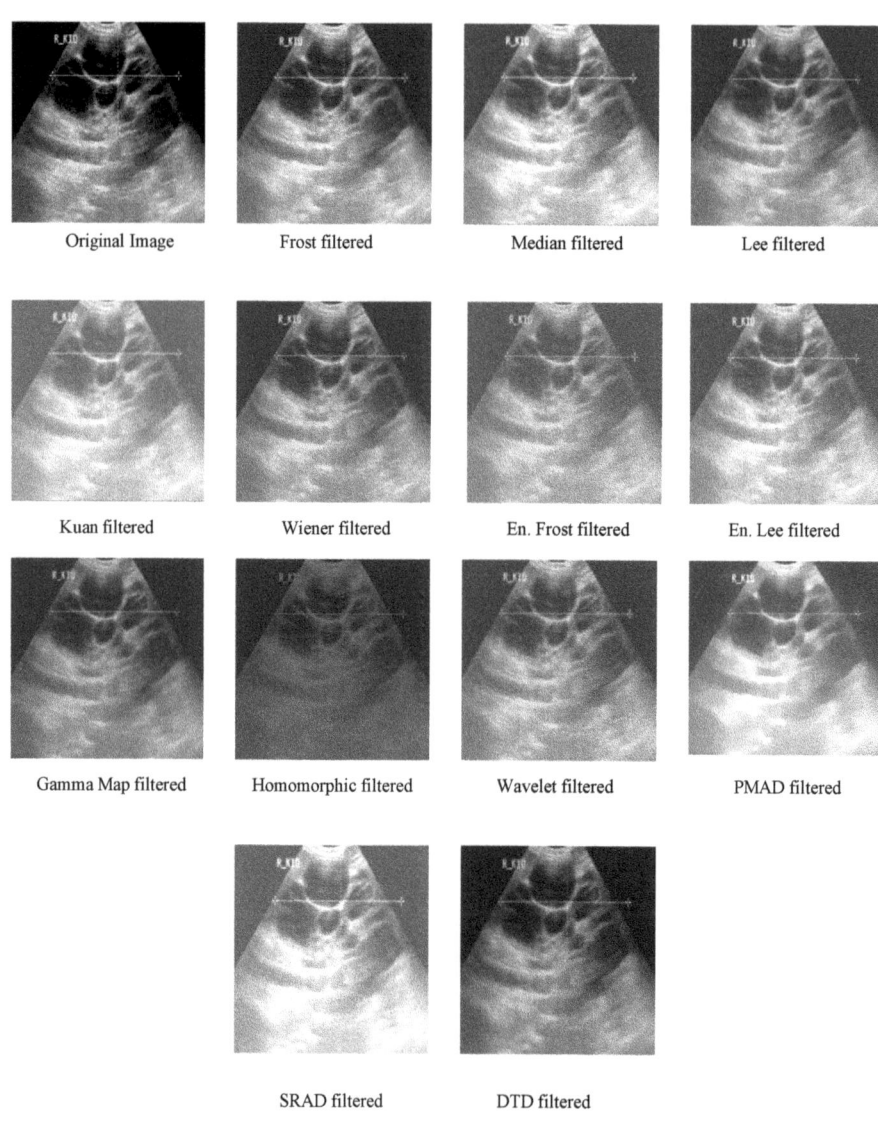

Fig 5.5 Original and despeckled images of kidney in the PCMAT system

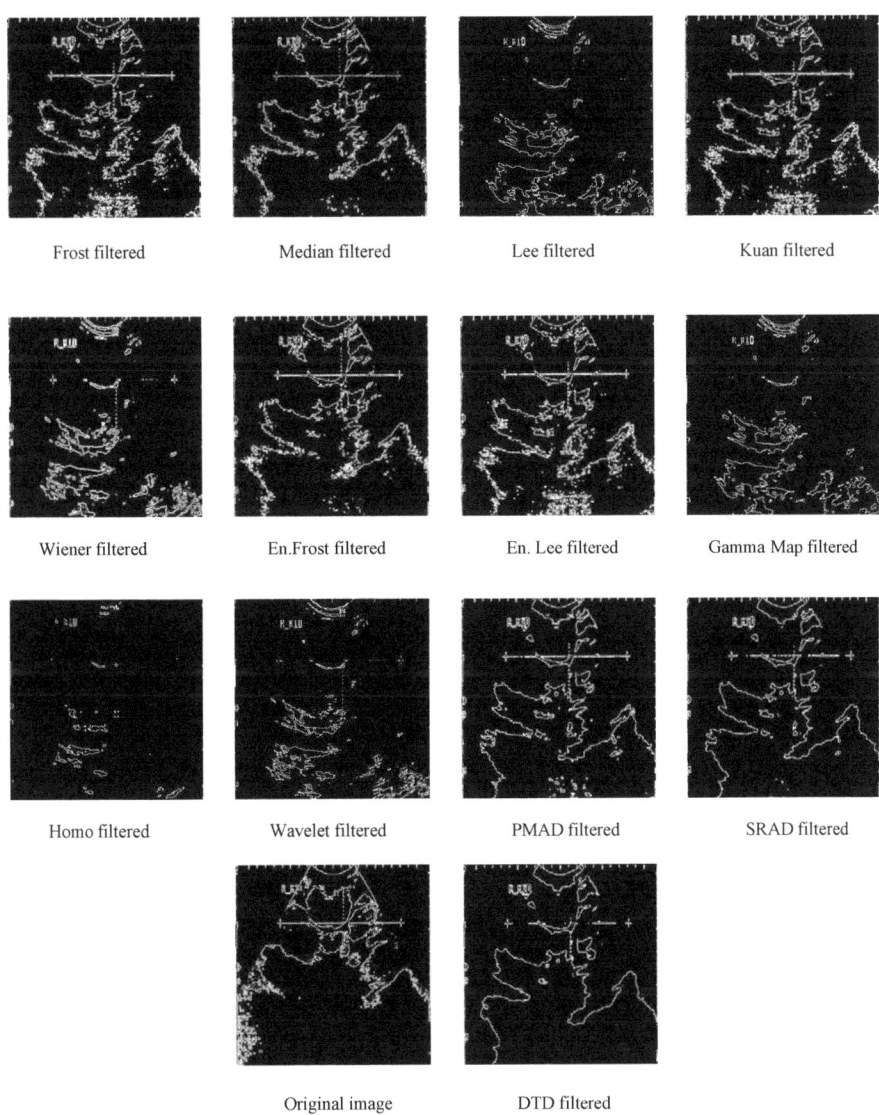

Fig 5.6 Canny edge detected images of kidney in the PCMAT system

Table 5.3 Calculated performance metrics of the despeckling filters applied on the kidney image in the PCMAT system

Group	Metrics	Frost	Median	Lee	Kuan	Homo morphic	Wiener	En. Frost	En Lee	GAM	Wavelet	PMAD	SRAD	DTD
Quality metrics	PSNR in dB	29.43	29.95	26.14	27.52	9.28	31.64	21.54	21.14	24.26	20.43	26.51	27.18	37.52
	PSNR (Canny) in dB	16.12	15.48	14.02	18.71	4.63	22.07	17.54	17.89	17.41	24.09	18.78	29.74	31.53
	AD	0.26	0.01	0.19	0.11	67.34	0.01	11.85	14.33	9.08	15.87	22.62	0.02	0.26
	MSE	117.43	121.54	148.25	132.45	8927.96	104.38	168.28	169.27	165.41	187.47	124.74	121.78	64.43
	MD	241	29	162	136	253.17	29	79	100	65	113	152	255	113
	NAE	0.04	0.04	0.06	0.05	0.97	0.04	0.17	0.28	0.13	0.23	0.32	0.11	0.09
	CNR	5.48	2.65	4.05	2.25	2.69	2.65	2.16	2.57	1.69	2.81	3.87	5.14	5.41
	FoM	0.51	0.49	0.47	0.48	0.09	0.54	0.49	0.51	0.52	0.55	0.38	0.51	0.57
Similarity metrics	SC	1.01	1.04	1.02	1.01	29.22	1.05	0.76	0.72	0.81	0.73	0.61	1.03	1.01
	CoC	0.99	0.99	0.98	0.99	0.94	0.99	0.97	0.97	0.98	0.96	0.94	0.96	0.98
	NCC	0.99	0.99	0.98	0.98	0.01	0.98	0.95	0.98	0.98	0.96	0.93	0.96	0.99
	IQI	0.97	0.88	0.86	0.87	0.00	0.97	0.92	0.92	0.97	0.96	0.88	0.92	0.98
	GAE	0.00	0.00	0.00	0.00	0.00	0.00	0.00	0.00	0.00	0.00	0.00	0.00	0.00
	NMSE	1.53	3.63	8.18	2.47	9.55	3.63	2.96	4.33	1.73	5.31	1.07	1.25	1.44
	MSSIM	0.90	0.91	0.88	0.91	0.05	0.95	0.77	0.71	0.84	0.68	0.56	0.63	0.72
Speckle metrics	SI	0.18	0.17	0.16	0.15	0.03	0.22	0.19	0.18	0.23	0.19	0.13	0.22	0.25
	ASNR	1.41	1.41	1.43	1.42	1.17	1.41	1.54	1.52	1.48	1.53	1.69	1.47	1.44
	IV	0.12	0.098	0.099	0.089	238.02	0.078	0.18	0.17	0.16	0.19	-0.18	0.23	0.19
	NSD	6.19	5.87	5.26	5.89	5.98	8.16	9.12	7.78	8.98	1.17	5.74	6.58	6.19
	ENL	2.06	2.04	2.05	2.03	4.03	2.04	1.48	1.44	1.59	1.35	1.15	2.04	2.02
	Execution time in sec	20.41	4.17	24.08	27.65	4.61	3.19	18.48	24.73	20.72	3.16	9.11	8.41	38.19

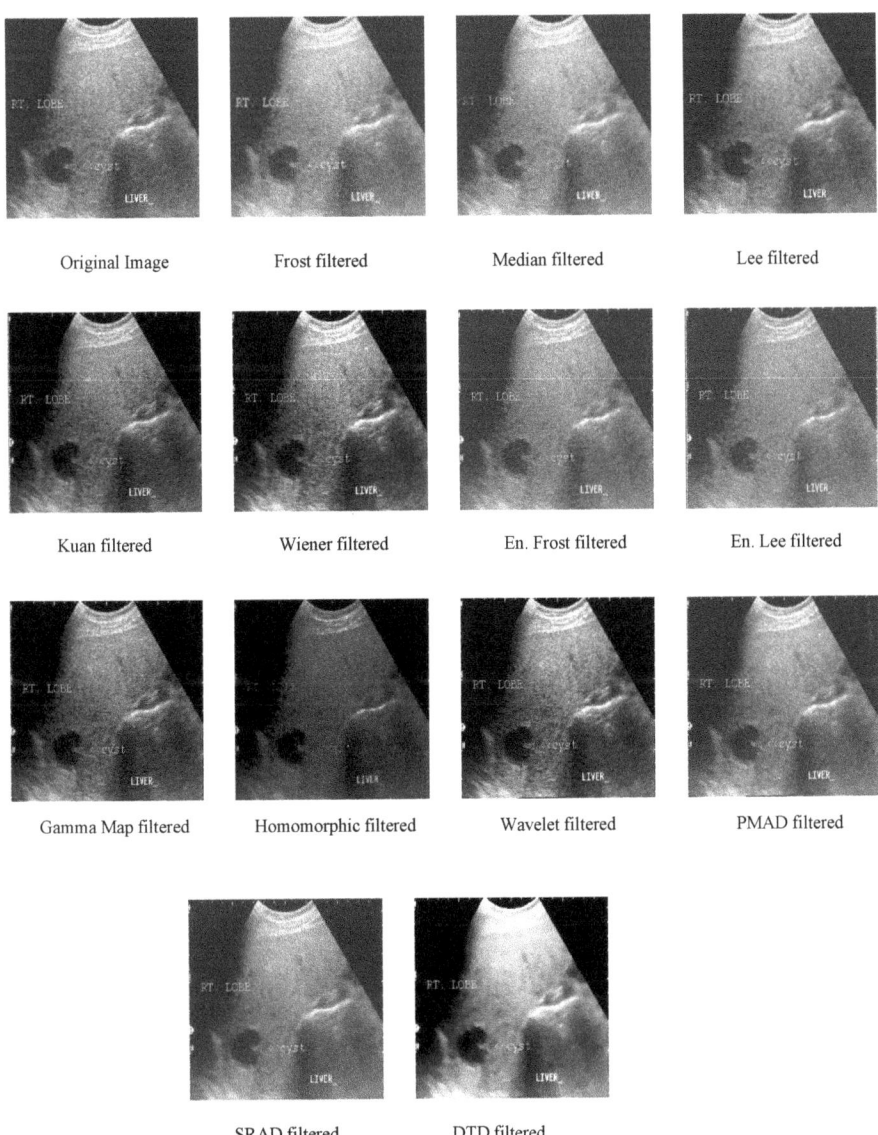

Fig 5.7 Original and despeckled images of liver in the PCMAT system

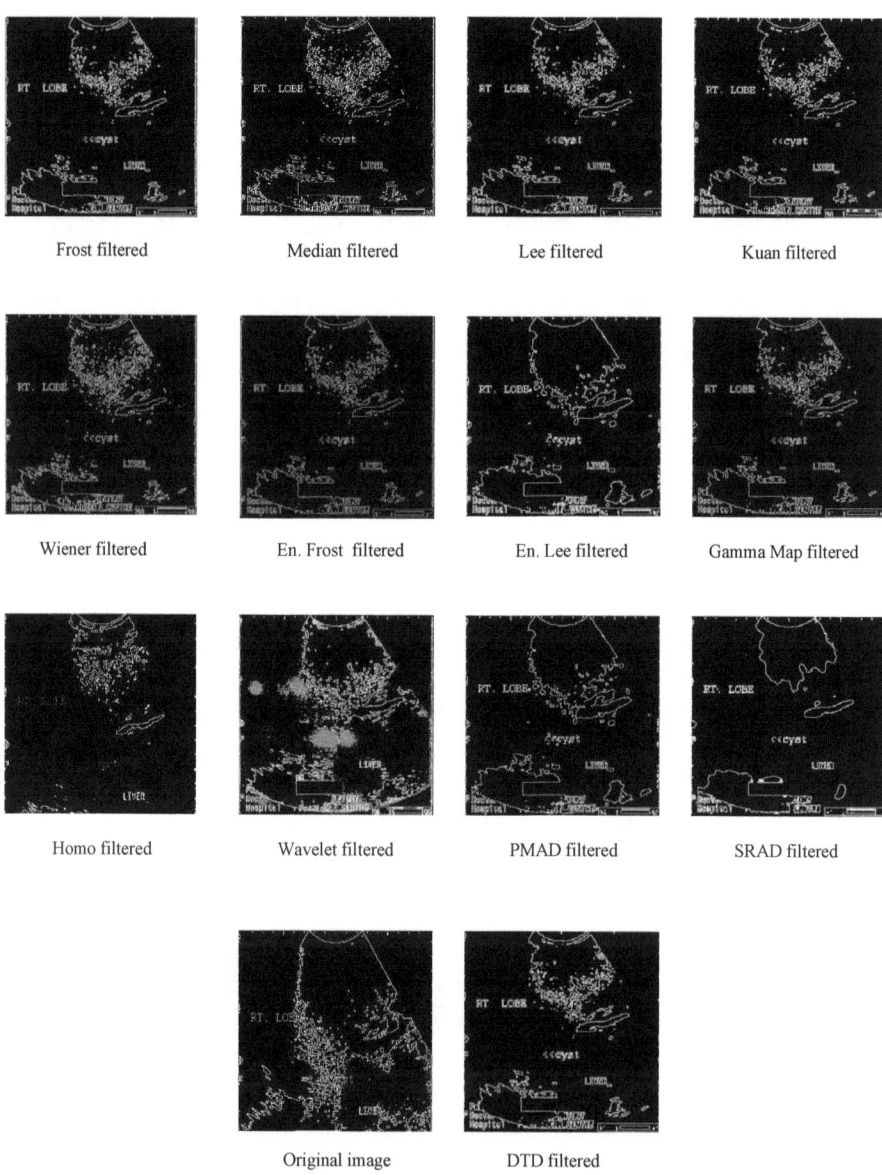

Fig 5.8 Canny edge detected images of liver in the PCMAT system

Table 5.4 Calculated performance metrics of the despeckling filters applied on the liver image in the PCMAT system

Group	Metrics	Frost	Median	Lee	Kuan	Homo morphic	Wiener	En. Frost	En Lee	GAM	Wavelet	PMAD	SRAD	DTD
Quality metrics	PSNR in dB	29.43	30.54	27.44	26.87	9.47	34.57	23.36	21.87	24.28	21.57	25.48	28.39	35.49
	PSNR (Canny) in dB	18.73	20.49	16.98	17.25	5.23	19.58	19.02	18.14	21.26	22.09	21.43	26.23	29.14
	AD	0.17	0.24	0.16	0.42	96.31	0.03	11.92	14.57	9.03	16.23	23.73	0.03	0.31
	MSE	121.61	107.31	138.15	138.75	8812.82	97.51	169.42	162.13	157.54	195.351	129.13	126.17	85.46
	MD	114	169	142	232	253.19	32	87	103	74	116	147	253	105
	NAE	0.037	0.03	0.08	0.049	0.98	0.03	0.12	0.14	0.09	0.165	0.24	0.08	0.06
	CNR	1.33	2.98	4.25	5.26	2.33	4.34	1.46	1.62	1.01	1.81	2.53	4.16	3.95
	FoM	0.48	0.49	0.48	0.46	0.14	0.51	0.45	0.44	0.52	0.55	0.49	0.52	0.57
	SC	1.07	1.01	1.02	1.01	5240.15	1.05	0.81	0.78	0.85	0.76	0.68	1.02	1.01
Similarity metrics	CoC	0.99	0.99	0.98	0.98	0.96	0.99	0.98	0.98	0.99	0.97	0.95	0.97	0.98
	NCC	0.99	0.99	0.98	0.98	0.01	0.99	0.96	0.98	0.98	0.94	0.92	0.97	0.99
	IQI	0.97	0.97	0.96	0.97	0.00	0.97	0.98	0.98	0.97	0.96	0.98	1.04	0.98
	GAE	0.00	0.00	0.00	0.00	0.00	0.00	0.00	0.00	0.00	0.00	0.00	0.00	0.00
	NMSE	1.72	6.56	7.89	2.56	7.58	0.058	0.09	0.021	0.08	0.07	4.98	1.62	1.72
	MSSIM	0.91	0.91	0.89	0.88	0.039	0.91	0.82	0.74	0.86	0.71	0.61	0.66	0.75
Speckle metrics	SI	0.18	0.17	0.16	0.16	0.09	0.23	0.21	0.19	0.22	0.18	0.14	0.28	0.31
	ASNR	1.57	1.56	1.44	1.56	1.12	1.56	1.62	1.64	1.62	1.65	1.77	1.62	159
	IV	0.19	0.21	0.098	0.097	179.24	0.23	0.21	0.22	0.19	0.21	-0.35	0.26	0.24
	NSD	6.28	6.19	5.08	5.78	5.97	8.17	8.57	7.57	9.14	2.18	6.56	6.17	6.47
	ENL	1.01	1.01	2.16	1.02	3.73	1.01	8.04	7.66	8.48	7.44	6.55	1.01	1.01
	Execution time in sec	17.77	4.39	21.48	23.58	3.74	4.63	17.39	22.56	18.44	3.48	7.67	6.63	38.24

5.7 DISCUSSION

In the PCMAT system, algorithms for twelve different standard speckle filters, the proposed DTD filter, five different edge detection methods, and calculation of twenty (including peak SNR of Canny edge detected image) metrics with execution time were developed in the MATLAB 7.1 version. The algorithms were tested on over 200 ultrasound images of several organs and the ultrasound B-scan images of the seven organs viz., abdomen, kidney, liver, gall bladder, heart, lungs, and pancreas-spleen (Figure 5.1) are presented as case studies based on the experts suggestions. In this chapter, only three case studies (for the abdomen, kidney and liver) and their respective outputs are presented in the form of images (Figures 5.3, 5.5 and 5.7), Canny edge detected images (Figures 5.4, 5.6 and 5.8) of the despeckling filters for visual inspection and twenty calculated metrics with execution time are tabulated (Table 5.2, 5.3 and 5.4) for estimating the performance of the despeckling filters quantitatively. The results of the remaining four case studies such as gall bladder, heart, lungs and pancreas-spleen are given in the Appendix-A.

Based on the visual inspection of the despeckled images and the Canny edge detected images by the trained sonologist/radiologist the following inferences have been arrived.

1. Frost and Median filters slightly improve the information of the edges, but the Lee filter improves the ability of preserving the edges/details.
2. Kuan and Lee filters despeckled the image to some extent, where as Lee filter is relatively better than the Kuan filter.
3. Enhanced Frost filter and enhanced Lee filter improve the performance of the Frost and Lee filters, respectively. But, the performance of the enhanced Frost filter is better than the enhanced Lee filter.
4. Performance of the Gamma Map filter is similar to the Kuan filter and the Lee filter.
5. Homomorphic filter is not considered as an advisable despeckling filter, since it sharpens the image and flattens the speckle variations that are evident from the despeckled as well as Canny edge detected images.
6. The PMAD filter enhances the speckle noise and distorted the images.

7. Wavelet despeckled images exhibits slight distortions when compared with the Frost and Median filtered images, since soft thresholding tends to smooth more as the decomposition level increases. An increase in the number of decomposition levels will always produce satisfactory noise speckle reduction but at the expense of more severe image smoothing in edges and fine details.
8. Wiener filter has comparable performance with the SRAD filter but the intra-region smoothing and edge preservation are not up to the level of SRAD filter.
9. The SRAD filter performs better intra-region smoothing of the image and preservation of edges in comparison with the other speckle reduction filters. The SRAD filtered images appears clearer and the boundaries/edges are better resolved in comparison with the other despeckling filters.
10. The proposed DTD filter preserves the edges and point targets relatively better than the SRAD and other traditional despeckling filter results. Also, the results of the Canny edge detected image of the DTD filtered image indicated that the DTD identifies and improves the variation of the hypoechoic and hyperechoic regions better over the other traditional filtering methods.

The calculated twenty performance metrics summarized in Tables 5.2, 5.3 and 5.4 are grouped into three difference categories for the purpose of comparison and discussion of the results arrived. They are,

1. Quality metrics Group: PSNR, peak SNR (Canny), AD, MSE, MD, NAE, CNR, and FoM.
2. Similarity metrics Group: SC, CoC, NCC, IQI, GAE, NMSE, and MSSIM
3. Speckle metrics Group: SI, ASNR, IV, NSD, and ENL

The calculated metrics values in the PCMAT system for the three case studies are presented as histogram plots as shown in Figures 5.9 to 5.26. Of the thirteen filters considered for this study, homomorphic filter is not considered for discussion, since it is not a suitable despeckling filter due to its high metrics values as well as complete flattening of the speckle variation on visual inspection. Therefore, the remaining twelve filters' performance metric values are classified as per the above grouping and comparative study was carried out from the metric values given in Tables 5.2 to 5.4 and from the histogram plots shown in Figures 5.9 to 5.26. Also, the metric GAE (Geometric

Average Error) is a measure of information between the original and despeckled image, which is approaching zero value for faithful transformation of information during filtering. The GAE value of all filters are found to be approaching zero value, therefore it is not taken for discussion. The inferences arrived out of this study are summarized as follows.

1. In the quality metrics group, PSNR and peak SNR (Canny) values of the DTD filter outperformed over the other standard filters, which is conspicuous from the Figure 5.9. In all the three cases studies, the PSNR and peak SNR (Canny) values of the DTD filter are found to be better than the other filters.
2. The quality metrics, Average Difference (AD) should be small for a faithful despeckling filter. The AD values found from the Tables 5.2 to 5.4 and histogram plots of the AD shown in Figure 5.10, it is found that DTD has less value comparable with that of the other standard filters.
3. From Tables 5.2 to 5.4 and Figure 5.11, DTD filter has lower mean square error (MSE) values than other standard filters, which clearly indicated that the DTD filter exhibited smaller difference between the original and denoised images when compared to other filters.
4. The maximum difference (MD) values of the DTD filter are found to be an optimum value, which is evident from the Tables 5.2 to 5.4 and Figure 5.12.
5. The normalized absolute error (NAE) values of the DTD filter have comparable value as that of the other filters that is evident from the Tables 5.2 to 5.4 and Figure 5.13. This suggested that the DTD filtered ultrasound images showed less error between the original and despeckled images.
6. The contrast noise ratio (CNR), a measure of contrast of the image with respect to the background, which shows the ability of the despeckling filter in detecting the low contrast lesion within the high contrast lesion or from the background. From the Tables 5.2 to 5.4 and Figure 5.14, it is noteworthy that the CNR values of the DTD filter have comparable values that of the standard SRAD filter.
7. The figure of merit (FoM), a measure of edge preservation of the despeckled image, of an ideal despeckling filter should be unity. In the case of DTD, it is found to be true from the values of FoM given in Tables 5.2 to 5.4 and Figure 5.15.

8. In the similarity metrics group, structural content (SC) should be unity for identical images. The DTD filter has unity value, which is evident from the Tables 5.2 to 5.4 and Figure 5.16.
9. The coefficient of correlation (CoC), a similarity metric, measures the edge preservation characteristics of despeckling filters, which has unity value when the original and despeckled images are identical. It is noteworthy from the Tables 5.2 to 5.4 and from the Figure 5.17, that the DTD filter has CoC value of unity.
10. The similarity metric, normalized cross correlation (NCC), a measure of image quality, has a value of unity for identical images. From the Table 5.2 to 5.4 and from the Figure 5.18, it is found that the DTD performed better than the other filters.
11. Image quality index (IQI), a member of similarity group, measures the degree of distortion between the original and despeckled images. Its value should be one for identical images. In the case of DTD, IQI value is found to be unity for all the three case studies given in Table 5.2 to 5.4 and Figure 5.19.
12. Normalized mean square error (NMSE) should be small or zero for identical original and despeckled images. From the values given in Tables 5.2 to 5.4 and Figure 5.20, it is clear that DTD has comparably smaller value.
13. The mean structure similarity index map (MSSIM) is used for comparing the luminance, contrast and structural contents of the original and despeckled images. Its value should be closer to unity for optimum similarity. The MSSIM values of the DTD filtered images for the three case studies given in Tables 5.2 to 5.4 and Figure 5.21exibited that the DTD posses optimum similarity metrics.
14. In the speckle metric group, the speckle index (SI) and average signal to noise ratio (ASNR), are the measures of speckle removal, has low and high value, respectively for improved image quality. But, from the case studies given in Tables 5.2 to 5.4 and Figures 5.22 and 5.23, the SI and ASNR values of DTD are slightly higher values than that of the other filters. This is because, the DTD filtered out only the speckle, but not the speckle like details such as hypo and hyper echoic regions.
15. The metrics IV (image variance), determines the contents of the speckle. A lower value of the IV smoothes the image heavily and reduces the speckle highly. But, from the Tables 5.2 to 5.4 and Figure 5.24, the IV value of DTD has optimum

value, which means that the DTD filter improves the image quality by optimally reducing the speckle.

16. The metrics, noise standard deviation (NSD), which determines the quantity of speckle in the processed image. It should be minimum for a good despeckling filter. From the Tables 5.2 to 5.4 and Figure 5.25, the DTD filter exhibited optimum NSD values, since it filtered the speckle noise instead of speckle information.

17. Finally, the effective number of looks (ENL), a measure of speckle level in the ultrasound B-scan image, should be less for good despeckling filter. In the case of DTD, the ENL values are comparably smaller than the other filters, which is evident from the Table 5.2 to 5.4 and Figure 5.26.

18. From the Table 5.2 to 5.4, the average execution time of the DTD algorithm is approximately five times more than the standard SRAD algorithm. This can be improved by using high speed DSPs and efficient coding schemes.

19. In summary, the DTD outperformed in the case of quality and similarity metrics groups, where as it optimally performed in the case of speckle metrics group. Therefore, the DTD should be recommended as a better choice for despeckling the ultrasound B-scan images than the other standard despeckling filter due to its effective despeckling and better visibility of the hypo and hyper echoic regions.

From the visual inspection of the despeckled and edge detected images and the calculated performance metrics values obtained from the PCMAT system, it is remarkable that the DTD filter performed well over the other filters both quantitatively as well as qualitatively.

Eventually, the DTD filter has taken much higher time for the execution of the algorithm in the PCMAT system, which is the bottle neck for its real-time implementation, but this could be improved by effective coding and memory mapping techniques.

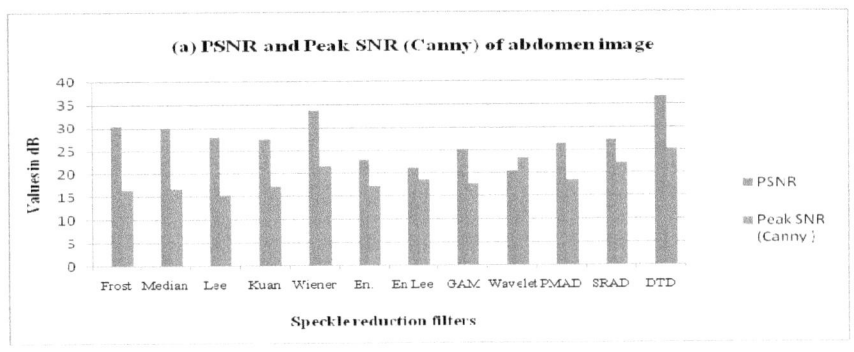

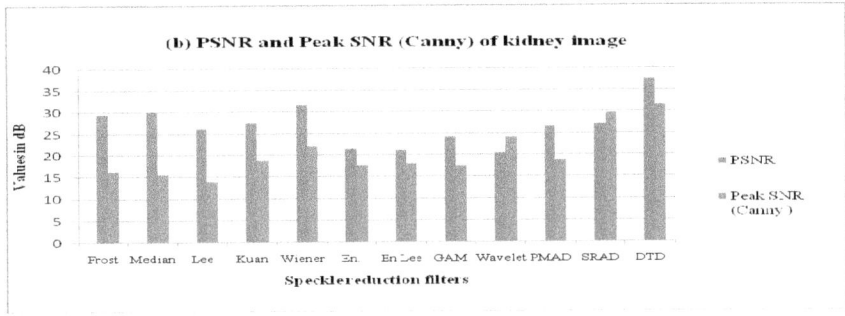

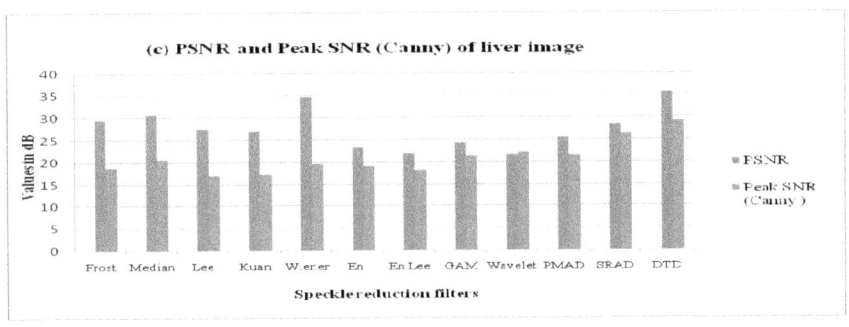

Fig 5.9 Histogram plot of the PSNR and Peak SNR (Canny) in the PCMAT system

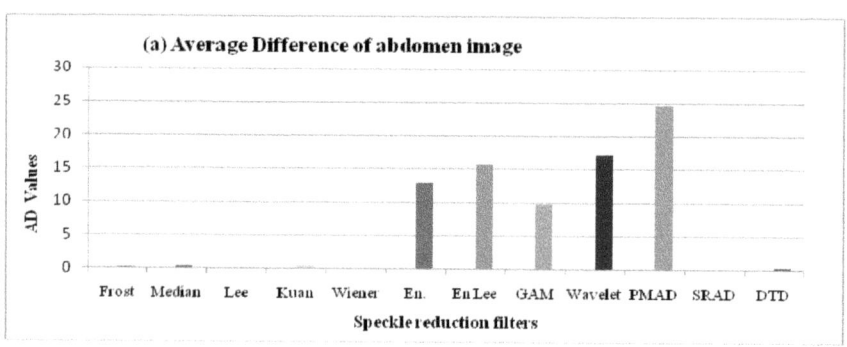

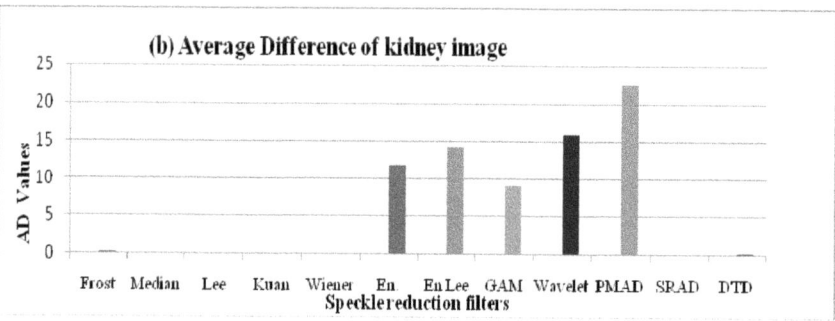

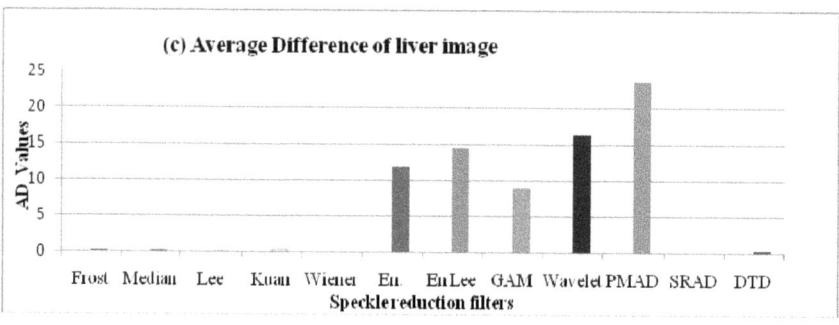

Fig 5.10 Histogram plot of the Average Difference (AD) in the PCMAT system

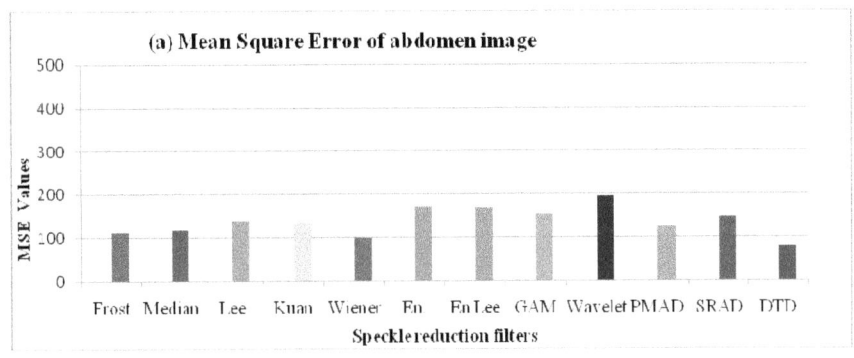

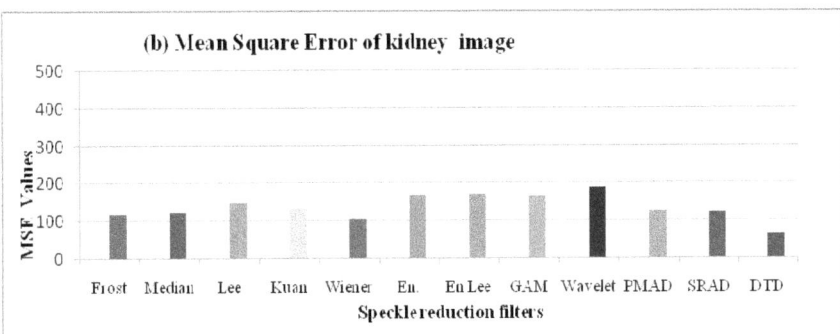

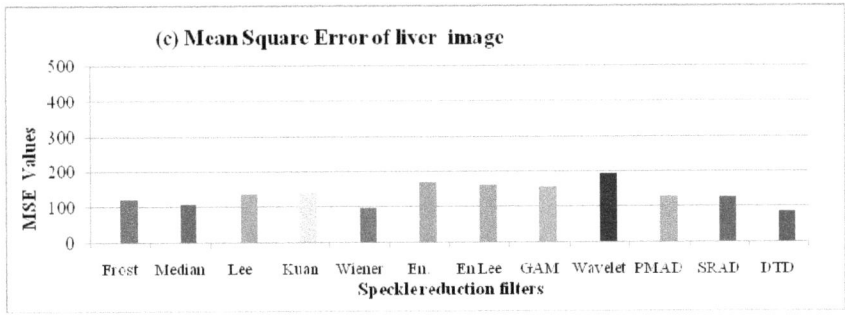

Fig 5.11 Histogram plot of the Mean Square Error (MSE) in the PCMAT system

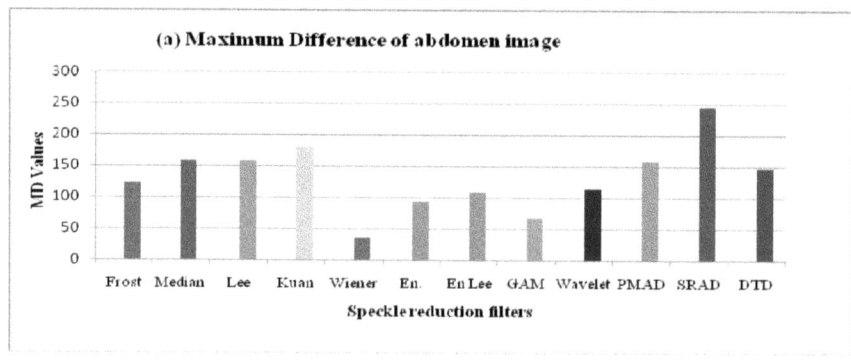

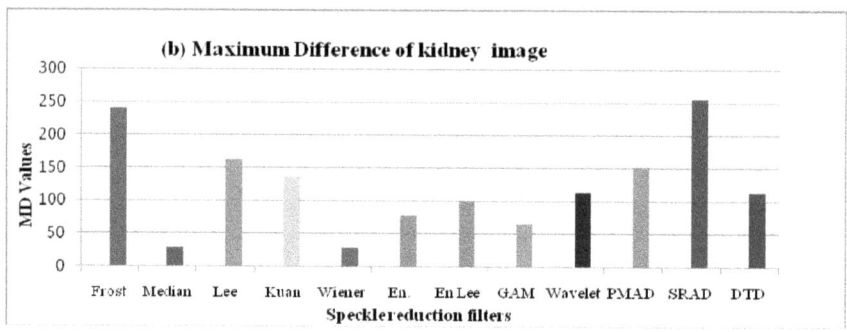

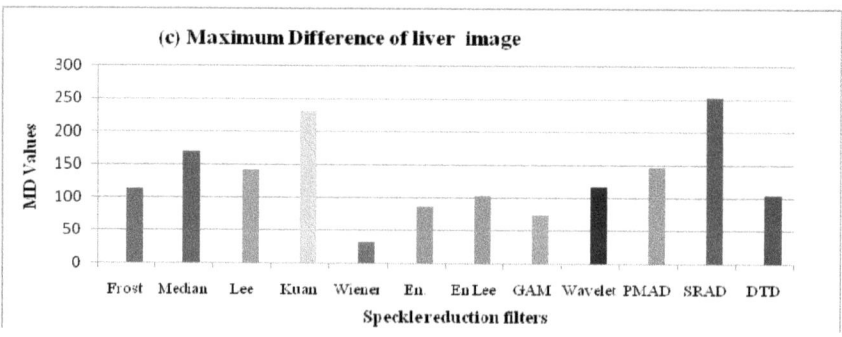

Fig 5.12 Histogram plot of the Maximum Difference (MD) in the PCMAT system

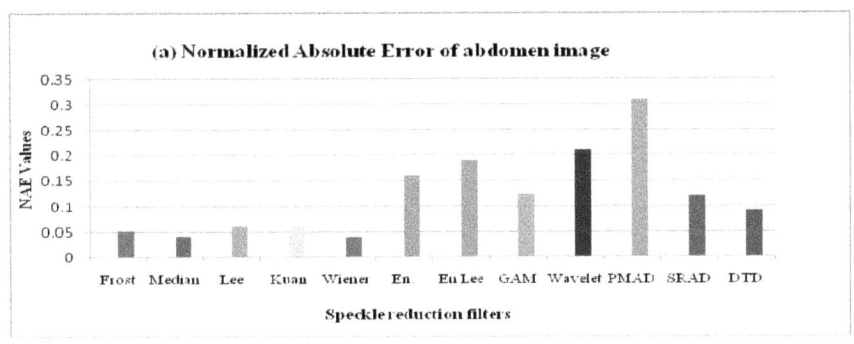

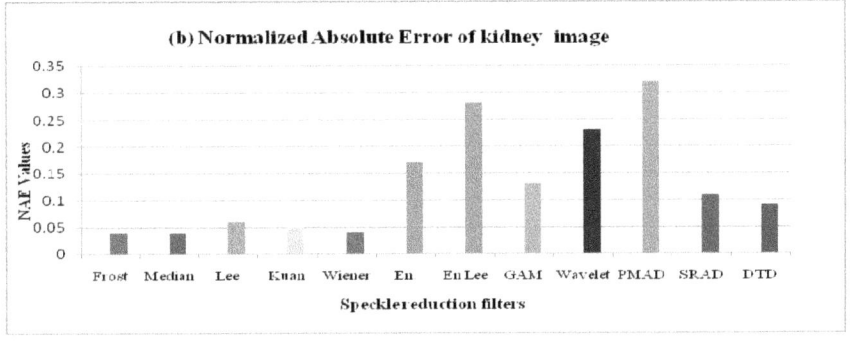

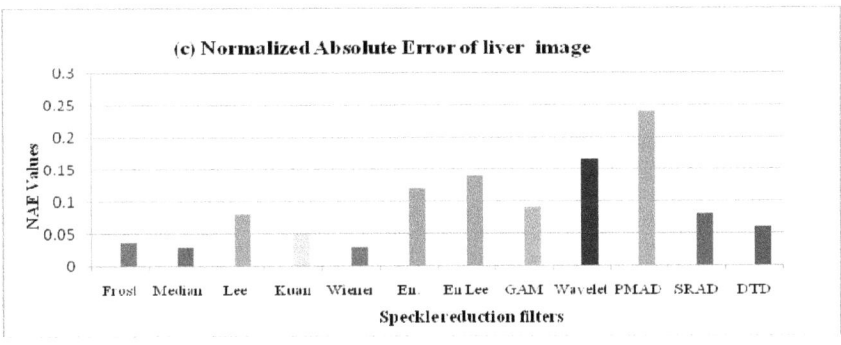

Fig 5.13 Histogram plot of the Normalized Absolute Error (NAE) in the PCMAT system

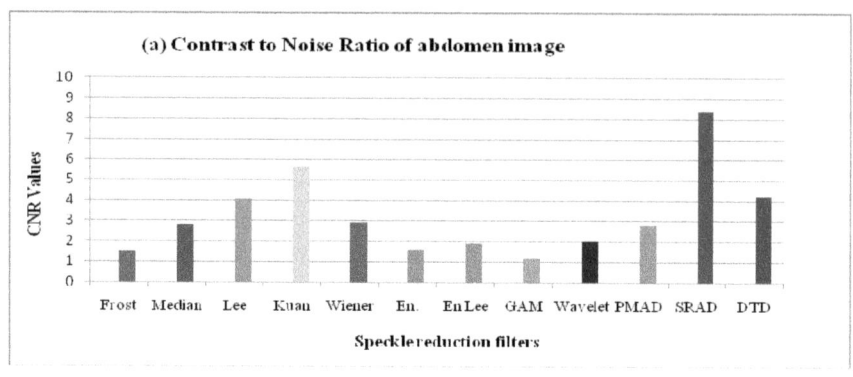

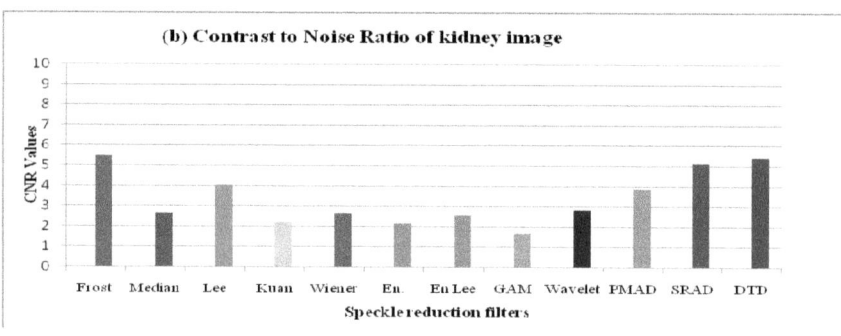

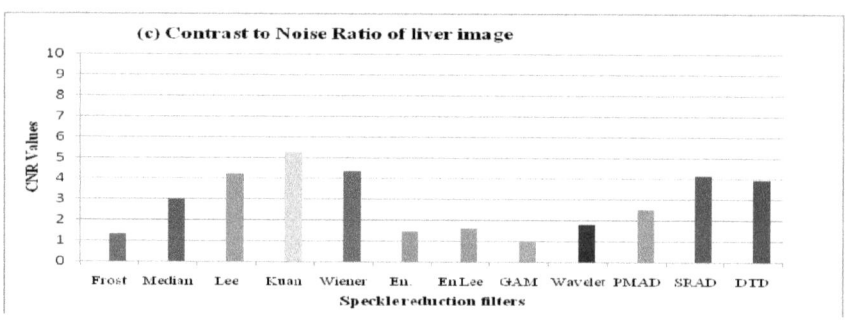

Fig 5.14 Histogram plot of the Contrast to Noise Ratio (CNR) in the PCMAT system

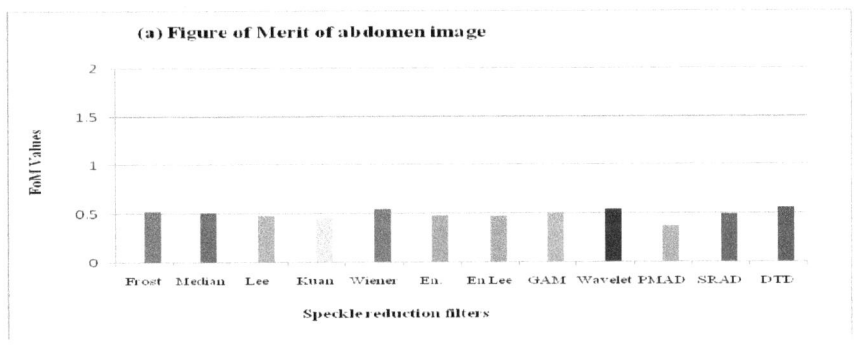

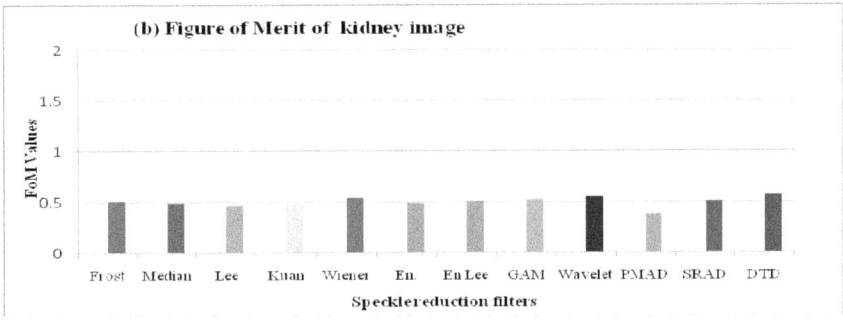

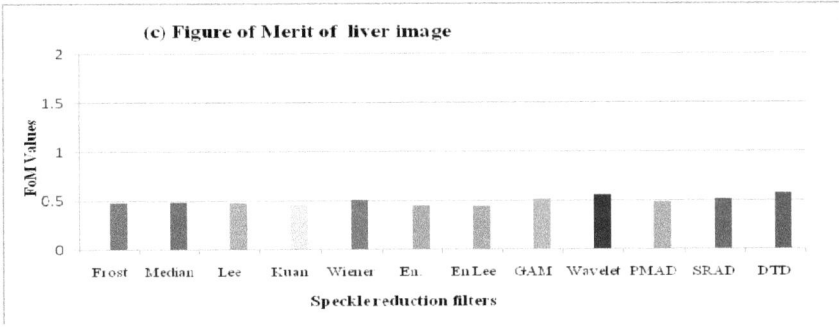

Fig 5.15 Histogram plot of the Figure of Merit (FoM) in the PCMAT system

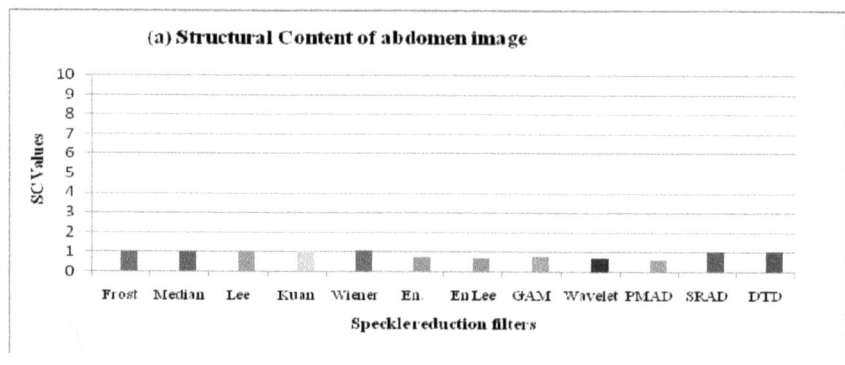

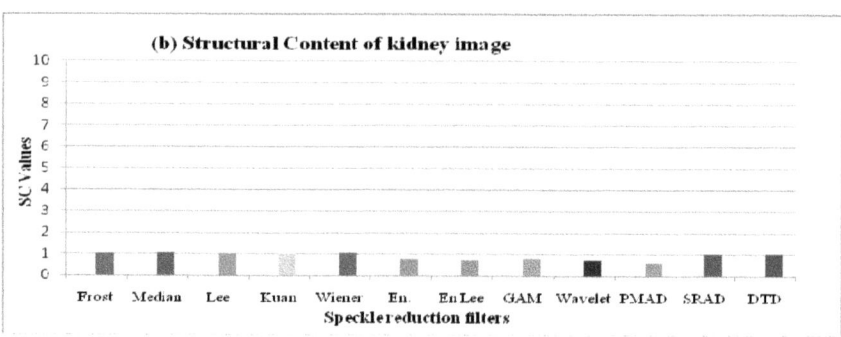

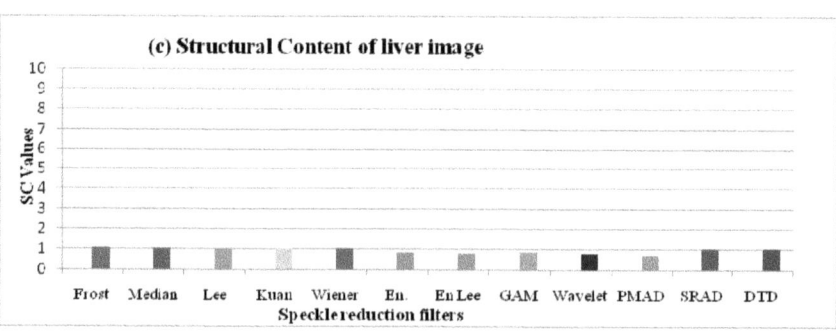

Fig 5.16 Histogram plot of the Structural Content (SC) in the PCMAT system

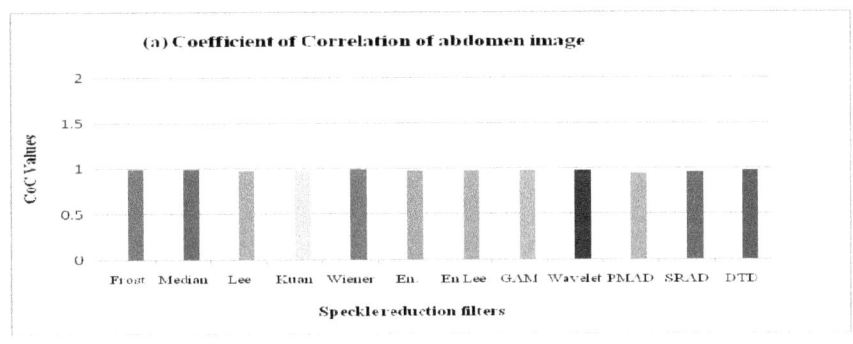

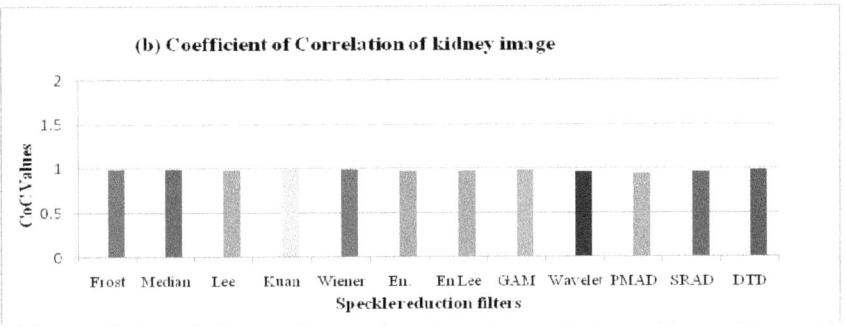

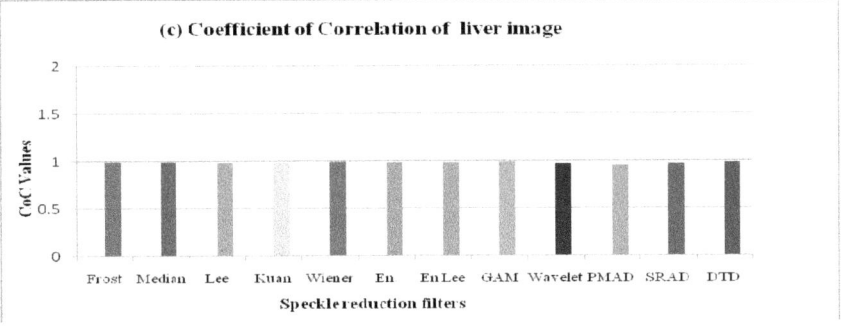

Fig 5.17 Histogram plot of the Coefficient of Correlation (CoC) in the PCMAT system

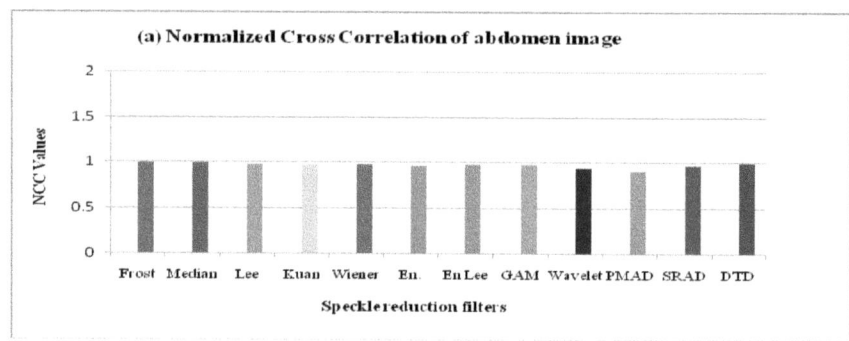

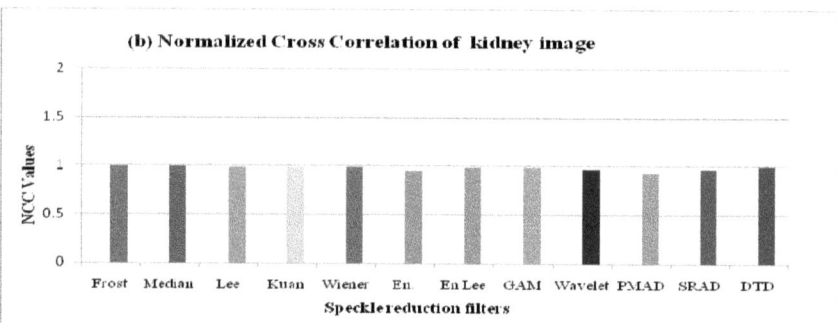

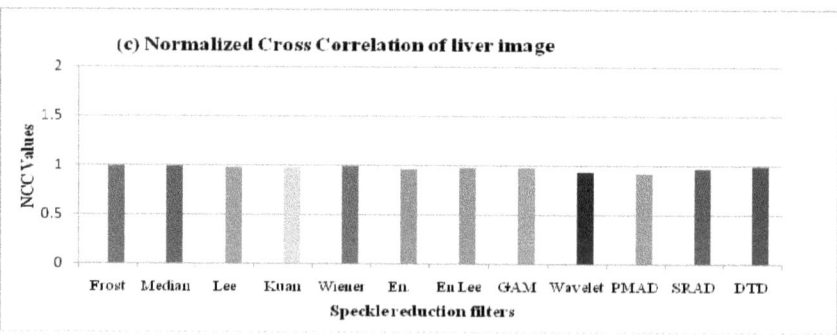

Fig 5.18 Histogram plot of the Normalized Cross Correlation (NCC) in the PCMAT system

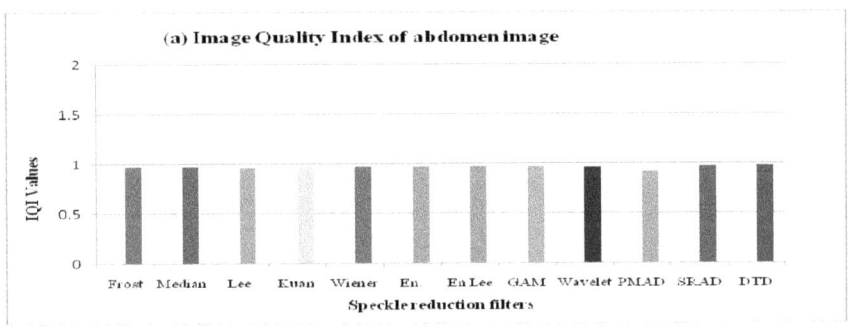

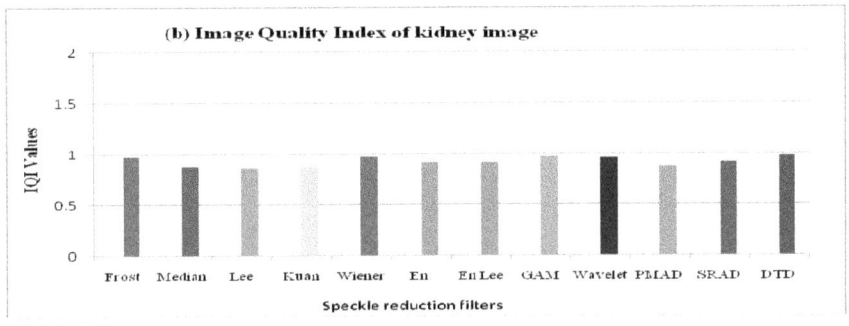

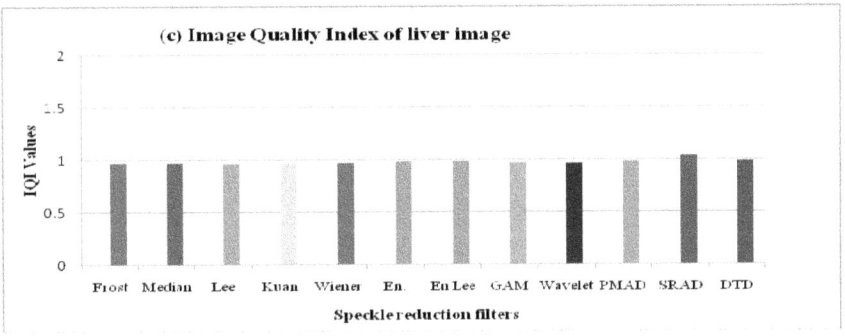

Fig 5.19 Histogram plot of the Image Quality Index (IQI) in the PCMAT system

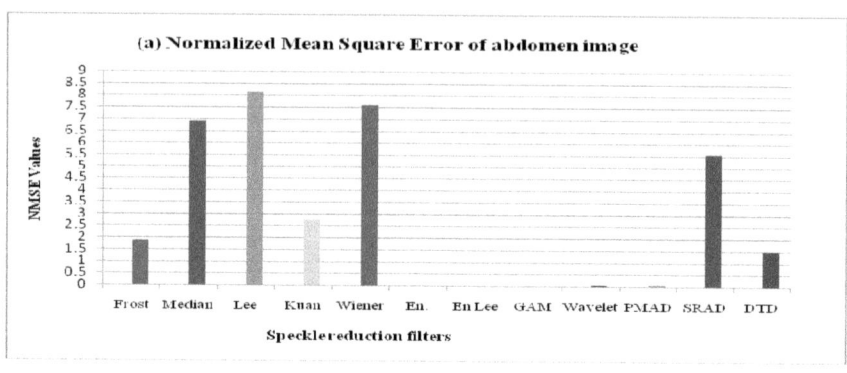

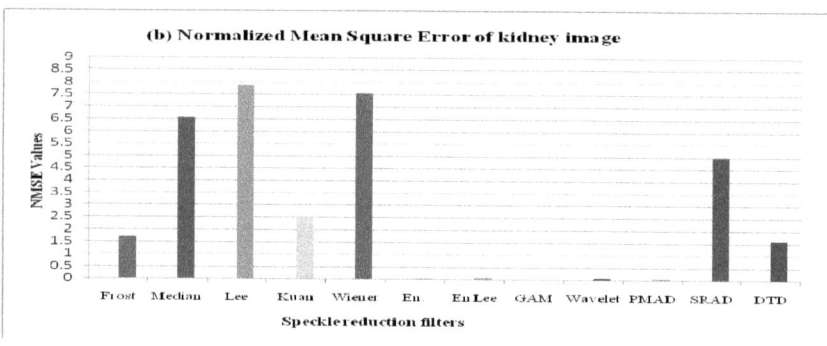

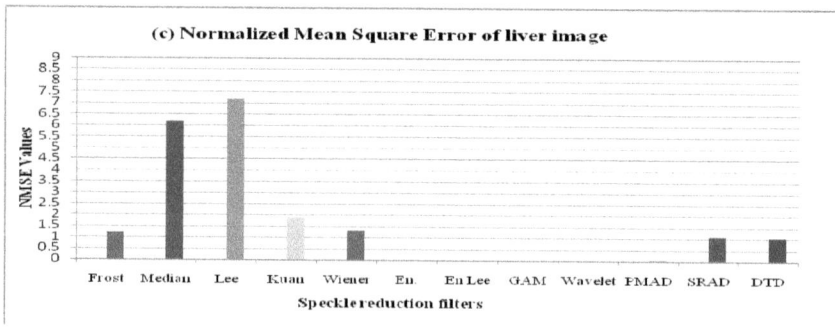

Fig 5.20 Histogram plot of the Normalized Mean Square Error (NMSE) in the PCMAT system

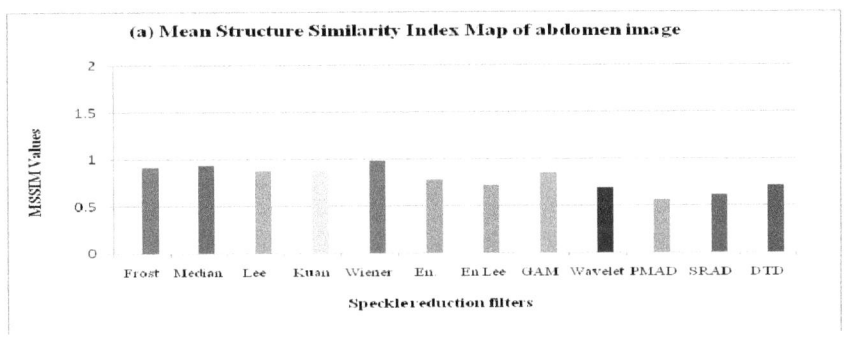

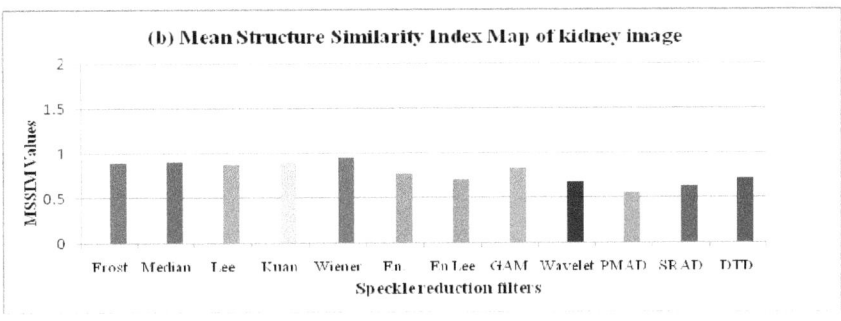

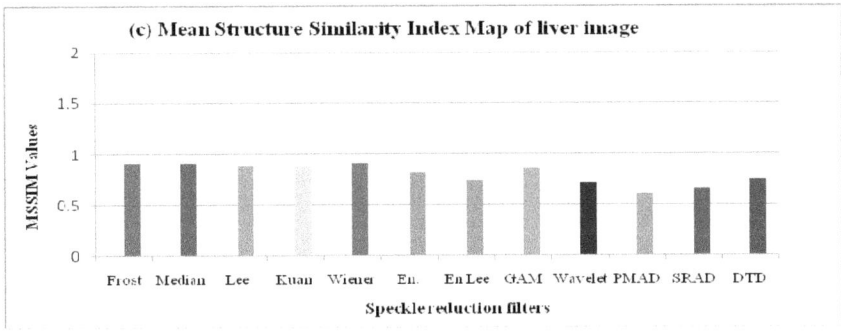

Fig 5.21 Histogram plot of the Mean Structure Similarity Index Map (MSSIM) in the PCMAT system

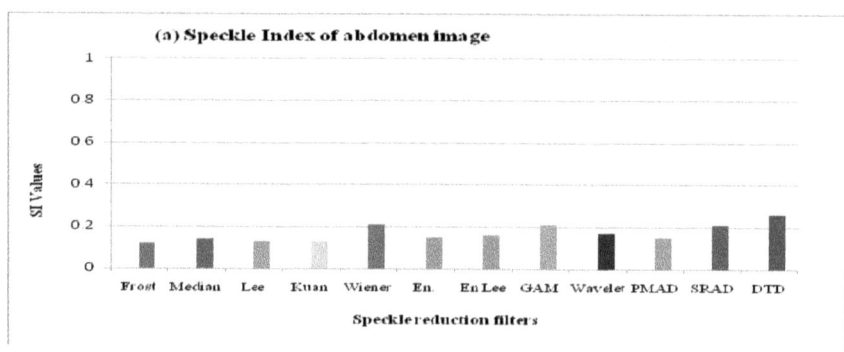

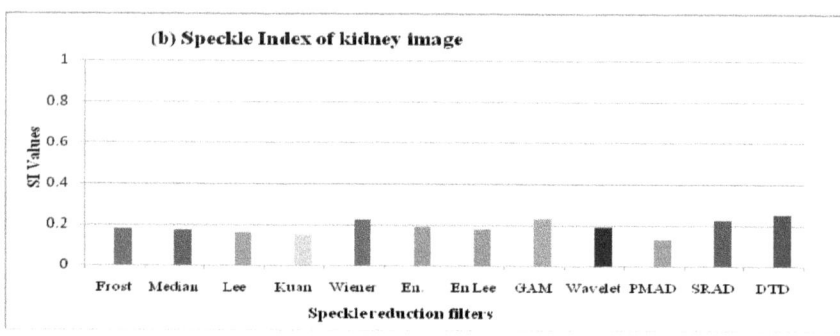

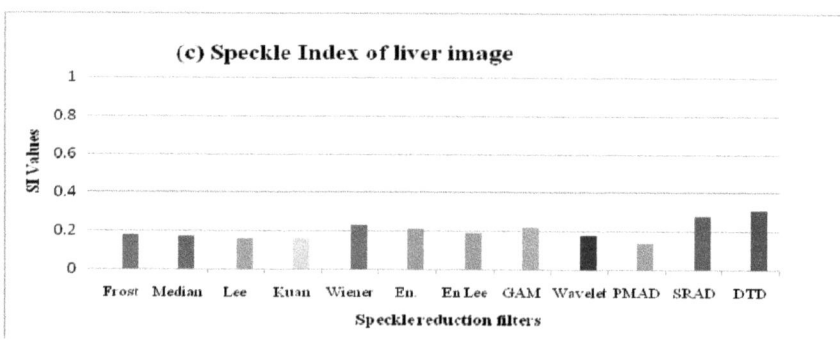

Fig 5.22 Histogram plot of the Speckle Index (SI) in the PCMAT system

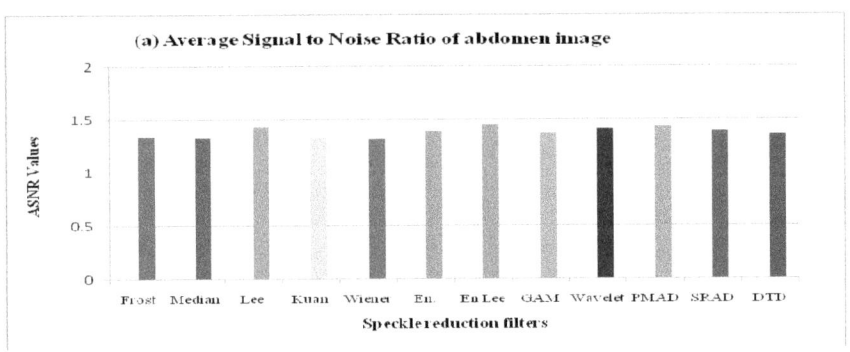

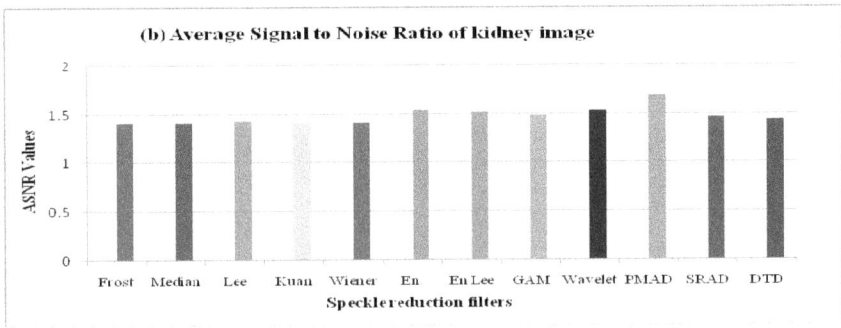

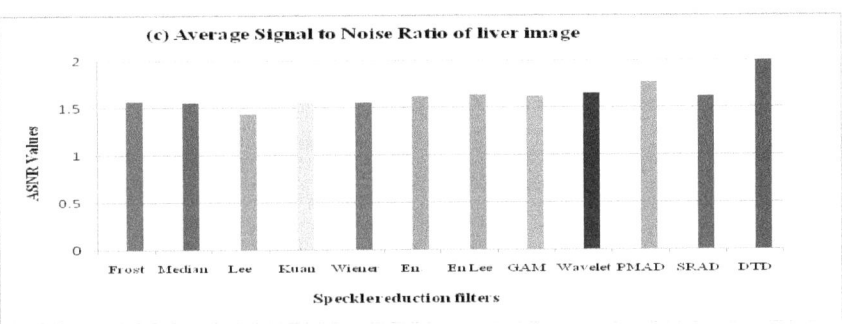

Fig 5.23 Histogram plot of the Average Signal to Noise Ratio (ASNR) in the PCMAT system

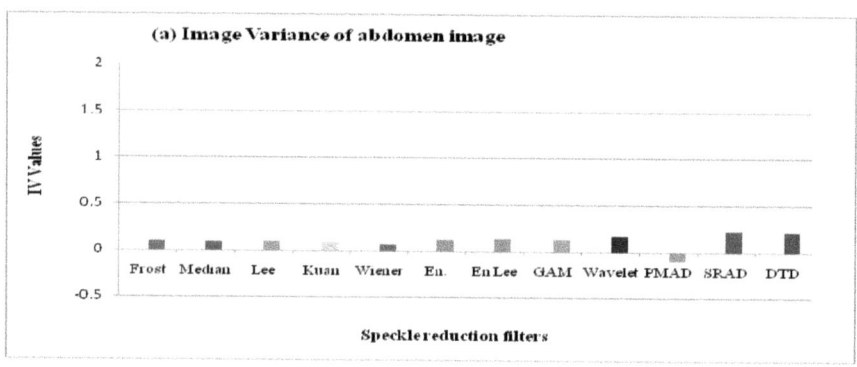

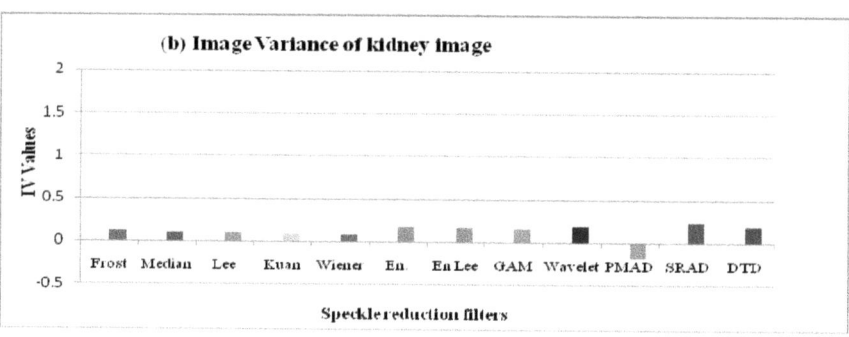

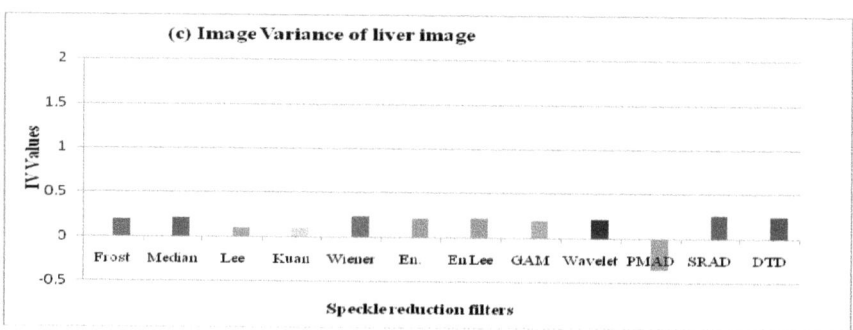

Fig 5.24 Histogram plot of the Image Variance (IV) in the PCMAT system

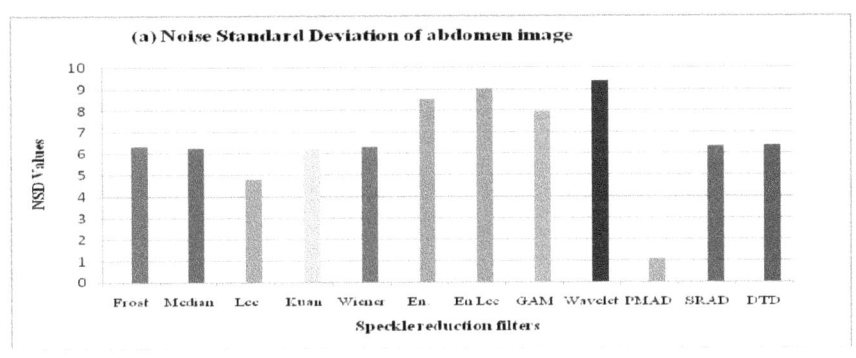

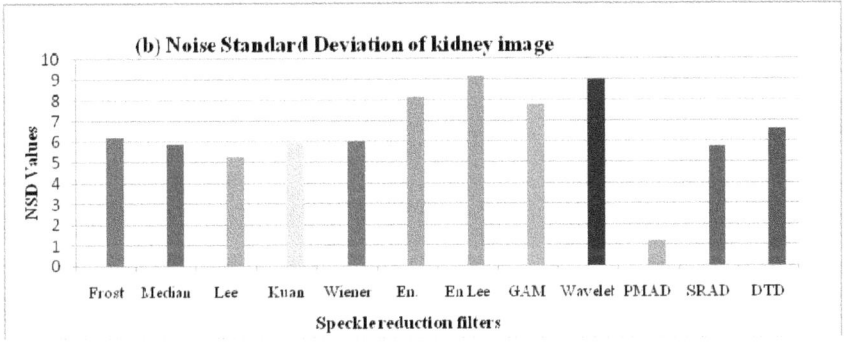

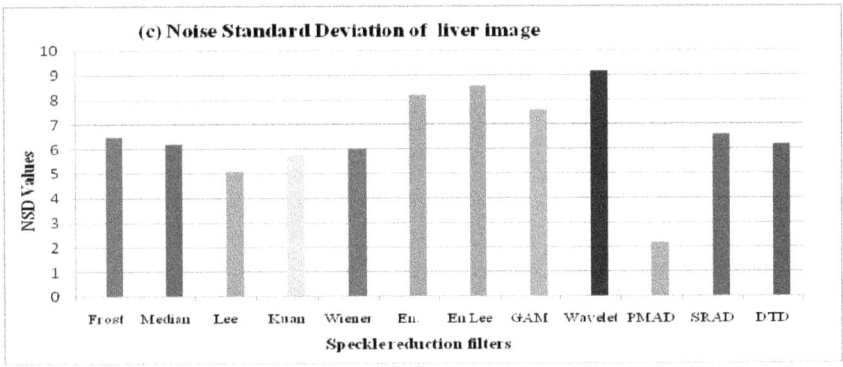

Fig 5.25 Histogram plot of the Noise Standard Deviation (NSD) in the PCMAT system

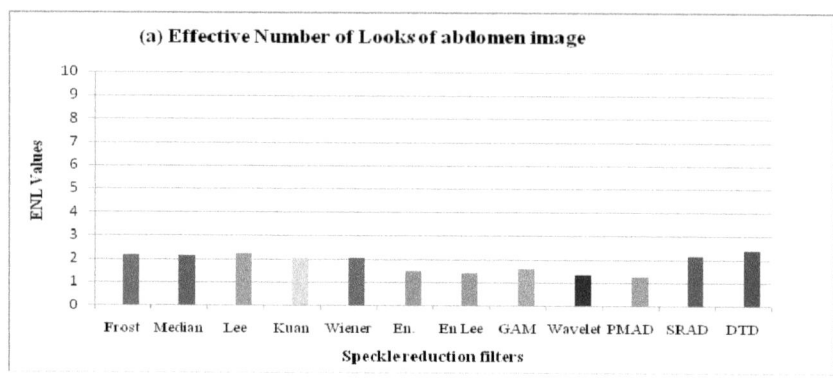

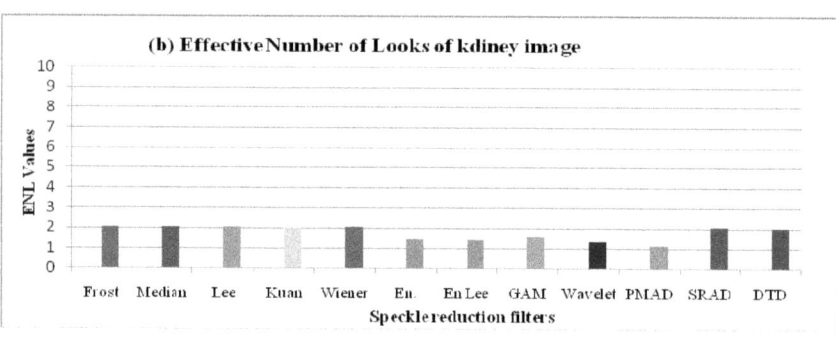

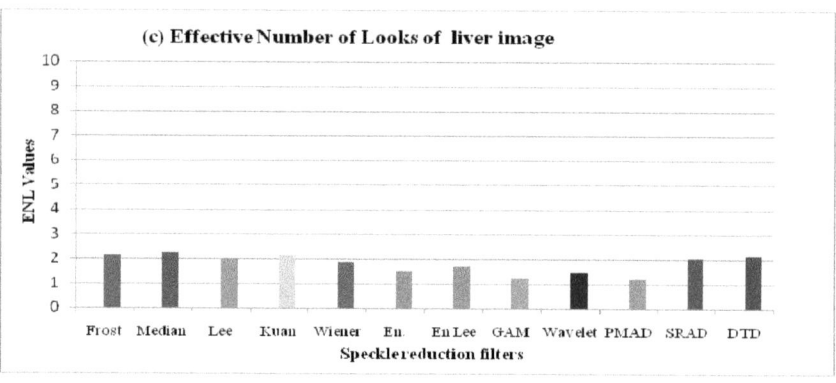

Fig 5.26 Histogram plot of the Effective Number of Looks (ENL) in the PCMAT system

REFERENCES

1. Sivakumar R., Gayathri M.K., and Nedumaran D., Speckle Filtering of Ultrasound B-Scan Images – A Comparative Study Between Spatial and Diffusion filter, IEEE Conference on Open Systems (ICOS 2010), Malaysia, 5-7 Dec. 2010, pp 80-85.
2. Sivakumar R., Gayathri M.K., and Nedumaran D., Speckle Filtering of Ultrasound B-scan Images - A Comparative Study of Single Scale Spatial Adaptive Filters, Multiscale Filter and Diffusion Filters, International Journal of Engineering and Technology, 2010, Vol.2, No.6, pp.514-523.
3. Sivakumar R., and Nedumaran D., Comparative Study of Speckle Noise Reduction of Ultrasound B-scan Images in Matrix Laboratory Environment, International Journal of Computer Applications, 2010, Vol.10, No.9, pp 46-50.
4. Sivakumar R., and Nedumaran D., Implementation of Wavelet Filters for Speckle Noise Reduction in Ultrasound Medical Images: A Comparative Study, Proceedings of the International conference on Signal, System and Communication (ICSSC2009), India, 21-23 Dec. 2009, pp.239-242.
5. Sivakumar R., and Nedumaran D., Performance study of Wavelet denoising techniques in Ultrasound images, Journal of Instrument Society of India, 2009,Vol. 39, No.30, pp. 194-196.
6. Nedumaran D., Sivakumar R., Sekar V., and Gayathri M.K., Speckle Noise Reduction in Ultrasound Biomedical B-Scan Images Using Discrete Topological Derivative, Ultrasound in Med. & Biol., 2012, Vol.38, No.2, pp. 276-286.
7. Maini J.R, and Aggarwal H., Study and comparison of various image edge detection techniques, International Journal of Image Processing, 2009, Vol.3, No.1, pp.1–12.
8. Bhadauria H.S., and Dewal M.L., Comparison of Edge Detection Techniques on Noisy Abnormal Lung CT Image Before and After Using Morphological Filter, International Journal of Advanced Engineering & Application, 2010, Vol.1, No.2, pp. 272–275.
9. Canny J.F., A Computational Approach to Edge Detection, IEEE Trans. on Pattern Analysis and Machine Intelligence, 1986, Vol. PAMI-8, No.6, pp. 679–697.
10. Roushdy M., Comparative Study of Edge Detection Algorithms Applying on the Grayscale Noisy Image Using Morphological Filter, GVIP Journal, 2006, Vol.6, No.4, pp.17–23.

CHAPTER - VI

IMPLEMENTATION AND PERFORMANCE STUDY OF DESPECKLING FILTER ALGORITHMS IN THE PCDSK SYSTEM

6.1 ALGORITHM INTRODUCTION

In the PCDSK system, all the despeckling algorithms were developed in the ANSI C using the code composer studio version 3.1 [1-5]. The algorithm comprises of all the thirteen speckle reduction filters including the proposed DTD filter, five-edge detection operators and twenty performance metrics. The methods for testing the algorithms and the case study details are described in Chapter-V, Section 5.2 and Section 5.3, respectively for the PCMAT system are adopted as such for the PCDSK system. In this chapter, the case study results for the abdomen, kidney and liver ultrasound B-scan images are presented for justifying the performance of the PCDSK system for real time application. The other four case studies tested in the PCDSK system are given in the Appendix-B.

6.2 DESCRIPTION OF DESPECKLING ALGORITHMS

The basic steps and concepts of all the despeckling and edge detection algorithms described in Chapter-V, Section 5.4 and 5.5 are common to both the PCMAT and the PCDSK system. Hence, those steps and concepts were not repeated in this Chapter. In the PCDSK system, all the programs (m-files) written in the MATLAB environment for the PCMAT system were converted into C code using the MATLAB code generator. The converted C files are integrated into a PCDSK system using Code Composer Studio. The basic steps involved in initializing the TMS320C6713 DSK and the program execution of all the despeckling and edge detection algorithms in the PCDSK system are summarized as follows:

Step 1	Initialize the code composer studio with the target (TMS320C6713 DSK)
Step 2	Open the project file (file name.pjt) and save it in a separate directory
Step 3	Add the source file (filter name.c), linker file (filter name.cmd) and run time support library (rts6701.lib)
Step 4	Build the project file to create the output file
Step 5	Load the program (file name.out)
Step 6	To process an image in the program (file name.out) it is necessary to load the image into memory. For this process, the image was resized and converted to a data file "image name.dat" in hex format, since the DSK supports dat format only. In this study, an image dimension of 256x256 pixels format is used amounting to (256x256)/4=16384 word/element, since each word/element contains four bytes
Step 7	For loading the image in (.dat) hex format, the input window is specified with the address (in_img) and data length (16384). After specifying this information, the image is loaded into the internal memory of the DSK
Step 8	The specific despeckling/edge detection program is executed on the loaded input image
Step 9	After the implementation of the despeckling/edge detection program, the processed image is saved in a specific folder using the address (out_img) and the data length (16384)
Step 10	The raw/original (in_img) and the processed (out_img) images are viewed separately in the Code Composer Studio using the view graph option

6.3 PERFORMANCE STUDY OF THE DESPECKLING FILTERS IN THE PCDSK SYSTEM

The basic steps adopted for testing the despeckling algorithm in the PCMAT system described in Chapter-V are followed as such for the PCDSK system. All the algorithms were tested on more than 200 different ultrasound B-scan images of various organs collected from four different sources (Given in Chapter-IV, Section 4.11, Table 4.3). Some of the important case studies (Abdomen, kidney and liver) suggested by the sonologist/radiologist are given in this Chapter for comparison of the results for estimating the performance of the proposed DTD despeckling filter. The results of the three case studies are presented in the following format for easy comparison.

1. The raw and the thirteen despeckled images are given for visual inspection of the images for estimating the performance of the speckle reduction filter in the PCDSK system.
2. Canny edge detected images of the raw and the thirteen despeckled images are presented for estimating the efficiency of preserving the details of the images before and after despeckling.
3. Nineteen performance metrics values calculated for the thirteen despeckling filters with the time for execution are summarized in a table format for easy comparison of results. Also, the peak SNR value calculated for the Canny edge detected images of all the despeckling filters are given for comparing the despeckling filter efficiency in identifying the edges in the PCDSK system.

In case study 1, ultrasound B-scan image of abdomen with calcified fibroid is used. Figure 6.1 shows the raw and thirteen despeckling filters output images of the abdomen in the PCDSK system. Figure 6.2 shows the Canny edge detected images of the thirteen despeckled output images obtained in the PCDSK system. The performance metrics calculated in the PCDSK system for the thirteen despeckling filters and their corresponding edge detected images with execution time are summarized in Table 6.1.

In case study 2, ultrasound B-scan image of kidney is utilized. The raw and its thirteen despeckled images in the PCDSK system are given in Figure 6.3. Figure 6.4 shows the Canny edge detected images obtained in the PCDSK system for the thirteen despeckling filters. Table 6.2 represents the calculated performance metrics and execution time with the calculated peak SNR values from the Canny edge detected images of the thirteen despeckling filters of kidney in the PCDSK system.

Similarly, in case study 3, ultrasound B-scan image of liver is used and its raw image with the thirteen despeckling filters output images in the PCDSK system are given in Figure 6.5. The Canny edge detected images of the thirteen despeckling filters obtained in the PCDSK system are given in Figure 6.6. The calculated performance metrics and execution time with the calculated peak SNR values of the Canny edge detected images of the thirteen despeckling filters for the liver image are presented in Table 6.3.

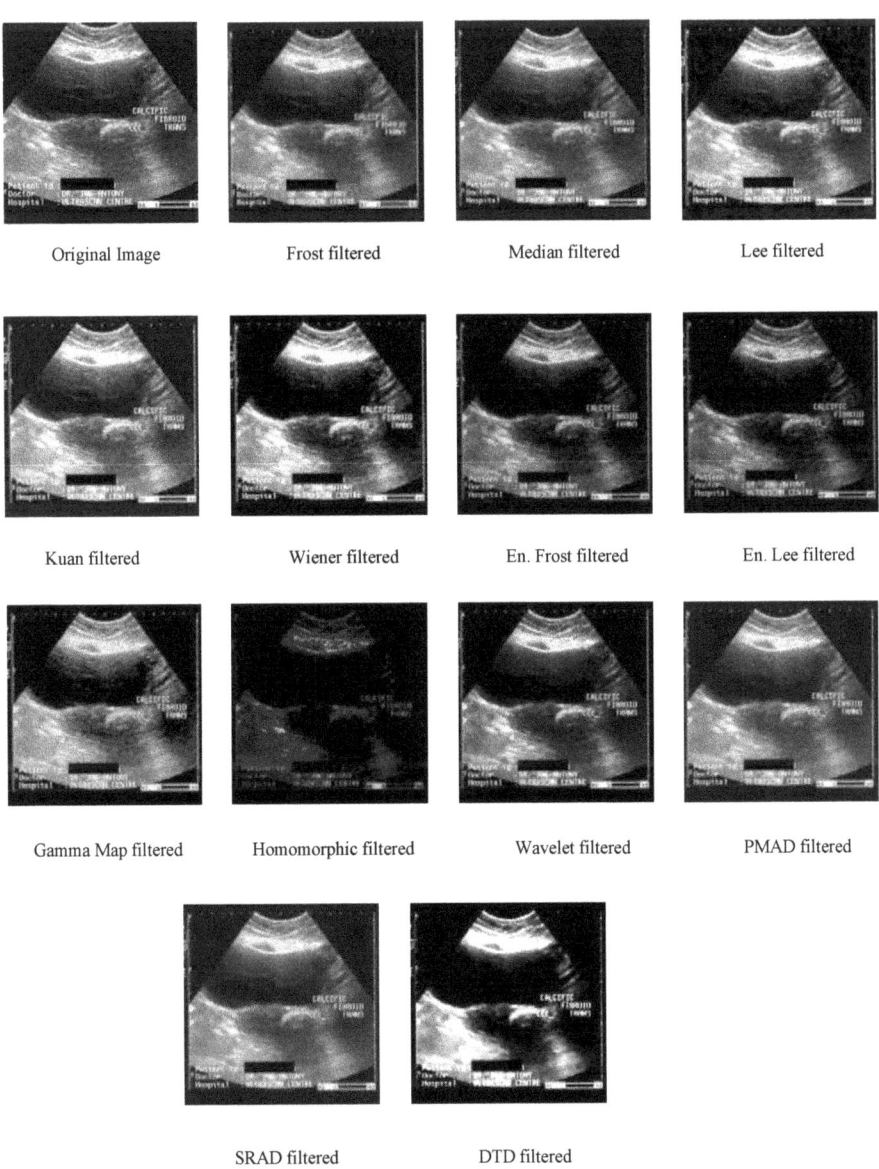

Fig 6.1 Original and despeckled images of abdomen in the PCDSK system

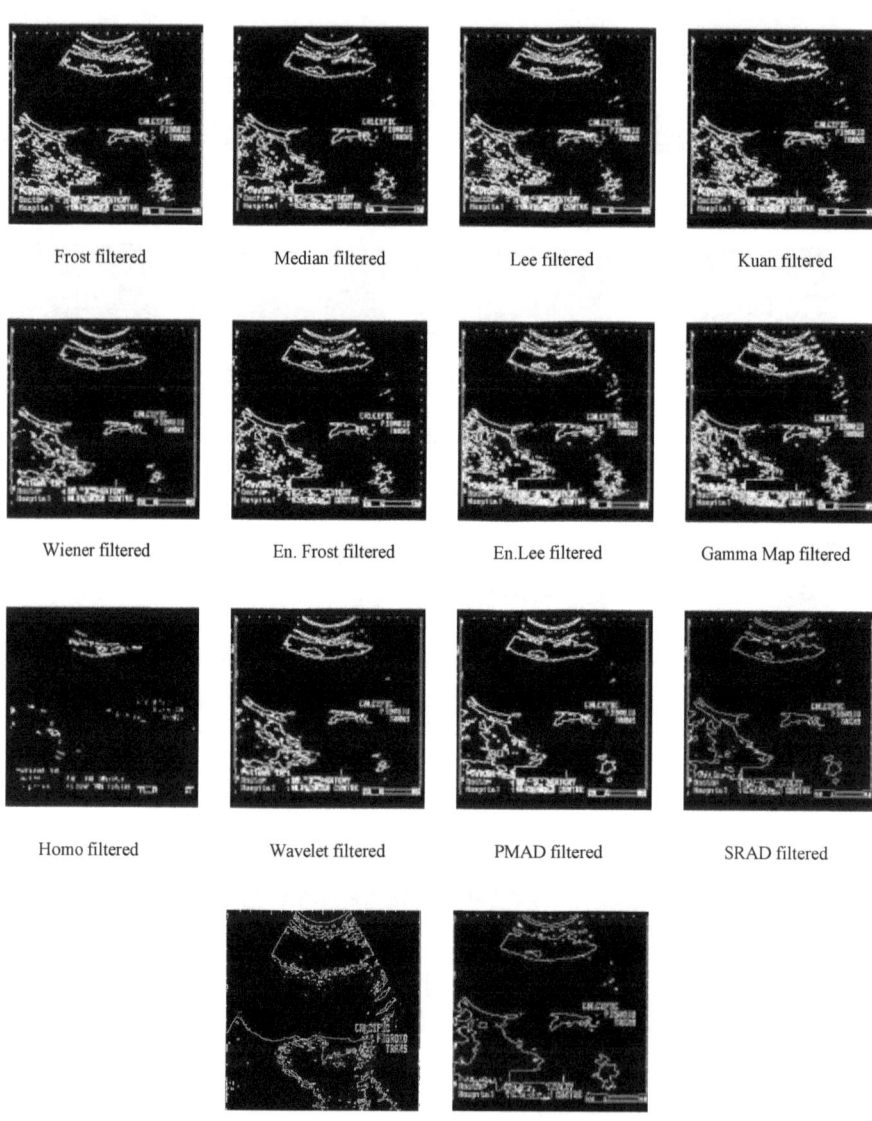

Fig 6.2 Canny edge detected images of abdomen in the PCDSK system

Table 6.1 Calculated performance metrics of the despeckling filters applied on the abdomen image in the PCDSK system

Group	Metrics	Frost	Median	Lee	Kuan	Homo morphic	Wiener	En. Frost	En Lee	GAM	Wavelet	PMAD	SRAD	DTD
Quality metrics	PSNR in dB	32.66	31.18	29.62	28.46	11.51	35.84	32..89	30.48	27.35	34.62	29.65	36.65	39.47
	PSNR (Canny)in dB	20.46	21.54	18.87	20.92	9.72	24.32	21.26	22.54	21.47	26.23	22.18	24.19	28.56
	AD	0.21	0.31	0.23	0.61	198.45	0.18	23.11	29.76	14.51	21.6	32.59	0.82	3.03
	MSE	113.55	119.49	139.46	135.19	7658.73	99.05	106.48	165.29	153.51	194.96	125.99	94.24	72.92
	MD	136.34	171.28	173.18	192.16	271.35	53.13	117.21	124.85	84.46	131.32	174.28	262.43	163.21
	NAE	0.04	0.01	0.02	0.05	1.75	0.01	0.13	0.16	0.094	0.18	0.28	0.09	0.06
	CNR	2.54	3.91	4.23	5.71	3.14	4.02	2.69	3.47	2.28	3.23	3.78	9.41	5.29
	FoM	0.62	0.59	0.52	0.56	0.24	0.68	0.53	0.57	0.59	0.62	0.43	0.59	0.72
	SC	1.15	1.15	1.16	1.16	3881.5	1.21	0.91	0.87	0.96	0.85	0.76	1.18	1.16
Similarity metrics	CoC	0.97	0.97	0.97	0.96	0.64	0.98	0.97	0.96	0.97	0.97	0.95	0.97	0.97
	NCC	0.98	0.99	0.98	0.98	0.02	0.98	0.96	0.98	0.98	0.94	0.91	0.97	0.99
	IQI	0.96	0.97	0.96	0.97	0.17	0.97	0.97	0.97	0.97	0.96	0.92	0.97	0.98
	GAE	0.00	0.00	0.00	0.00	0.00	0.00	0.00	0.00	0.00	0.00	0.00	0.00	0.00
	NMSE	2.02	7.06	8.27	2.88	1.09	7.75	0.156	0.16	0.145	0.17	0.22	5.71	1.61
	MSSIM	0.83	0.89	0.73	0.72	0.082	0.97	0.64	0.58	0.68	0.43	0.39	0.42	0.59
Speckle metrics	SI	0.29	0.27	0.25	0.18	0.22	0.23	0.29	0.39	0.41	0.26	0.29	0.46	0.36
	ASNR	1.43	1.42	1.52	1.42	1.11	1.41	1.48	1.54	1.46	1.5	1.52	1.48	1.45
	IV	0.109	0.103	0.117	0.098	253.165	0.085	0.137	0.157	0.146	0.189	-0.084	0.218	0.242
	NSD	6.48	6.43	4.98	6.4	2.66	6.46	8.71	9.2	8.13	9.53	1.27	6.47	6.51
	ENL	2.08	2.48	2.52	2.48	2.21	1.78	1.14	1.56	1.18	1.45	2.05	2.35	2.08
	Execution time in sec	10.04	2.56	12.73	13.58	18.57	3.28	4.25	5.38	2.17	1.26	2.19	3.26	29.24

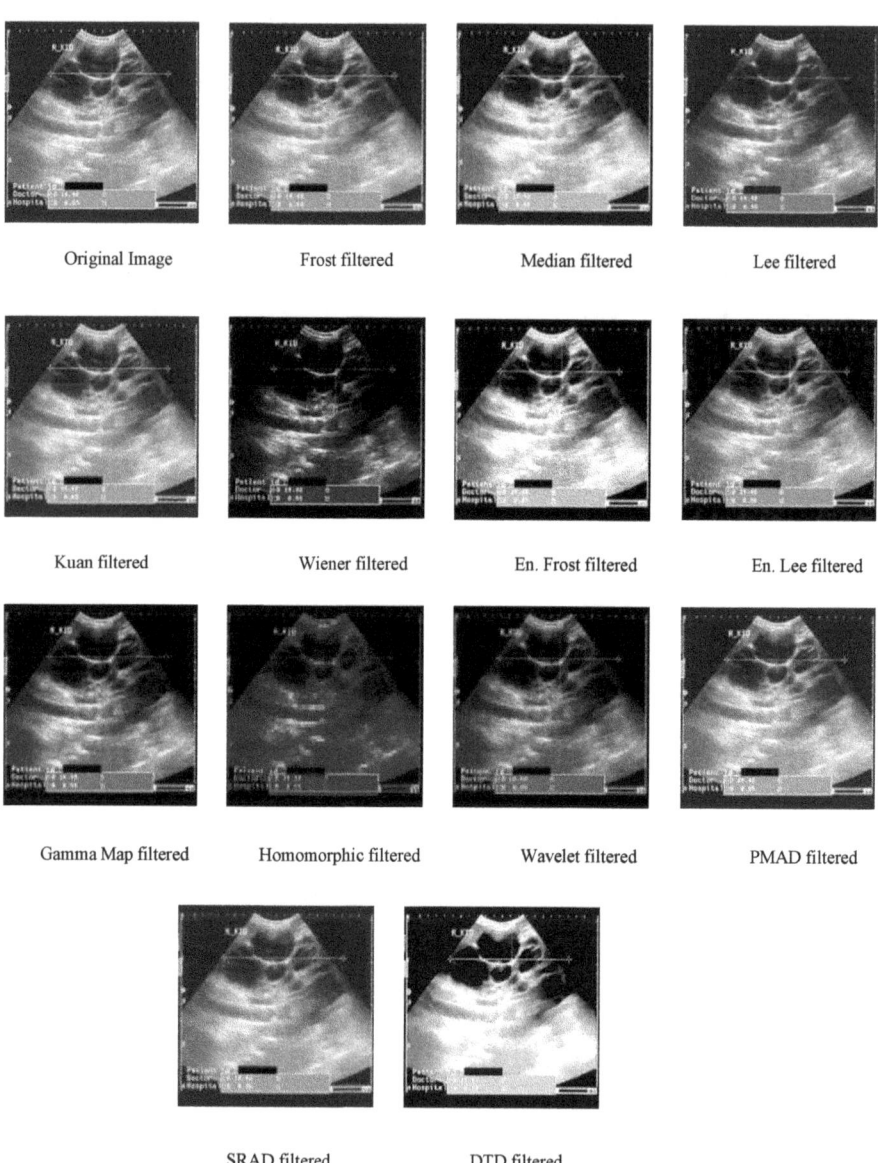

Fig 6.3 Original and despeckled images of kidney in the PCDSK system

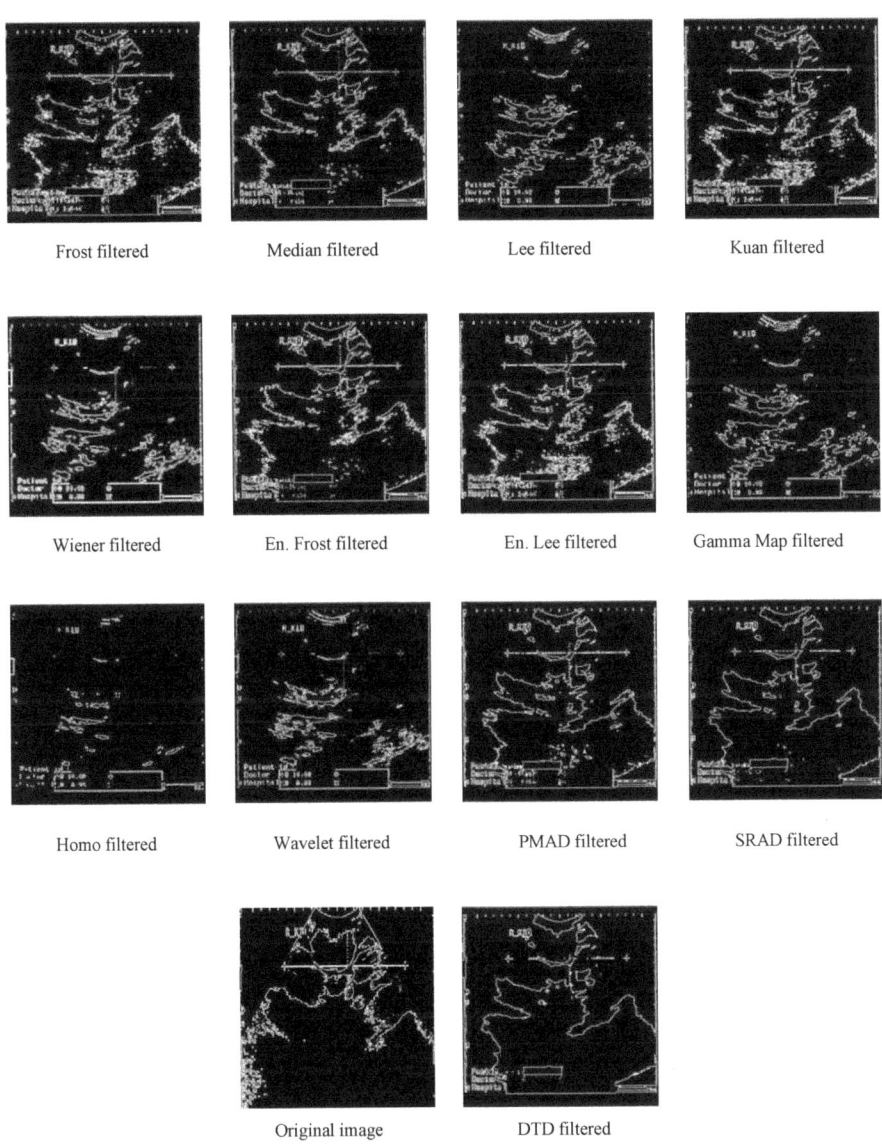

Fig 6.4 Canny edge detected images of kidney in the PCDSK system

Table 6.2 Calculated performance metrics of the despeckling filters applied on the kidney image in PCDSK system

Group	Metrics	Frost	Median	Lee	Kuan	Homo morphic	Wiener	En. Frost	En Lee	GAM	Wavelet	PMAD	SRAD	DTD
Quality metrics	PSNR in dB	32.66	33.18	29.37	30.75	2.51	34.87	24.77	24.37	26.49	23.66	29.74	30.41	39.18
	PSNR (Canny)in dB	19.83	19.46	17.52	22.08	8.39	25.17	21.78	22.56	21.17	27.45	22.54	33.50	35.29
	AD	0.39	0.16	0.38	0.24	72.47	0.18	11.98	14.46	9.21	16.00	22.16	0.15	0.42
	MSE	118.87	122.28	148.76	133.47	8974.72	105.42	169.19	170.32	164.15	188.42	125.48	122.51	64.17
	MD	218.27	46.56	179.18	153.45	210.33	46.19	96.23	117.17	82.43	130.12	169.24	272.31	130.12
	NAE	0.01	0.01	0.03	0.02	0.94	0.01	0.14	0.25	0.10	0.20	0.29	0.08	0.06
	CNR	6.56	3.73	5.13	3.33	3.77	3.73	3.24	3.65	2.77	3.89	4.95	6.22	6.49
	FoM	0.58	0.61	0.55	0.58	0.17	0.73	0.52	0.53	0.62	0.63	0.42	0.53	0.65
Similarity metrics	SC	1.15	1.18	1.16	1.15	29.36	1.19	0.90	0.86	0.95	0.87	0.75	1.17	1.15
	CoC	0.98	0.98	0.98	0.96	0.47	0.98	0.97	0.96	0.97	0.97	0.95	0.97	0.99
	NCC	0.97	0.98	0.98	0.98	0.04	0.98	0.96	0.98	0.98	0.94	0.91	0.97	0.98
	IQI	0.97	0.98	0.96	0.97	0.32	0.97	0.97	0.97	0.98	0.96	0.92	0.97	0.98
	GAE	0.00	0.00	0.00	0.00	0.00	0.00	0.00	0.00	0.00	0.00	0.00	0.00	0.00
	NMSE	1.48	6.19	7.58	2.12	9.74	1.42	0.14	0.28	0.17	0.19	0.21	1.16	1.28
	MSSIM	0.82	0.86	0.74	0.68	0.043	0.96	0.63	0.62	0.71	0.47	0.32	0.47	0.62
Speckle metrics	SI	0.31	0.30	0.29	0.28	0.16	0.35	0.32	0.31	0.36	0.32	0.26	0.35	0.38
	ASNR	1.50	1.50	1.52	1.51	1.26	1.50	1.63	1.61	1.57	1.62	1.78	1.56	1.53
	IV	0.14	0.12	0.12	0.11	238.04	0.10	0.20	0.19	0.18	0.21	-0.16	0.25	0.21
	NSD	4.97	5.01	4.98	5.02	2.63	5.01	6.80	7.22	6.36	7.48	8.71	5.01	5.04
	ENL	2.56	2.27	1.98	2.26	2.05	2.14	2.08	1.98	1.78	1.24	2.52	2.89	2.56
	Execution time in sec	10.46	2.41	11.56	13.24	17.62	2.12	4.13	5.74	3.38	2.26	5.62	4.26	32.52

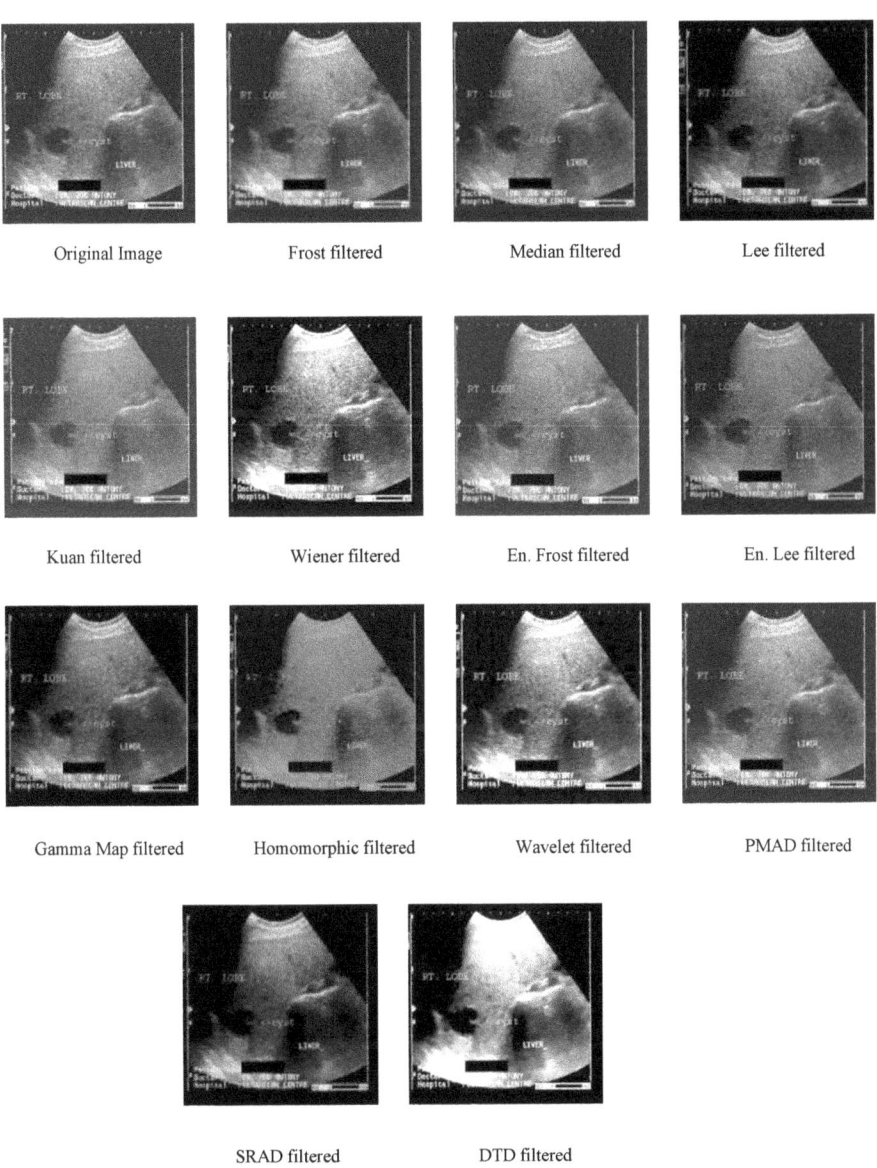

Fig 6.5 Original and despeckled images of liver in the PCDSK system

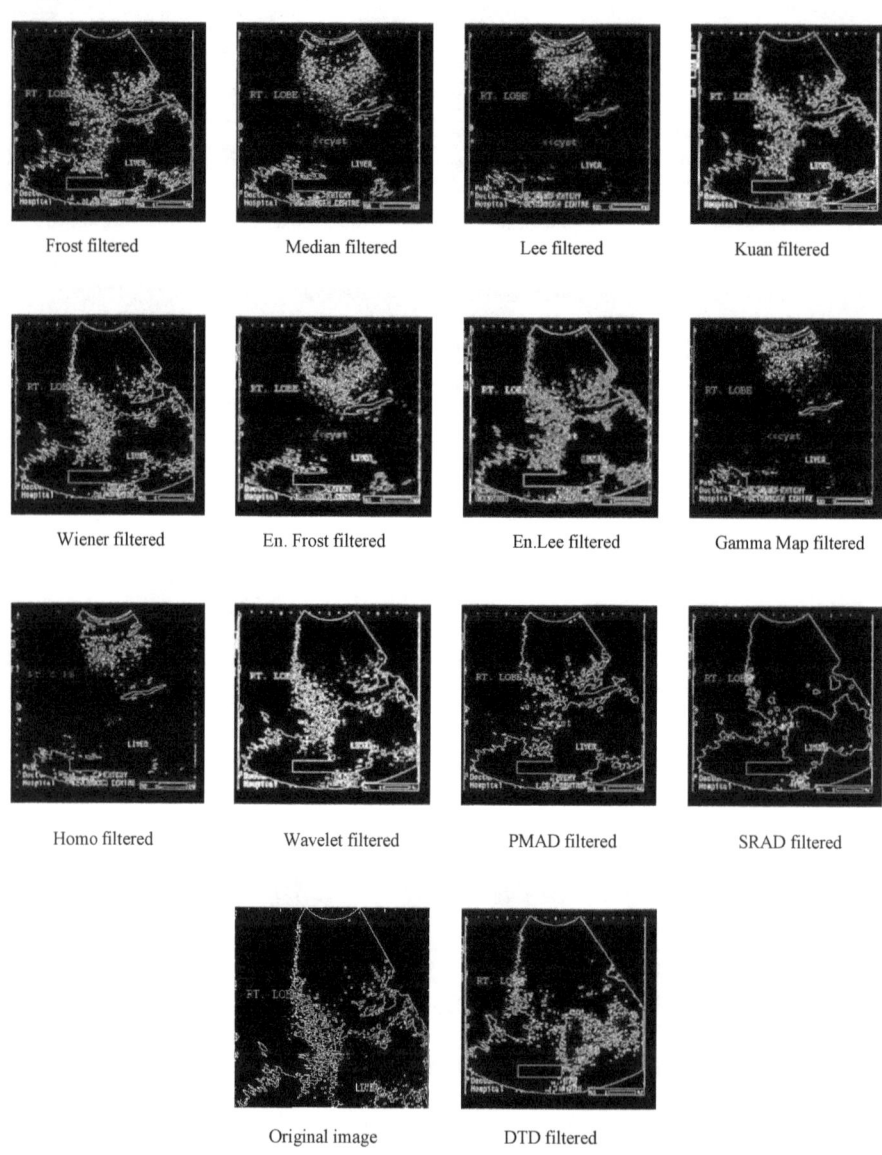

Fig 6.6 Canny edge detected images of liver in the PCDSK system

Table 6.3 Calculated performance metrics of the despeckling filters applied on the liver image in PCDSK system

Group	Metrics	Frost	Median	Lee	Kuan	Homo morphic	Wiener	En. Frost	En Lee	GAM	Wavelet	PMAD	SRAD	DTD
Quality metrics	PSNR in dB	32.61	33.77	30.69	30.23	12.52	37.23	26.59	24.12	27.54	24.72	28.51	31.46	38.72
	PSNR (Canny)in dB	22.49	24.25	20.74	21.01	8.99	23.34	22.78	21.90	25.02	25.85	25.19	29.99	32.90
	AD	0.34	0.37	0.28	0.54	196.44	0.18	11.05	13.75	9.23	16.36	22.86	0.24	3.52
	MSE	126.35	112.05	142.89	143.49	7251.56	102.25	174.16	166.87	162.28	200.09	133.87	130.91	90.20
	MD	131.42	186.32	159.24	149.08	208.35	49.16	104.52	120.23	91.31	133.78	164.48	190.29	122.36
	NAE	0.01	0.02	0.05	0.02	0.95	0.00	0.09	0.11	0.06	0.14	0.21	0.05	0.03
	CNR	2.41	4.86	5.32	6.34	3.48	5.52	2.53	2.71	2.09	2.89	3.61	7.24	5.12
	FoM	0.56	0.57	0.56	0.54	0.22	0.59	0.53	0.52	0.60	0.63	0.57	0.60	0.65
	SC	1.21	1.15	1.16	1.15	5240.29	1.19	0.95	0.92	0.99	0.90	0.82	1.16	1.15
Similarity metrics	CoC	0.96	0.97	0.96	0.95	0.32	0.98	0.97	0.96	0.97	0.97	0.95	0.96	0.98
	NCC	0.98	0.98	0.98	0.98	0.03	0.98	0.96	0.98	0.96	0.96	0.94	0.97	0.98
	IQI	0.98	0.98	0.96	0.97	0.26	0.97	0.97	0.97	0.98	0.96	0.92	0.97	0.98
	GAE	0.00	0.00	0.00	0.00	0.00	0.00	0.00	0.00	0.00	0.00	0.00	0.00	0.00
	NMSE	1.33	6.28	7.42	2.05	9.83	1.42	0.14	0.15	0.13	0.15	0.18	1.24	1.18
	MSSIM	0.89	0.87	0.72	0.68	0.026	0.92	0.65	0.62	0.69	0.48	0.34	0.43	0.66
	SI	0.31	0.30	0.29	0.29	0.22	0.36	0.34	0.32	0.35	0.31	0.27	0.41	0.44
Speckle metrics	ASNR	1.66	1.65	1.53	1.65	1.21	1.65	1.71	1.73	1.71	1.74	1.86	1.71	159.09
	IV	0.36	0.38	0.27	0.27	179.41	0.40	0.38	0.39	0.36	0.38	-0.18	0.43	0.41
	NSD	9.94	9.87	4.70	9.83	2.82	9.91	1.41	1.47	1.35	1.51	1.72	9.91	10.00
	ENL	2.56	2.27	1.98	2.26	2.05	2.14	2.08	1.98	1.78	1.24	2.52	2.89	2.56
	Execution time in sec	10.09	3.58	14.26	13.52	17.28	2.79	3.52	4.19	1.23	2.18	1.54	3.48	28.34

The execution time of each algorithm tested on the three case study images in both the PCMAT and PCDSK systems are summarized in Table 6.4.

Table 6.4 Comparison of execution time of algorithms tested on the three images in the PCMAT and PCDSK systems

Images	System	Frost	Median	Lee	Kuan	Homo morphic	Wiener	En. Frost	En Lee	GAM	Wavelet	PMAD	SRAD	DTD
Abdomen	PCMAT	18.16	4.28	22.36	25.38	4.58	4.18	18.14	24.48	19.18	2.49	8.26	6.98	37.46
	PCDSK	10.04	2.56	12.73	13.58	18.57	3.28	4.25	5.38	2.17	1.26	2.19	3.26	29.24
Kidney	PCMAT	20.41	4.17	24.08	27.65	4.61	3.19	18.48	24.73	20.72	3.16	9.11	8.41	38.19
	PCDSK	10.46	2.41	11.56	13.24	17.62	2.12	4.13	5.74	3.38	2.26	5.62	4.26	32.52
Liver	PCMAT	17.77	4.39	21.48	23.58	3.74	4.63	17.39	22.56	18.44	3.48	7.67	6.63	38.24
	PCDSK	10.09	3.58	14.26	13.52	17.28	2.79	3.52	4.19	1.23	2.18	1.54	3.48	28.34
Average execution time (sec)	PCMAT	18.78	4.28	22.64	25.536	4.31	4.00	18.003	23.923	19.446	3.043	8.346	7.34	37.963
	PCDSK	10.196	2.85	12.85	13.446	17.823	2.73	3.966	5.103	2.26	1.9	3.116	3.666	30.03
Difference in Average execution time in sec		8.583	1.43	9.79	12.09	-13.513	1.27	14.036	18.82	17.186	1.143	5.23	3.673	7.93

6.4 DISCUSSION

All the despeckling algorithms were developed in the Code Composer Studio (Version 3.1) and tested in the TMS320C6713 based PCDSK system. Similar to the PCMAT system performance study, all the algorithms were tested more than 200 ultrasound B-scan images of various organs and the images of seven organs viz., abdomen, kidney, liver, gall bladder, heart, lungs and pancreas-spleen as suggested by the sonologist/radiologist due to marked improvements in the hypoechoic and hyperechoic regions were presented as case studies. In this chapter, only three case studies (for the abdomen, kidney and liver) and their respective outputs are presented in the form of images (Figures 6.1, 6.3 and 6.5) and Canny edge detected images (Figures 6.2, 6.4 and 6.6) for visual inspection. The despeckling filters' twenty calculated metrics with execution time are tabulated (Table 6.1, 6.2 and 6.3) for estimating the performance of the despeckling filters. The results of the remaining four organs such as gall bladder, heart, lungs and pancreas-spleen are given in the Appendix-B.

The despeckled images obtained from the PCDSK system were scrutinized by trained sonologist/radiologist. They found that the images were very similar to the results obtained by the PCMAT system and hence, the inferences arrived for the PCMAT system is applicable for the results obtained from the PCDSK system. But, in the case of the PCDSK system, both the raw and despeckled images appeared to be less resolved when zoomed to higher levels, which may be due to the quantization effect of the image data format supported by the TMS320C6713 DSK.

From the three case studies conducted for the PCDSK system, similar trends have been observed for the calculated performance metrics as that of the PCMAT system, which has been portrayed in the Tables 6.1 to 6.3 and the Figures 6.7 to 6.24. Therefore, all the points arrived from the calculated performance metrics of the PCMAT system described in Chapter-V, Section 5.7 can be considered as same for the PCDSK system.

Like the PCMAT system, the DTD filter implemented in the PCDSK system also showed similar performance characteristics for the quality and similarity metrics groups (mentioned in Chapter-V, Section 5.7). Also, the DTD filter performance in the PCDSK system showed similar trends as that of the speckle metrics group found for the PCMAT system. As a result, the DTD filter performance study in the PCDSK system confirms similar trends in the performance characteristic results obtained for the PCMAT system. Hence, the DTD filter is a better method for despeckling the ultrasound B-scan images over the other standard despeckling filters.

From the Table 6.4, it is found that the DTD algorithm consumed approximately 19, 12 times more execution time than the existing outperformed SRAD filter in the PCMAT and PCDSK systems, respectively. But, the DTD algorithm execution time in the PCDSK system is reduced approximately by 8 sec (~21% reduction in execution time), when compared to the PCMAT system. This can be further improved by using efficient coding and high speed DSPs for real-time implementation.

The calculated metric values (given in Tables 6.1 to 6.3) of the three case studies performed in the PCDSK system are presented as histogram plots as shown in Figures 6.7 to 6.24.

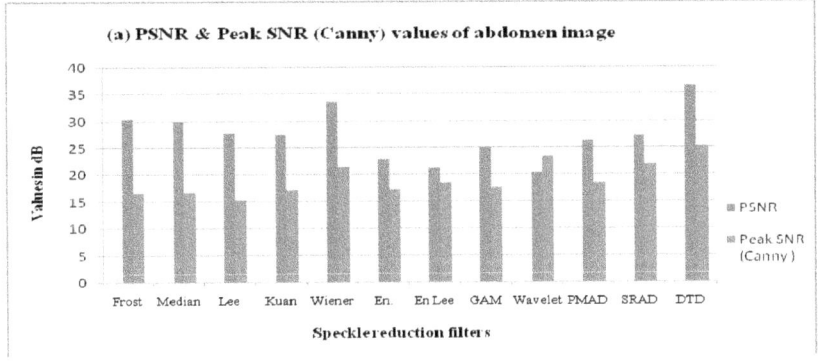

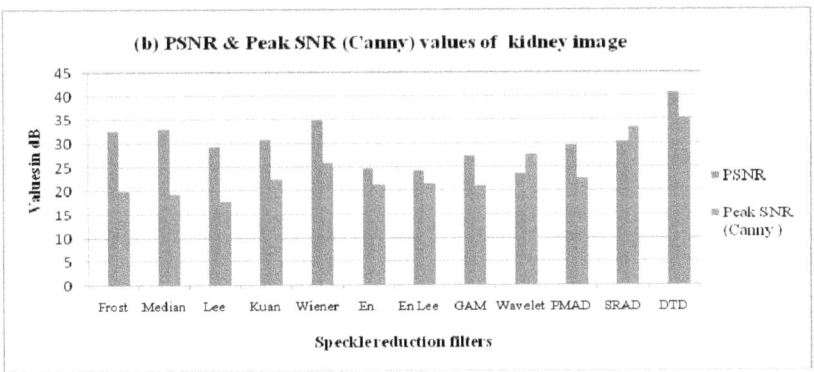

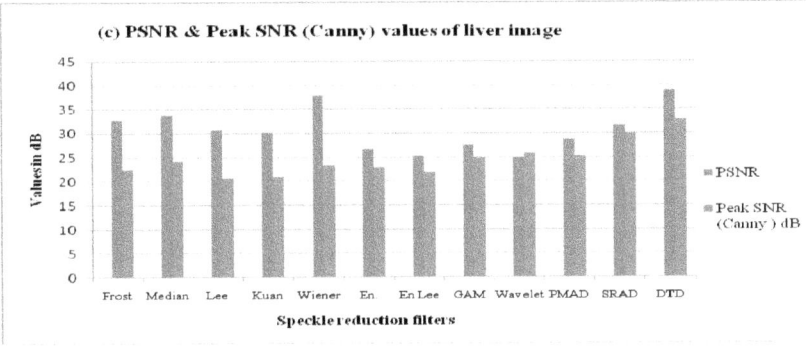

Fig 6.7 Histogram plot of the PSNR and Peak SNR (Canny) in the PCDSK system

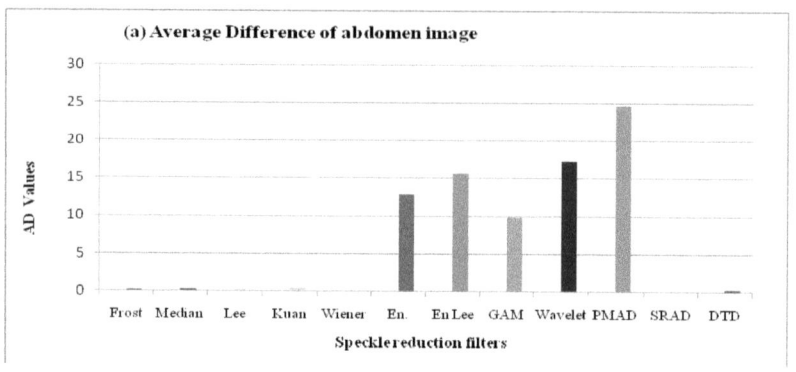

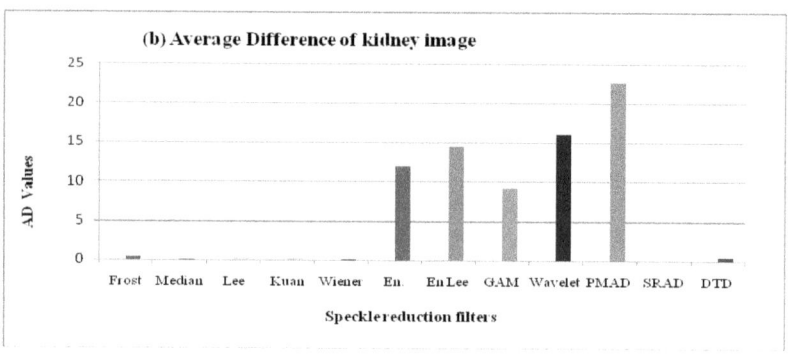

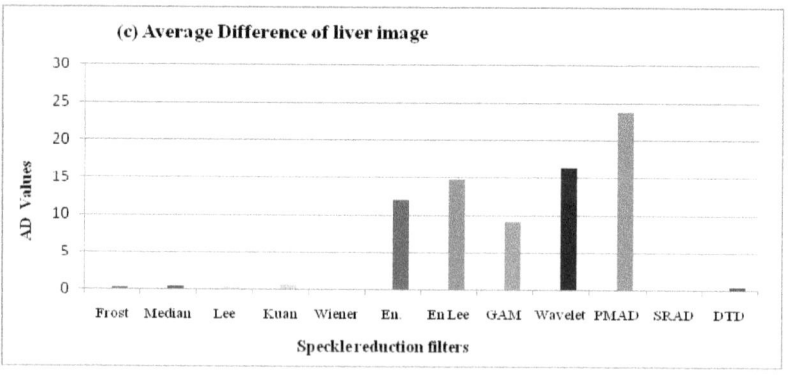

Fig 6.8 Histogram plot of the Average Difference (AD) in the PCDSK system

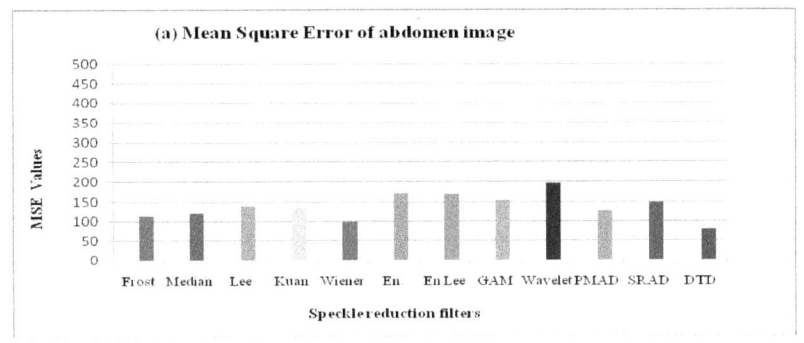

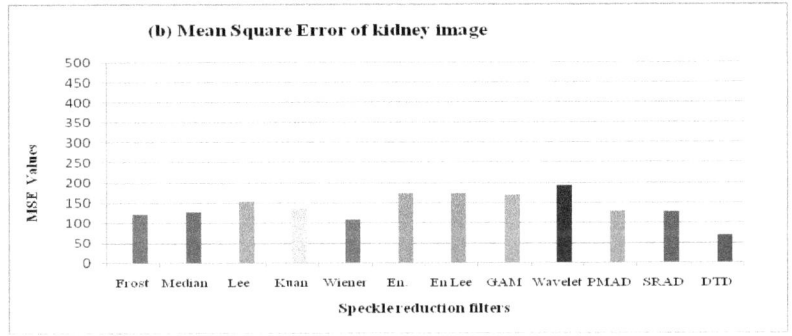

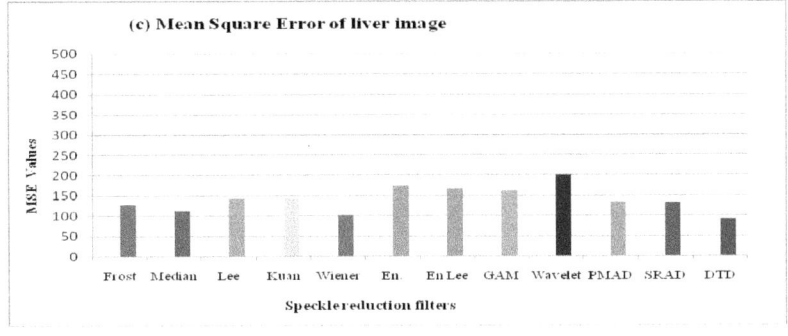

Fig 6.9 Histogram plot of the Mean Square Error (MSE) in the PCDSK system

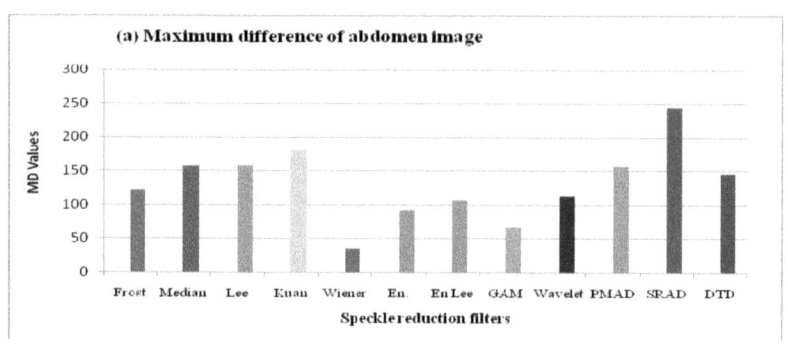

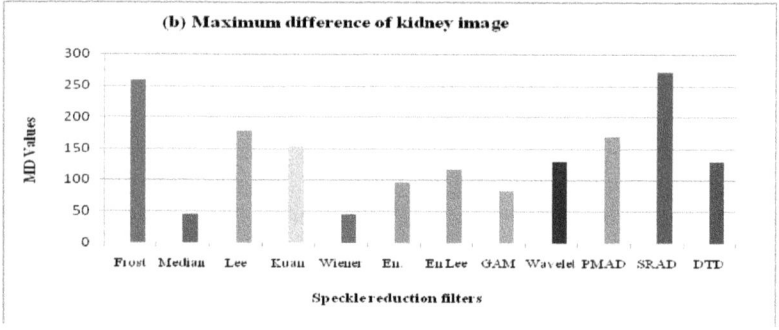

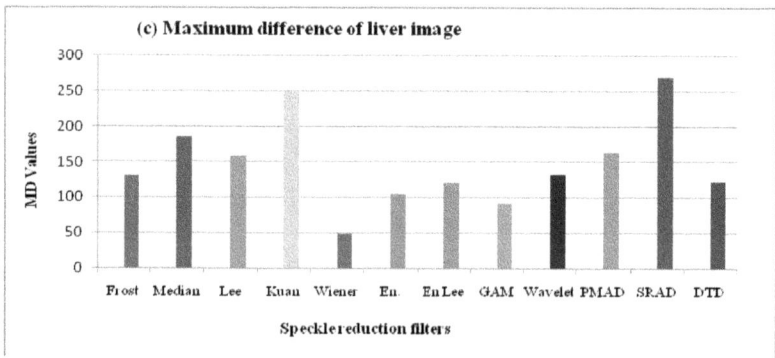

Fig 6.10 Histogram plot of the Maximum Difference (MD) in the PCDSK system

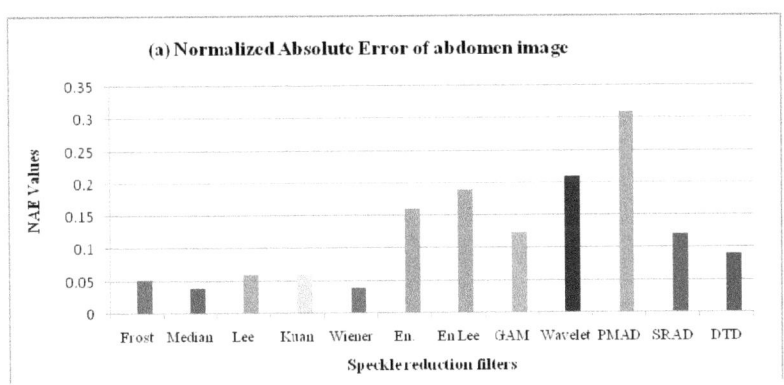

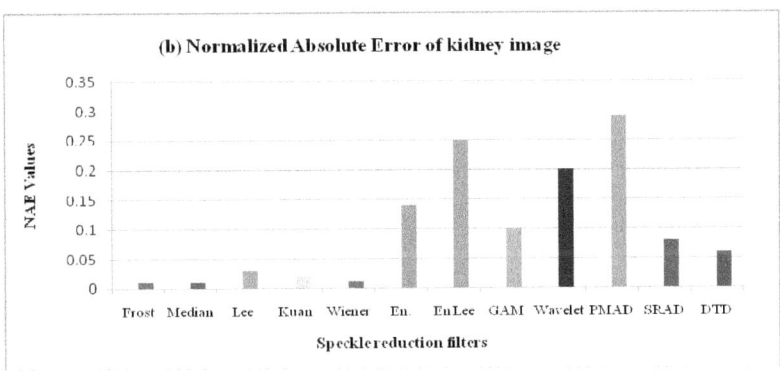

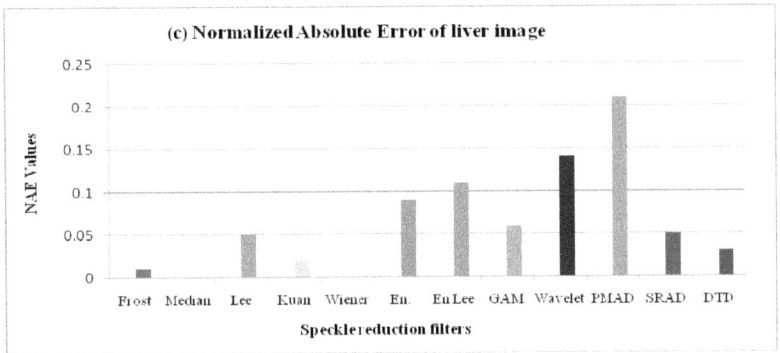

Fig 6.11 Histogram plot of the Normalized Absolute Error (NAE) in the PCDSK system

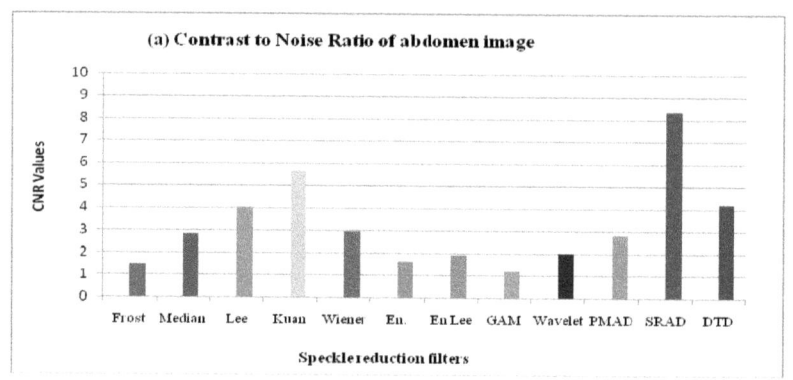

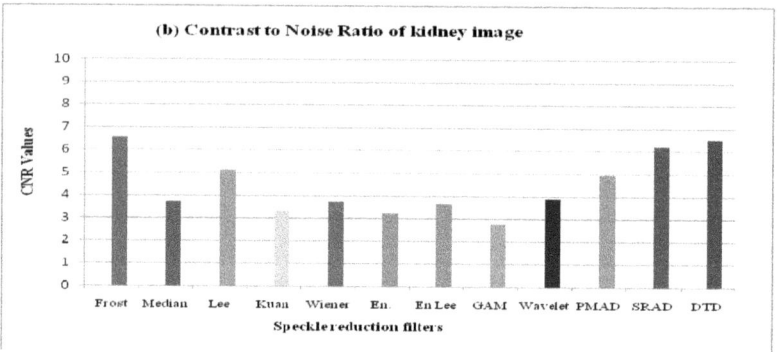

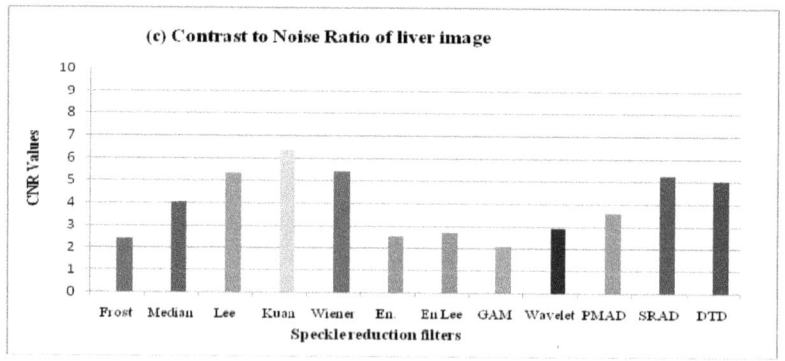

Fig 6.12 Histogram plot of the Contrast to Noise Ratio (CNR) in the PCDSK system

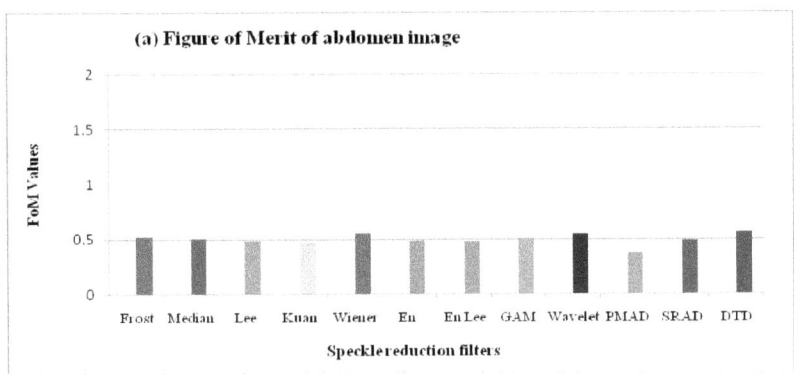

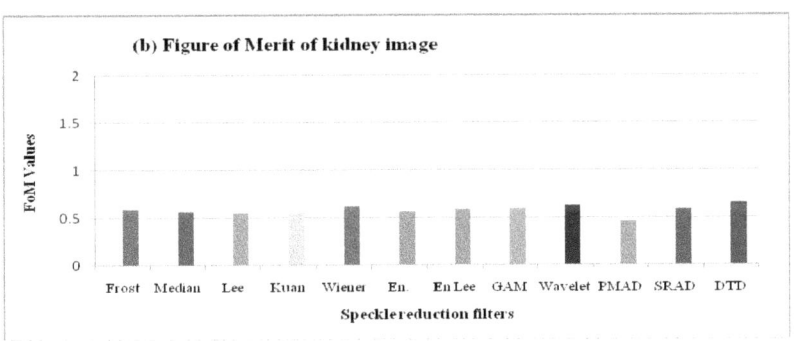

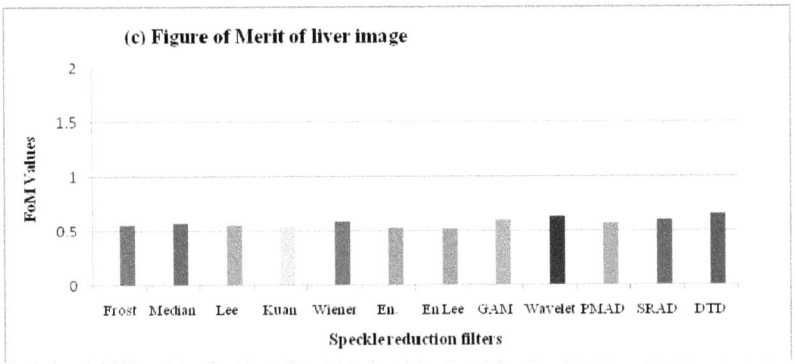

Fig 6.13 Histogram plot of the Figure of Merit (FoM) in the PCDSK system

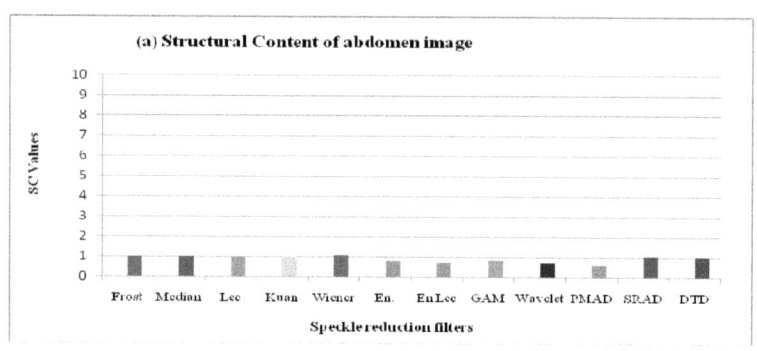

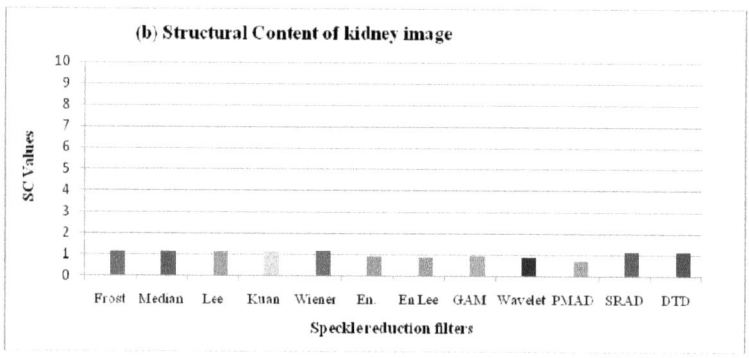

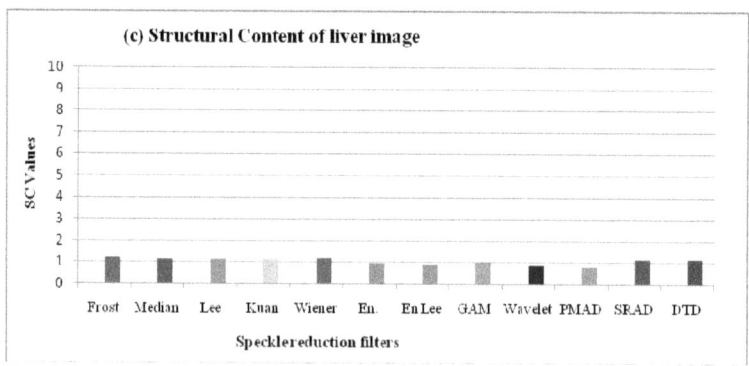

Fig 6.14 Histogram plot of the Structural Content (SC) in the PCDSK system

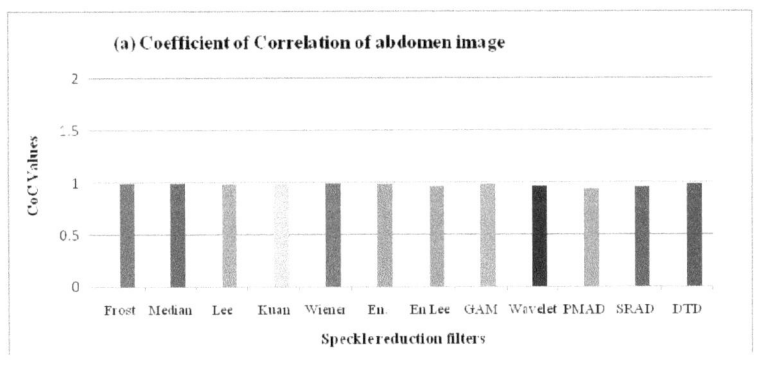

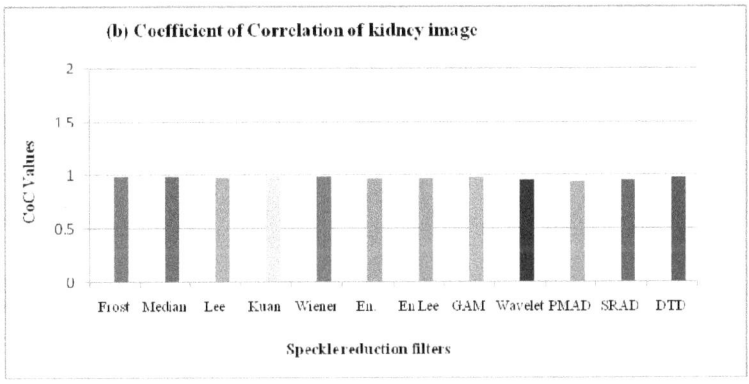

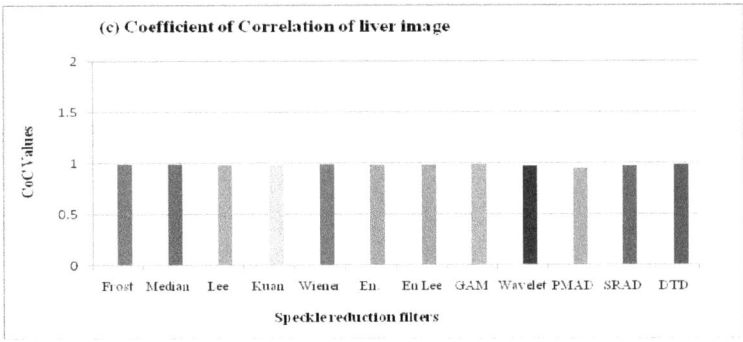

Fig 6.15 Histogram plot of the Coefficient of Correlation (CoC) in the PCDSK system

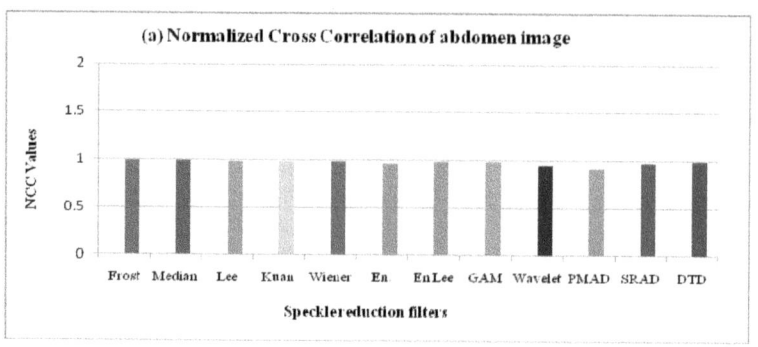

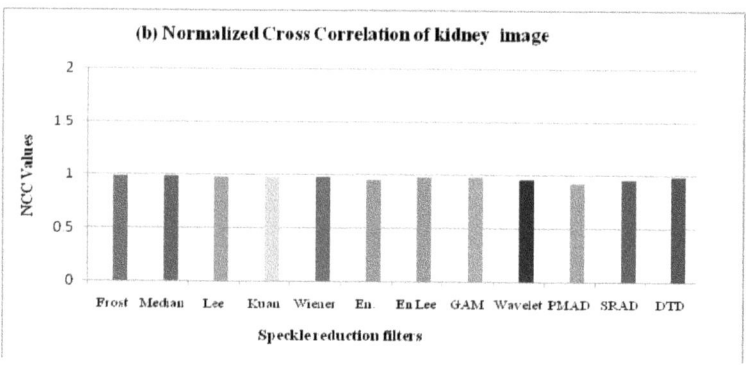

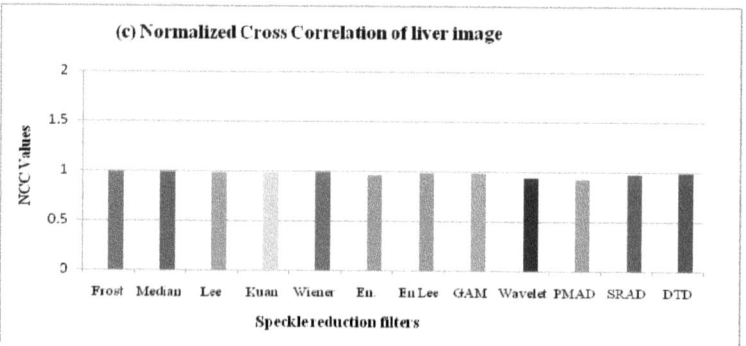

Fig 6.16 Histogram plot of the Normalized Cross Correlation (NCC) in the PCDSK system

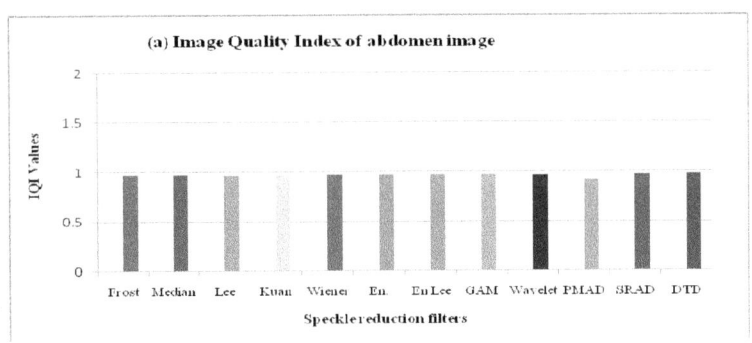

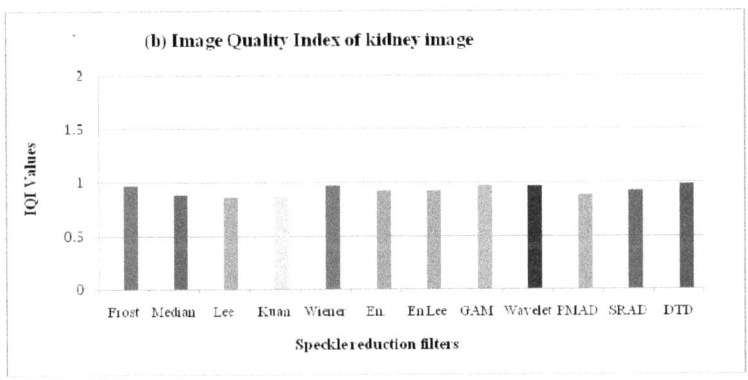

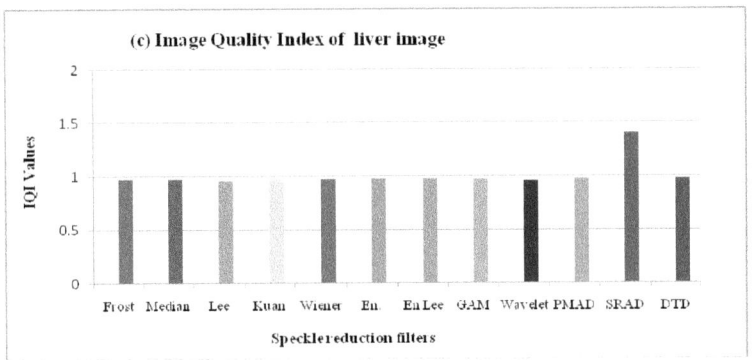

Fig 6.17 Histogram plot of the Image Quality Index (IQI) in the PCDSK system

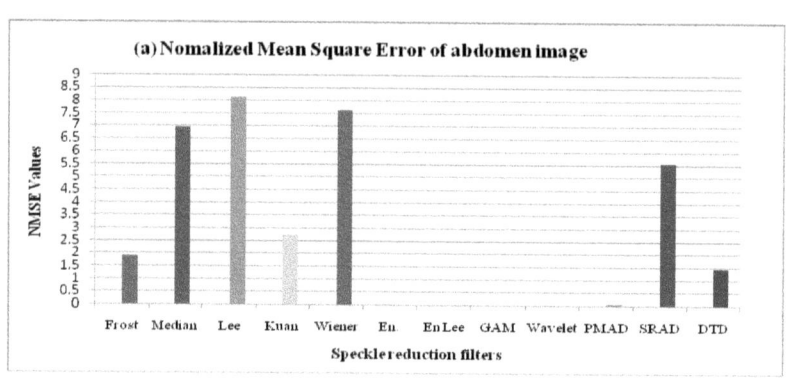

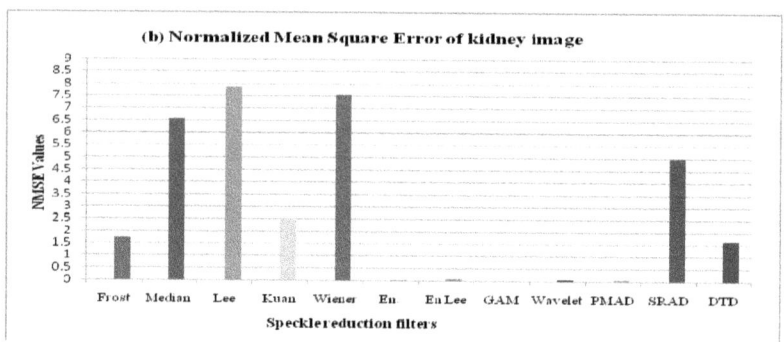

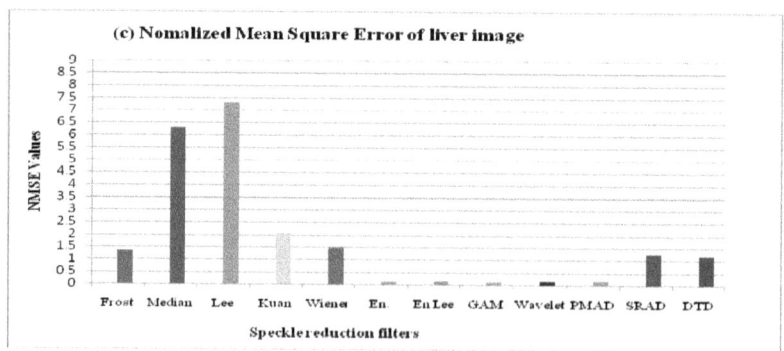

Fig 6.18 Histogram plot of the Normalized Mean Square Error (NMSE) in the PCDSK system

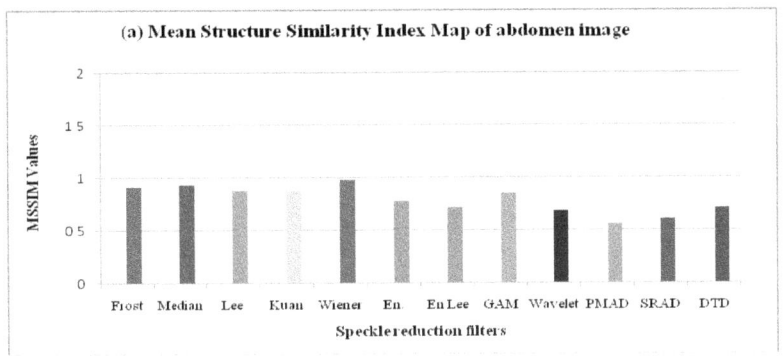

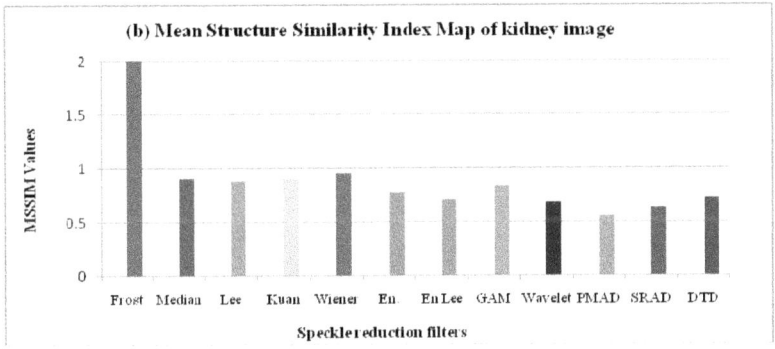

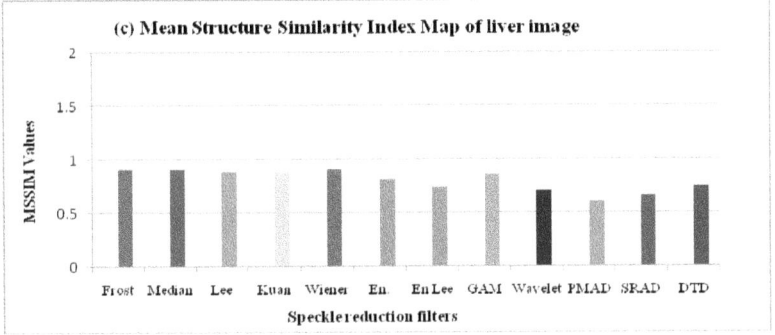

Fig 6.19 Histogram plot of the Mean Structure Similarity Index Map (MSSIM) in the PCDSK system

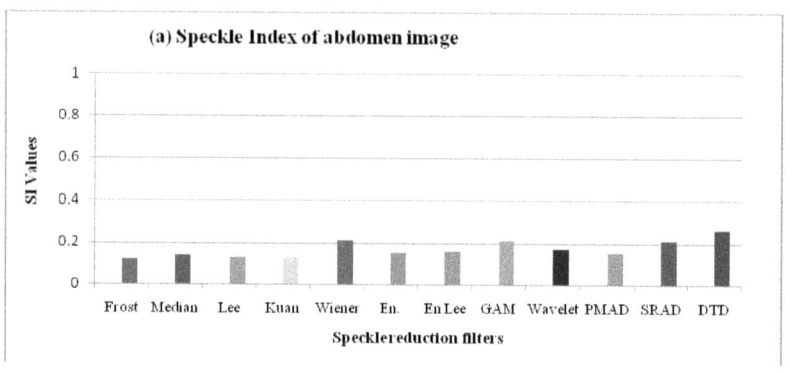

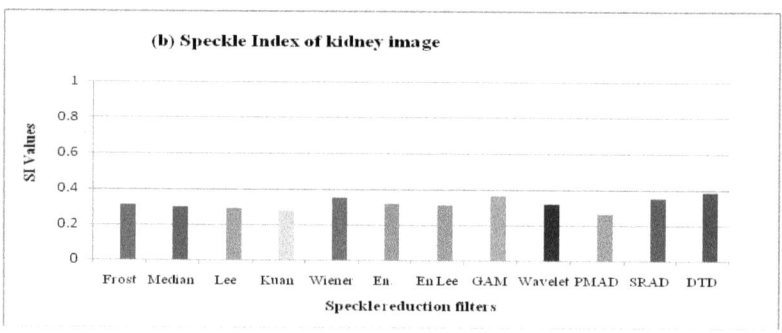

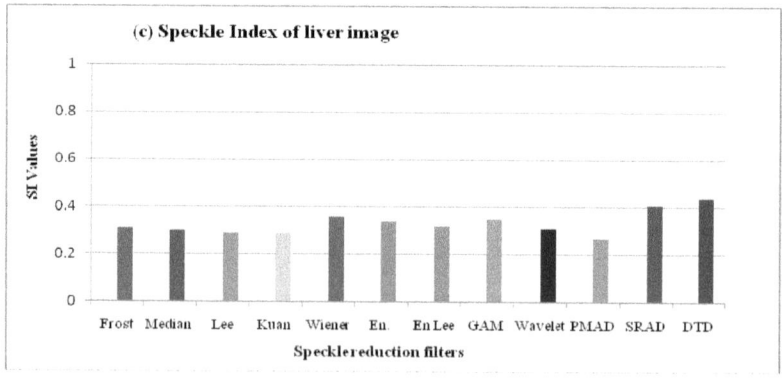

Fig 6.20 Histogram plot of the Speckle Index (SI) in the PCDSK system

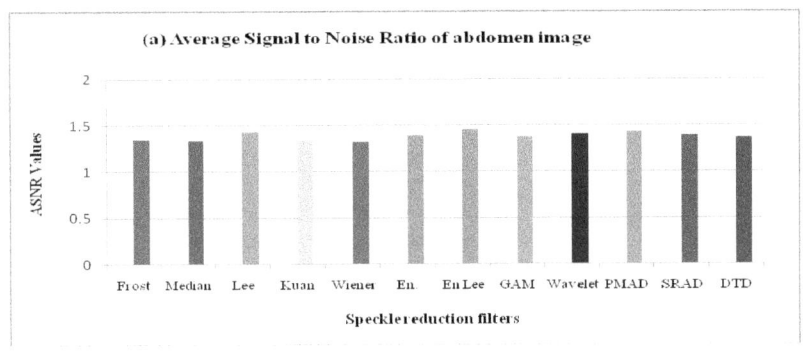

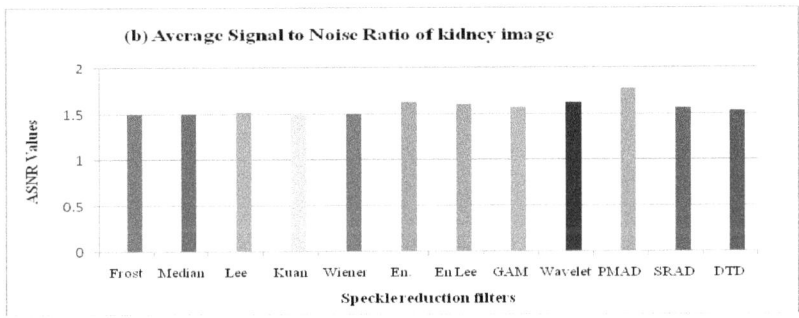

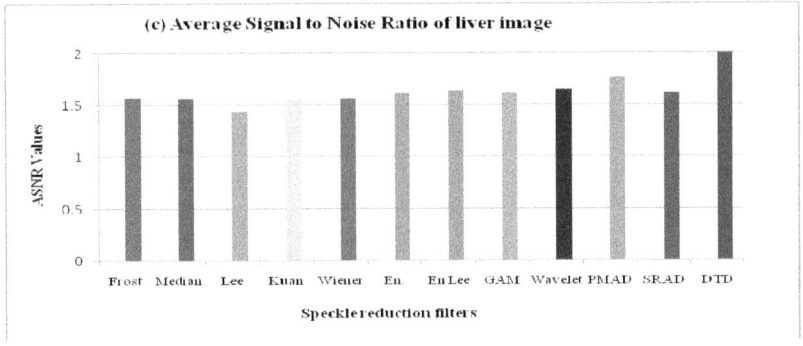

Fig 6.21 Histogram plot of the Average Signal to Noise Ratio (ASNR) in the PCDSK system

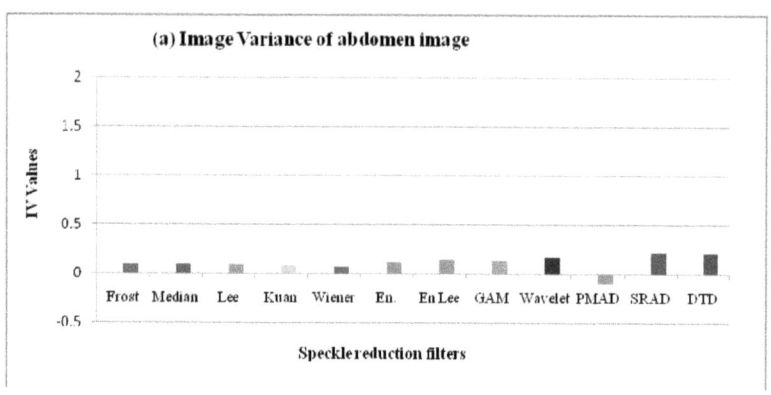

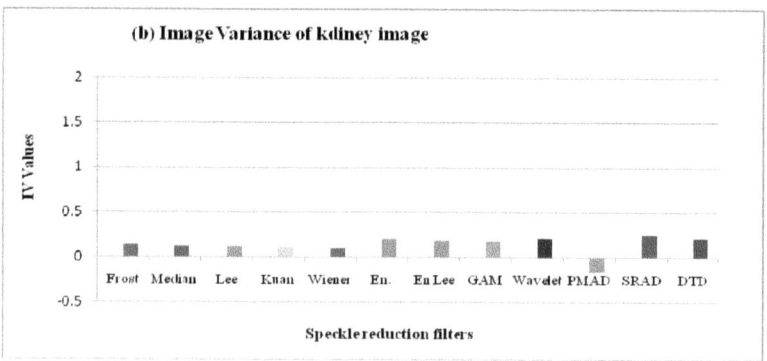

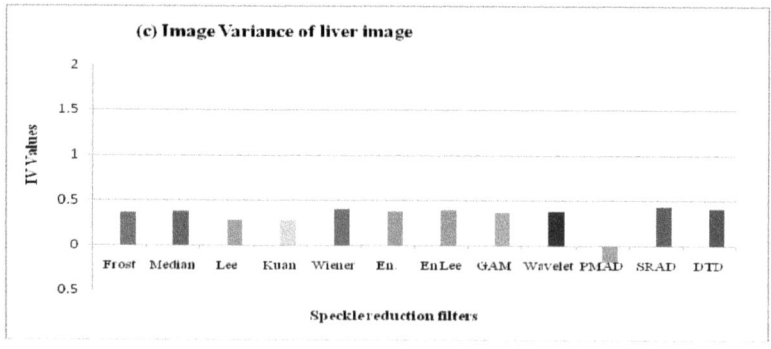

Fig 6.22 Histogram plot of the Image Variance (IV) in the PCDSK system

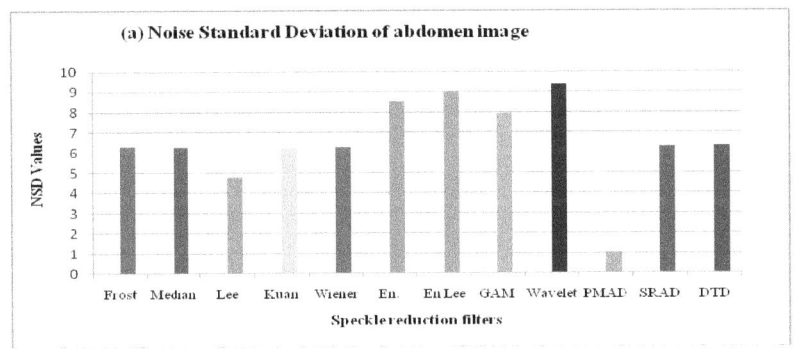

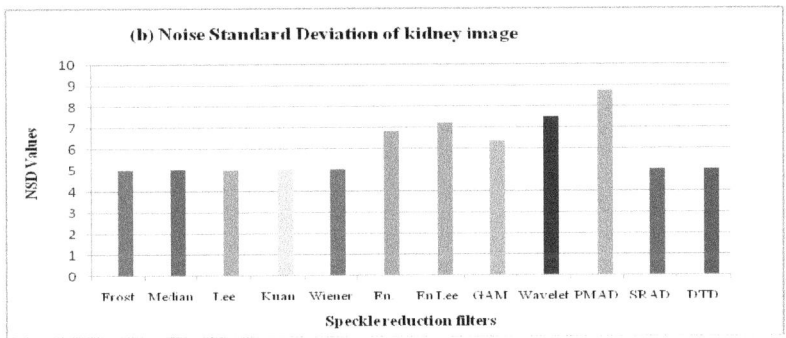

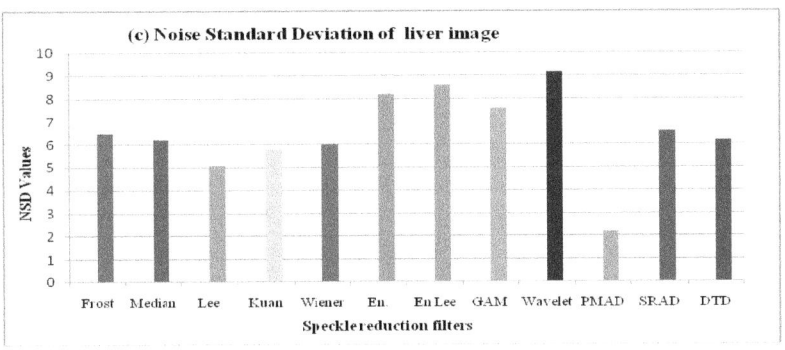

Fig 6.23 Histogram plot of the Noise Standard Deviation (NSD) in the PCDSK system

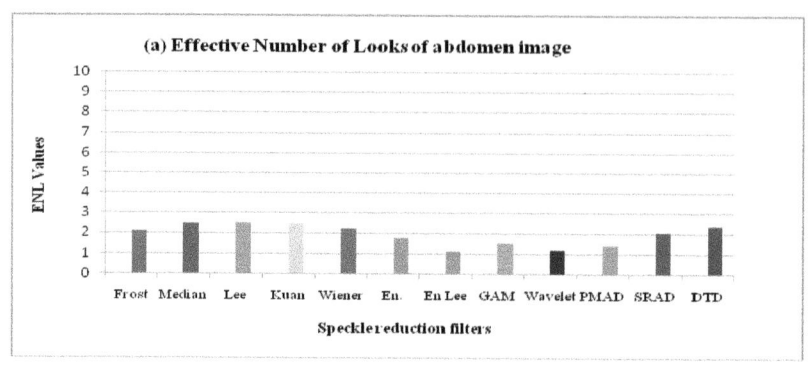

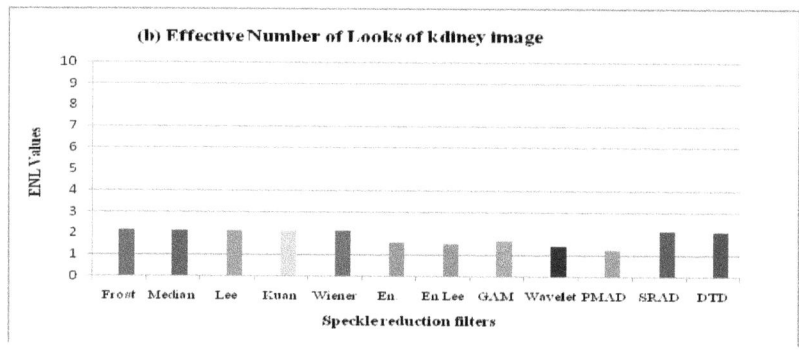

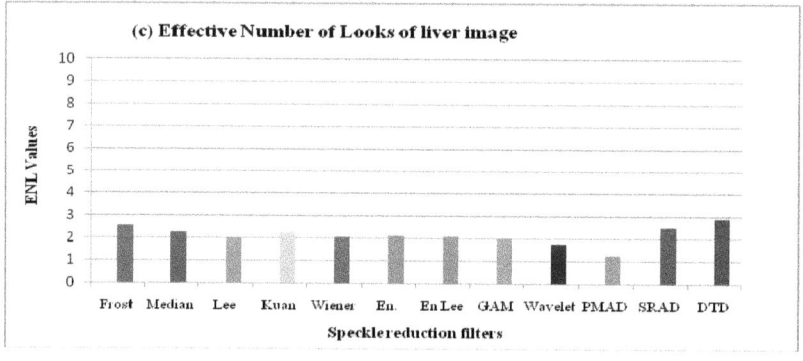

Fig 6.24 Histogram plot of the Effective Number of Looks (ENL) in the PCDSK system

REFERENCES

1. Qureshi S., Embedded Image Processing on the TMS320C6000 DSP, Labcyte Inc., Palo Alto, CA, USA, 2005.
2. Chassaing R., Digital Signal Processing and Applications with the C6713 and C6416, Wiley Inter Science, New Jersey, USA, 2005.
3. Chassaing R., DSP Applications Using C and the TMS320C6x DSK, John Wiley & Sons, Inc., USA, 2002.
4. Kehtarnavaz N., Real Time Digital Signal Processing Based on the TMS320C6000, Elsevier, Newnes, USA, 2005.
5. Tretter S.A., Communication System Design Using DSP Algorithms with Laboratory Experiments for the TMS320C6713 DSK, Springer, New York, USA, 2008.

CHAPTER-VII

CONCLUSIONS AND FUTURE SCOPE

Ultrasound B-scan imaging is the most efficient non-invasive technique that has been potentially and increasingly used for diagnosis over five decades. Unfortunately, the quality of the ultrasound B-scan image is degraded by the presence of speckle noise that reduces the visual evaluation of ultrasound images. Speckle reduction is a delicate and difficult task, since speckle is not a pure noise and it may carry some useful diagnostic information. Over the years, biomedical researchers have developed several despeckling techniques to suppress the speckle noise without losing the valuable diagnostic details. Also, recent developments in ultrasound device technology due to the advancements in digital image processing techniques and chip technology paves ways for developing more robust despeckling techniques for improving the quality of the ultrasound images for routine clinical practice.

Presently, ultrasound equipment manufacturers incorporated the speckle reduction algorithms like averaging by several scans, eliminating outliers and ensemble averaging in their machines for suppressing the speckle noise during real-time and routine clinical trials. In addition to this, a number of post-processing techniques such as adaptive median filters, adaptive diffusion filters and wavelet filters have been developed. Although the aforementioned techniques have had some success, speckle noise removal is still a very challenging problem and requires new approaches to solve this problem. Nowadays, such challenging problems are strategically solved by transforming ideas from other domain by making use of the advancements in information technology and merging of ideas within the interdisciplinary fields. One such attempt was made in this research work by transforming the discrete topological derivative (DTD) method, originally conceived as a structural mechanics concept, for solving the speckle reduction problem in ultrasound B-scan images.

This thesis is aimed at developing a novel DTD filter method for speckle reduction in ultrasound B-scan images and testing and validation of the proposed method by comparing with the existing despeckling techniques. With this goal, the basic concepts of speckle formation in ultrasound B-scan images, mathematical modelling of speckle and its implications in diagnostics were studied and recorded in this thesis. Further, several speckle reduction techniques, performance metrics and edge detection methods reported in the literature since 1970 were reviewed in Chapter-II of this thesis for the thorough understanding and experimentation of the existing and proposed despeckling concepts.

The basic concepts of the proposed DTD method and its discrete implementation for speckle reduction in ultrasound B-scan images are discussed in Chapter-III. The proposed DTD method was implemented in two different systems viz., a PC based MATLAB (PCMAT) system for easy algorithm development and PC based TMS320C6713 DSK (PCDSK) system for studying the real-time implementation possibilities of the proposed algorithm. The configuration of the PCMAT and PCDSK systems and the details of the ultrasound B-scan image data used for this study are briefed in Chapter-IV.

In this research work, algorithm for existing despeckling filters such as Frost, Median, Lee, Kuan, Homomorphic, Wiener, enhanced Frost, enhanced Lee, Gamma Map, Wavelet, PMAD, SRAD and the proposed DTD filter were developed both in the PCMAT and PCDSK system and are described in Chapters V and VI, respectively. The developed algorithms were tested on more than 200 ultrasound B-scan images collected from four different sources in both the PCMAT and PCDSK systems. The results obtained in both the systems were validated through visual inspection by trained sonologist/radiologist and comparison of calculated performance metrics. The important results arrived out of this study are discussed in Chapter V, Section 5.7 and Chapter VI, Section 6.4, respectively for the PCMAT and PCDSK systems.

The concluding remarks of this research work are summarized as follows:

1. Visual inspection of original and despeckled images by trained sonologist /radiologist (Certificate of Testing is given in Appendix-C) certified that the DTD algorithm improves the resolution of the image and edge detection over the traditional methods. Also, the DTD method improved differentiation of the hypoechoic and hyperechoic regions resulting in better diagnosis. Further, the DTD improves the tissue contrast, so that exact size of the lesions can be measured.

2. The calculated nineteen metrics were grouped into quality, similarity and speckle metrics and compared the different parameters in each group. In this comparative study, DTD filter is outperformed in the case of quality and similarity metrics groups, whereas it is optimally performed in the case of speckle metrics group. Comparison of performance metrics calculated for the existing standard filters and the proposed DTD filters in both the PCMAT and PCDSK systems exhibited similar trends and are discussed in Chapter V and VI, respectively. Thus, the DTD method is found to be an efficient method in terms of the quantitative measures.
3. Canny edge detection with peak SNR value calculation of the DTD despeckling shows that the DTD method preserves the diagnostic details well over the other traditional methods.
4. The comparison of execution time of the algorithms in both the systems exhibits that the proposed DTD algorithm in the PCDSK system took approximately 21% reduction in the execution time than the PCMAT system, which shows a ray of hope for real-time implementation of the algorithm in the commercial ultrasound machines for routine clinical practices.

In summary, the proposed DTD method for ultrasound B-scan speckle reduction has addressed the qualitative aspects of despeckling over existing methods through improvements in preserving the hypoechoic and hyperechoic regions and the performance of the DTD algorithms was demonstrated quantitatively through the calculated parametric values, which shows a considerable improvement in quality and similarity metrics. **The only drawback of the DTD method is its computational/execution time, i.e., it took around 19 and 12 times more execution time than the existing outperformed SRAD filter in the PCMAT and PCDSK systems, respectively, which can be improved through efficient coding schemes and using high speed DSPs.**

At the outset, the DTD method has several advantageous features viz., the performance is robust to noise and iterative, overall image resolution is retained and improves both the hypo and hyper echoic regions. Hence, the proposed DTD algorithm might be useful in reducing the speckle noise and improving the contrast details of soft tissues and structures visible in the B-scan images to look at the image features obscured by the speckle noise.

Further, the proposed DTD technique has demonstrated that it is competitive with the existing despeckling techniques and may have useful role in future medical ultrasound systems. With the advent of the new generation digital signal processor technology, the DTD method may be feasible for real time diagnosis and routine clinical practices.

FUTURE SCOPE

The present DTD algorithm needs user intervention for finding out the right iteration for identifying the optimum topological derivative value. **Also, the DTD algorithm requires more time than the other standard methods.** Therefore, further work will concentrate on improvement of the algorithm without user intervention and efficient coding for reducing the execution time of the algorithm for real-time implementation. Further, the DTD method should be attempted for efficient characterization of the microstructures/soft tissues in ultrasound imaging.

LIST OF PUBLICATIONS

International Publications

1. Nedumaran D., **Sivakumar R.**, Sekar V., and Gayathri M.K., Speckle Noise Reduction in Ultrasound Biomedical B-Scan Images Using Discrete Topological Derivative, ELSEVIER, Ultrasound in Med. & Biol., 2012, Vol.38, No.2, pp. 276-286. ISSN: 0301-5629.
www.sciencedirect.com/science/article/pii/S0301562911014554

2. **Sivakumar R.**, Gayathri M.K., and Nedumaran D., Speckle Filtering of Ultrasound B-Scan Images – A Comparative Study Between Spatial and Diffusion filter, IEEE Conference on Open Systems (ICOS 2010), Malaysia, 5-7 Dec. 2010, pp 80-85. ISBN: 978-1-4244-9193-3.
ieeexplore.ieee.org/iel5/5714409/5719958/05720068.pdf

3. **Sivakumar R.**, Gayathri M.K., and Nedumaran D., Speckle Filtering of Ultrasound B-scan Images - A Comparative Study of Single Scale Spatial Adaptive Filters, Multiscale Filter and Diffusion Filters, International Journal of Engineering and Technology, 2010, Vol.2, No.6, pp.514-523. ISSN: 1793-8236. http://www.ijetch.org/abstract/174-E803.htm

4. **Sivakumar R.**, and Nedumaran D., Comparative Study of Speckle Noise Reduction of Ultrasound B-scan Images in Matrix Laboratory Environment, International Journal of Computer Applications, 2010, Vol.10, No.9, pp 46-50. ISSN: 0975-8887.
www.ijcaonline.org/volume10/number9/pxc3872024.pdf

National Publication

1. **Sivakumar R.**, and Nedumaran D., Performance Study of Wavelet Denoising Techniques in Ultrasound Images, Journal of Instrument Society of India, 2009,Vol. 39, No.30, pp. 194-196. ISSN: 0970-9983.

International Conferences

1. **Sivakumar R.**, and Nedumaran D., Development of Despeckle Algorithms for Medical Ultrasound Images – A Comparative Study, Proceedings of the International conference on Instrumentation and National Symposium on Instrumentation-34, 2010, Pune, pp. 73.

2. **Sivakumar R.**, and Nedumaran D., Implementation of Wavelet Filters for Speckle Noise Reduction in Ultrasound Medical Images: A Comparative Study, Proceedings of the International conference on Signal, System and Communication (ICSSC2009), India, 21-23 Dec. 2009, pp.239-242.

National Conferences

1. **Sivakumar R.,** and Nedumaran D., Performance study of Wavelet Denoising Techniques in Ultrasound Images, Proceedings of the National Symposium on Instrumentation-33, 2008, Vishakapatnam, pp.50.

2. **Sivakumar R.,** Balasubramaniam D., and Nedumaran D., Study of Discrete Wavelet Transform Techniques in Biomedical Image Processing, Proceedings of the National Symposium on Instrumentation-31, 2006, CP-71, Gwalior, pp.52.

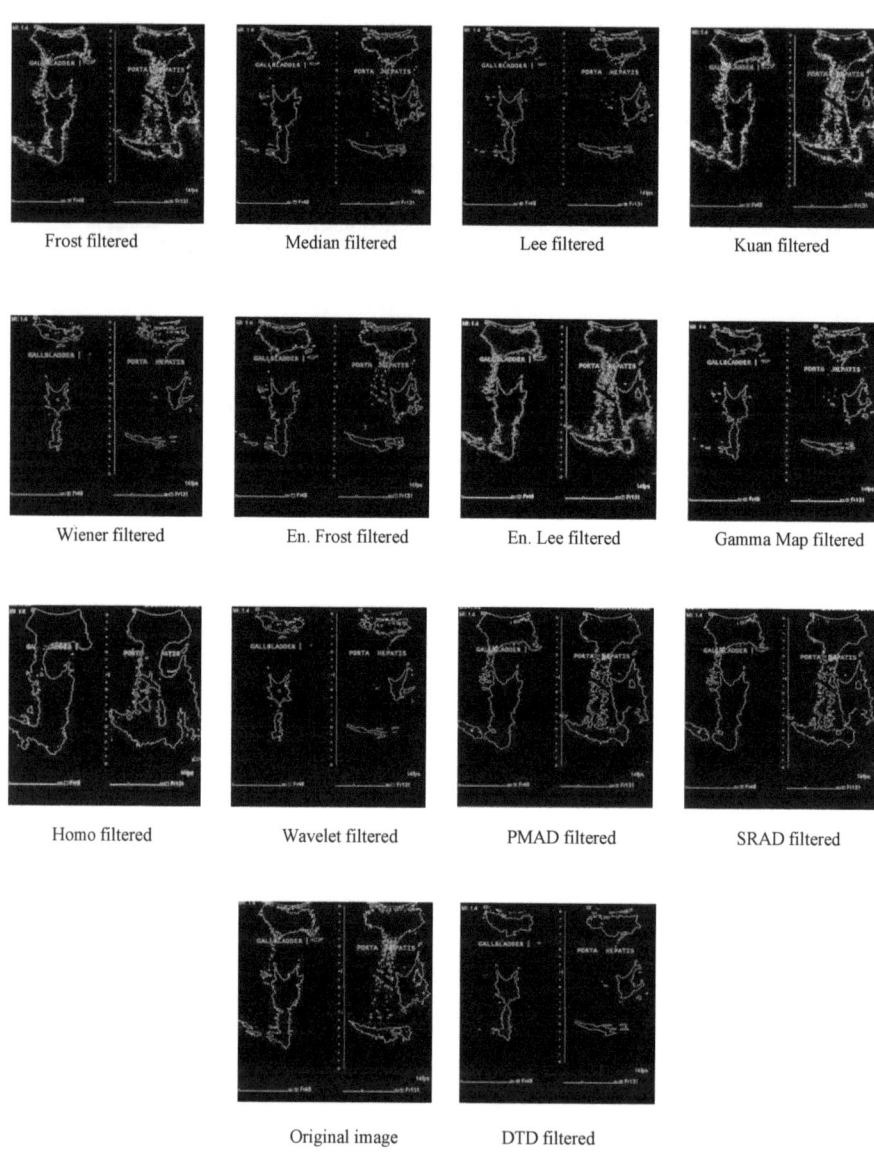

Fig A2 Canny edge detected images of gall bladder in the PCMAT system

Table A1 Calculated performance metrics of the despeckling filters applied on the gall bladder image in the PCMAT system

Group	Metrics	Frost	Median	Lee	Kuan	Homo morphic	Wiener	En. Frost	En Lee	GAM	Wavelet	PMAD	SRAD	DTD
Quality metrics	PSNR in dB	31.72	31.24	29.21	28.78	9.57	34.90	24.16	22.54	26.41	21.68	27.71	28.55	37.81
	PSNR (Canny)in dB	17.62	17.86	16.31	18.22	7.56	22.55	18.33	19.54	18.66	24.53	19.50	23.13	26.29
	AD	0.23	0.35	0.26	0.56	77.15	0.10	12.95	15.75	9.90	17.36	24.75	0.13	0.38
	MSE	116.23	122.17	141.67	137.87	9652.38	101.73	174.16	171.97	156.26	197.63	128.67	150.64	81.85
	MD	131.18	166.18	167.18	190.18	212.37	44.18	102.18	116.18	76.18	123.18	166.18	210.18	155.18
	NAE	0.07	0.06	0.08	0.08	1.00	0.06	0.18	0.21	0.14	0.23	0.33	0.14	0.11
	CNR	1.56	2.91	4.13	5.72	2.15	3.02	1.69	2.00	1.28	2.10	2.89	8.44	4.29
	FoM	0.57	0.56	0.53	0.51	0.16	0.60	0.53	0.52	0.56	0.59	0.42	0.54	0.61
	SC	1.07	1.07	1.08	1.08	4023.11	1.13	0.83	0.79	0.88	0.77	0.68	1.10	1.08
Similarity metrics	CoC	0.99	0.99	0.98	0.98	0.93	0.99	0.98	0.97	0.98	0.97	0.94	0.96	0.98
	NCC	0.99	0.99	0.98	0.98	0.02	0.98	0.96	0.98	0.98	0.94	0.91	0.97	0.99
	IQI	0.97	0.97	0.96	0.97	0.00	0.97	0.97	0.97	0.97	0.96	0.92	0.97	0.98
	GAE	0.00	0.00	0.00	0.00	0.00	0.00	0.00	0.00	0.00	0.00	0.00	0.00	0.00
	NMSE	1.97	7.01	8.22	2.83	1.04	7.70	0.11	0.11	0.10	0.12	0.17	5.66	1.56
	MSSIM	0.94	0.96	0.91	0.91	0.09	1.01	0.81	0.75	0.88	0.71	0.59	0.64	0.74
Speckle metrics	SI	0.21	0.23	0.22	0.22	0.19	0.30	0.24	0.25	0.30	0.26	0.24	0.30	0.35
	ASNR	1.38	1.37	1.47	1.37	1.06	1.36	1.43	1.49	1.41	1.45	1.47	1.43	1.40
	IV	0.23	0.23	0.23	0.23	118.60	0.21	0.26	0.28	0.27	0.31	0.04	0.36	0.35
	NSD	6.41	6.36	4.91	6.33	2.59	6.39	8.64	9.13	8.06	9.46	1.20	6.40	6.44
	ENL	1.60	1.61	2.09	1.62	1.28	1.61	1.19	1.13	1.28	1.09	1.13	1.60	1.59
	Execution time in sec	17.82	4.57	23.78	26.12	5.16	4.52	18.52	25.89	20.45	2.59	8.74	7.16	38.56

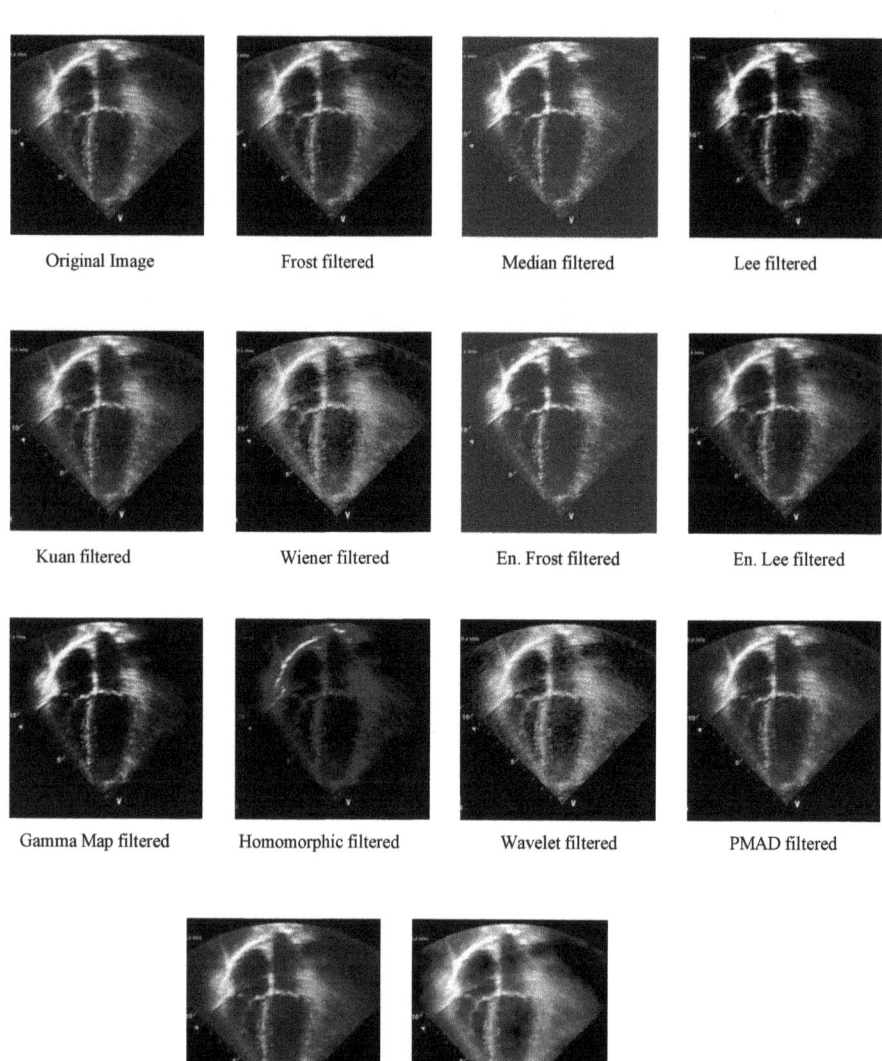

Fig A3 Original and despeckled images of heart in the PCMAT system

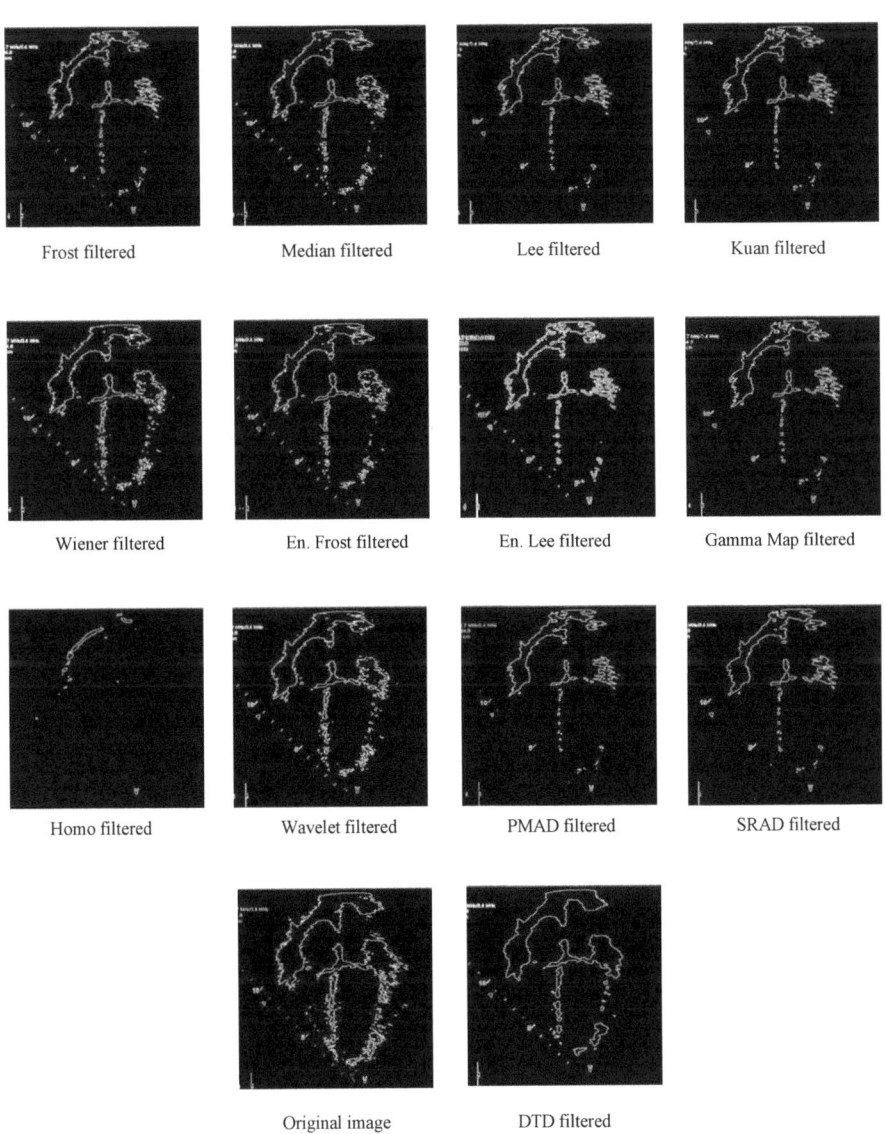

Fig A4 Canny edge detected images of heart in the PCMAT system

Table A2 Calculated performance metrics of the despeckling filters applied on the heart image in the PCMAT system

Group	Metrics	Frost	Median	Lee	Kuan	Homo morphic	Wiener	En. Frost	En Lee	GAM	Wavelet	PMAD	SRAD	DTD
Quality metrics	PSNR in dB	30.72	31.24	27.43	28.81	10.57	32.93	22.83	22.43	25.55	21.72	27.80	28.47	38.81
	PSNR (Canny)in dB	17.20	16.56	15.10	19.79	5.71	23.15	18.62	18.97	18.49	25.17	19.86	30.82	32.61
	AD	0.34	0.09	0.27	0.19	67.42	0.09	11.93	14.41	9.16	15.95	22.70	0.10	0.34
	MSE	120.85	124.96	151.67	135.87	8931.38	107.80	171.70	172.69	168.83	190.89	128.16	125.20	67.85
	MD	182.18	38.18	171.18	145.18	212.35	38.18	88.18	109.18	74.18	122.18	161.18	124.18	122.18
	NAE	0.06	0.06	0.08	0.07	0.99	0.06	0.19	0.30	0.15	0.25	0.34	0.13	0.11
	CNR	5.56	2.73	4.13	2.33	2.77	2.73	2.24	2.65	1.77	2.89	3.95	5.22	5.49
	FoM	0.56	0.54	0.52	0.53	0.14	0.59	0.54	0.56	0.57	0.60	0.43	0.56	0.62
	SC	1.07	1.10	1.08	1.07	29.28	1.11	0.82	0.78	0.87	0.79	0.67	1.09	1.07
Similarity metrics	CoC	0.99	0.99	0.98	0.99	0.94	0.99	0.97	0.97	0.98	0.96	0.94	0.96	0.98
	NCC	0.99	0.99	0.98	0.98	0.01	0.98	0.95	0.98	0.98	0.96	0.93	0.96	0.99
	IQI	0.97	0.88	0.86	0.87	0.00	0.97	0.92	0.92	0.97	0.96	0.88	0.92	0.98
	GAE	0.00	0.00	0.00	0.00	0.00	0.00	0.00	0.00	0.00	0.00	0.00	0.00	0.00
	NMSE	1.89	6.86	8.08	3.01	7.61	0.15	0.11	0.12	0.14	0.19	6.22	2.14	1.89
	MSSIM	0.93	0.94	0.91	0.94	0.08	0.98	0.80	0.74	0.87	0.71	0.59	0.66	0.75
	SI	0.27	0.26	0.25	0.24	0.12	0.31	0.28	0.27	0.32	0.28	0.22	0.31	0.34
Speckle metrics	ASNR	1.45	1.45	1.47	1.46	1.21	1.45	1.58	1.56	1.52	1.57	1.73	1.51	1.48
	IV	0.26	0.24	0.24	0.23	238.16	0.22	0.32	0.31	0.30	0.33	-0.04	0.37	0.33
	NSD	4.90	4.94	4.91	4.95	2.56	4.94	6.73	7.15	6.29	7.41	8.64	4.94	4.97
	ENL	2.10	2.08	2.09	2.07	4.07	2.08	1.52	1.48	1.63	1.39	1.19	2.08	2.06
	Execution time in sec	18.57	4.52	23.35	26.14	4.74	3.89	19.12	25.08	21.19	3.52	9.57	8.78	37.41

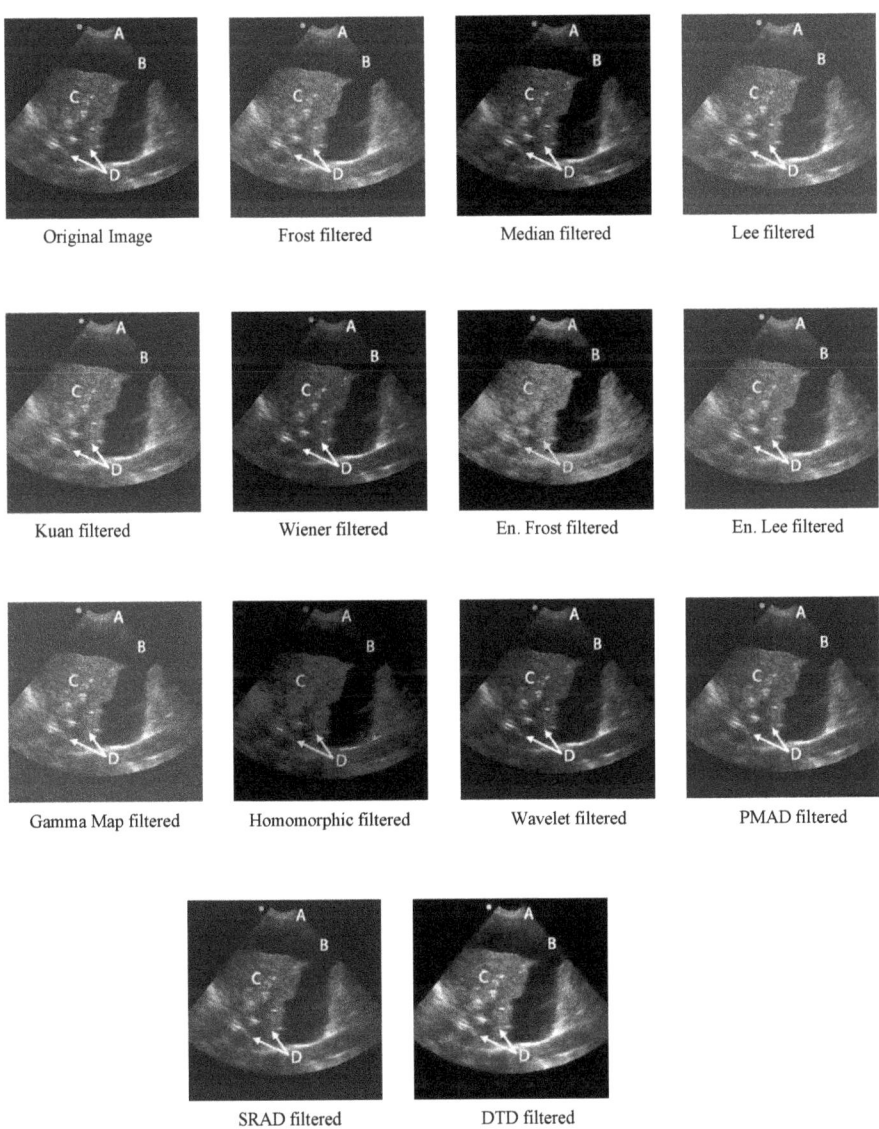

Fig A5 Original and despeckled images of lungs in the PCMAT system

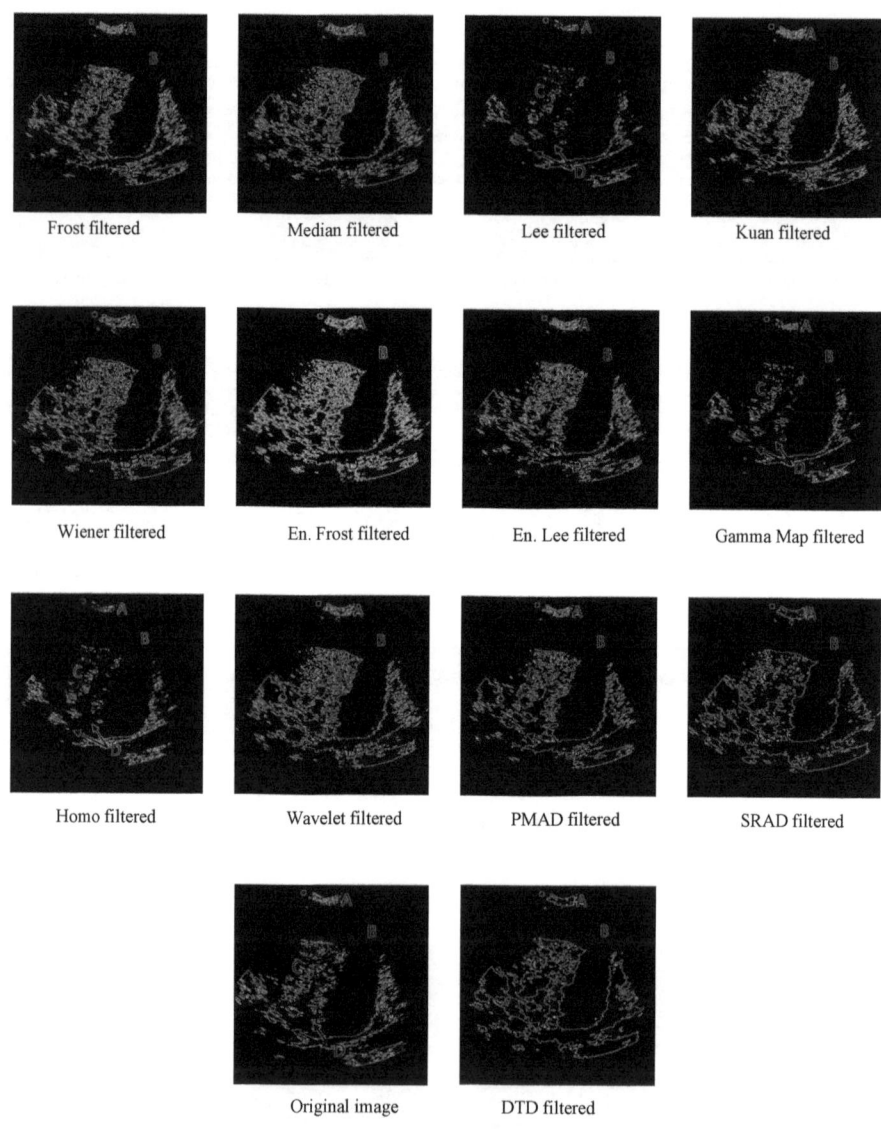

Fig A6 Canny edge detected images of lungs in the PCMAT system

Table A3 Calculated performance metrics of the despeckling filters applied on the lungs image in the PCMAT system

Group	Metrics	Frost	Median	Lee	Kuan	Homo morphic	Wiener	En. Frost	En Lee	GAM	Wavelet	PMAD	SRAD	DTD
Quality metrics	PSNR in dB	30.72	31.83	28.73	28.16	10.76	35.86	24.65	23.16	25.57	22.86	26.77	29.68	36.78
	PSNR (Canny) in dB	19.81	21.57	18.06	18.33	6.31	20.66	20.10	19.22	22.34	23.17	22.51	27.31	30.22
	AD	0.25	0.32	0.24	0.50	96.39	0.11	12.00	14.65	9.11	16.31	23.81	0.11	0.39
	MSE	125.03	110.73	141.57	142.17	8816.24	100.93	172.84	165.55	160.96	198.77	132.55	129.59	88.88
	MD	123.18	178.18	151.18	141.18	232.37	41.18	96.18	112.18	83.18	125.18	156.18	182.18	114.18
	NAE	0.06	0.05	0.10	0.07	1.00	0.05	0.14	0.16	0.11	0.19	0.26	0.10	0.08
	CNR	1.41	3.06	4.33	5.34	2.41	4.42	1.54	1.70	1.09	1.89	2.61	4.24	4.03
	FoM	0.53	0.54	0.53	0.51	0.19	0.56	0.50	0.49	0.57	0.60	0.54	0.57	0.62
Similarity metrics	SC	1.13	1.07	1.08	1.07	5240.21	1.11	0.87	0.84	0.91	0.82	0.74	1.08	1.07
	CoC	0.99	0.99	0.98	0.98	0.96	0.99	0.98	0.98	0.99	0.97	0.95	0.97	0.98
	NCC	0.99	0.99	0.98	0.98	0.01	0.99	0.96	0.98	0.98	0.94	0.92	0.97	0.99
	IQI	0.97	0.97	0.96	0.97	0.00	0.97	0.98	0.98	0.97	0.96	0.98	1.04	0.98
	GAE	0.00	0.00	0.00	0.00	0.00	0.00	0.00	0.00	0.00	0.00	0.00	0.00	0.00
	NMSE	1.30	6.24	7.26	2.00	9.75	1.39	0.09	0.10	0.08	0.10	0.13	1.19	1.13
	MSSIM	0.94	0.94	0.92	0.91	0.07	0.94	0.85	0.77	0.89	0.74	0.64	0.69	0.78
	SI	0.27	0.26	0.25	0.25	0.18	0.32	0.30	0.28	0.31	0.27	0.23	0.37	0.40
Speckle metrics	ASNR	1.61	1.60	1.48	1.60	1.16	1.60	1.66	1.68	1.66	1.69	1.81	1.66	159.04
	IV	0.33	0.35	0.24	0.24	179.38	0.37	0.35	0.36	0.33	0.35	-0.21	0.40	0.38
	NSD	4.78	4.53	4.79	4.14	5.12	6.61	6.98	6.29	7.14	8.56	5.21	5.36	4.78
	ENL	1.05	1.05	2.20	1.06	2.77	1.05	1.08	1.70	1.52	1.48	1.59	1.05	1.05
	Execution time in sec	16.83	4.19	22.32	24.17	4.11	4.28	17.89	23.14	19.08	3.52	7.42	6.43	37.08

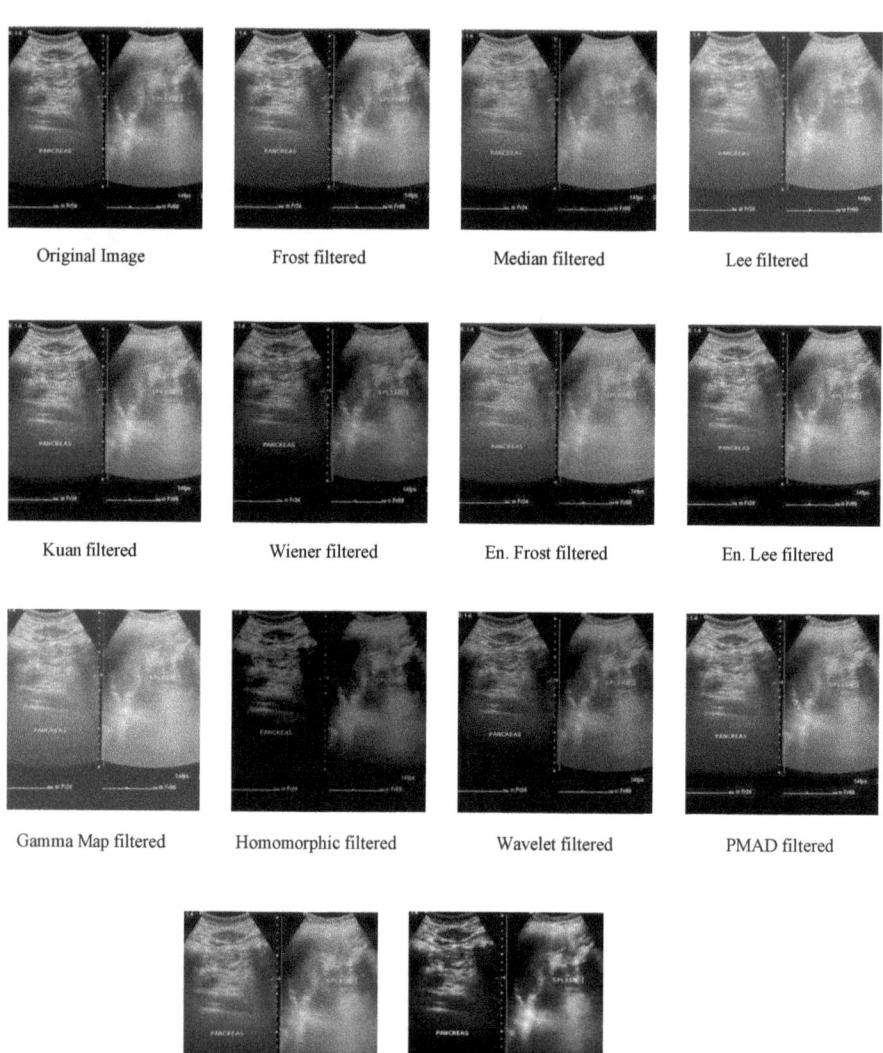

Fig A7 Original and despeckled images of pancreas - spleen in the PCMAT system

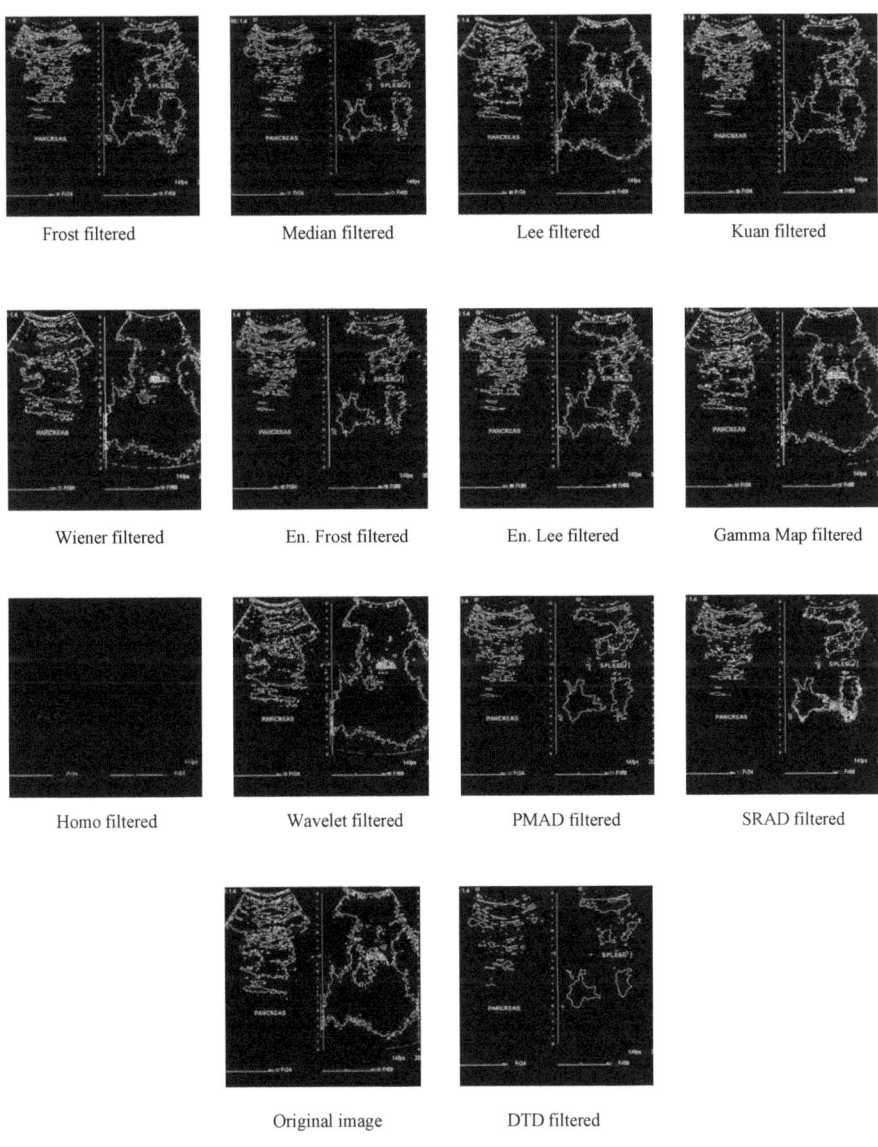

Fig A8 Canny edge detected images of pancreas - spleen in the PCMAT system

Table A4 Calculated performance metrics of the despeckling filters applied on the pancreas - spleen image in the PCMAT system

Group	Metrics	Frost	Median	Lee	Kuan	Homomorphic	Wiener	En. Frost	En Lee	GAM	Wavelet	PMAD	SRAD	DTD
Quality metrics	PSNR in dB	29.43	29.95	26.14	27.52	9.28	31.64	21.54	21.14	24.26	20.43	26.51	27.18	37.52
	PSNR (Canny) in dB	16.12	15.48	14.02	18.71	4.63	22.07	17.54	17.89	17.41	24.09	18.78	29.74	31.53
	AD	0.26	0.01	0.19	0.11	67.34	0.01	11.85	14.33	9.08	15.87	22.62	0.02	0.26
	MSE	117.43	121.54	148.25	132.45	8927.96	104.38	168.28	169.27	165.41	187.47	124.74	121.78	64.43
	MD	241	29	162	136	253.17	29	79	100	65	113	152	255	113
	NAE	0.04	0.04	0.06	0.05	0.97	0.04	0.17	0.28	0.13	0.23	0.32	0.11	0.09
	CNR	5.48	2.65	4.05	2.25	2.69	2.65	2.16	2.57	1.69	2.81	3.87	5.14	5.41
	FoM	0.51	0.49	0.47	0.48	0.09	0.54	0.49	0.51	0.52	0.55	0.38	0.51	0.57
Similarity metrics	SC	1.01	1.04	1.02	1.01	29.22	1.05	0.76	0.72	0.81	0.73	0.61	1.03	1.01
	CoC	0.99	0.99	0.98	0.99	0.94	0.99	0.97	0.97	0.98	0.96	0.94	0.96	0.98
	NCC	0.99	0.99	0.98	0.98	0.01	0.98	0.95	0.98	0.98	0.96	0.93	0.96	0.99
	IQI	0.97	0.88	0.86	0.87	0.98	0.97	0.92	0.92	0.97	0.96	0.88	0.92	0.98
	GAE	0.00	0.00	0.00	0.00	0.00	0.00	0.00	0.00	0.00	0.00	0.00	0.00	0.00
	NMSE	1.53	3.63	2.18	2.47	2.55	3.63	2.96	2.33	1.73	3.31	1.07	1.25	1.44
	MSSIM	0.9	0.91	0.88	0.91	0.05	0.95	0.77	0.71	0.84	0.68	0.56	0.63	0.72
Speckle metrics	SI	0.18	0.17	0.16	0.15	0.03	0.22	0.19	0.18	0.23	0.19	0.13	0.22	0.25
	ASNR	1.41	1.41	1.43	1.42	1.17	1.41	1.54	1.52	1.48	1.53	1.69	1.47	1.44
	IV	0.12	0.098	0.099	0.089	238.02	0.078	0.18	0.17	0.16	0.19	-0.18	0.23	0.19
	NSD	4.78	4.818	4.79	4.83	2.44	4.818	6.61	7.03	6.17	7.29	8.52	4.82	4.85
	ENL	2.06	2.04	2.05	2.03	4.03	2.04	1.48	1.44	1.59	1.35	1.15	2.04	2.02
	Execution time in sec	18.23	4.17	23.78	26.52	4.81	3.89	18.13	24.89	20.73	3.74	8.92	7.56	38.17

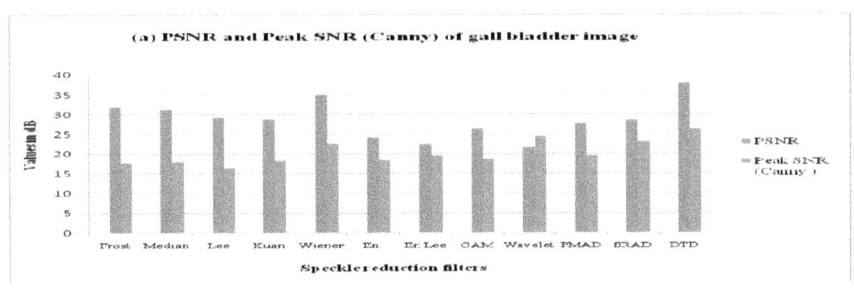
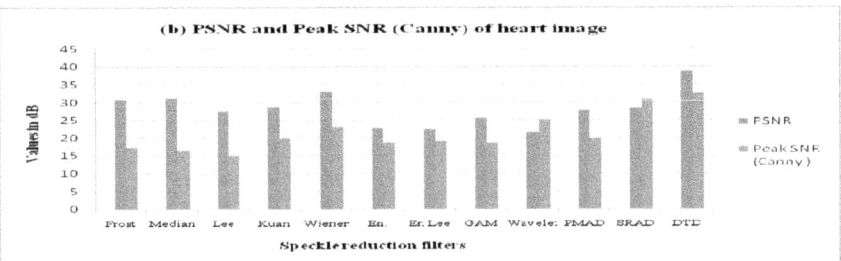
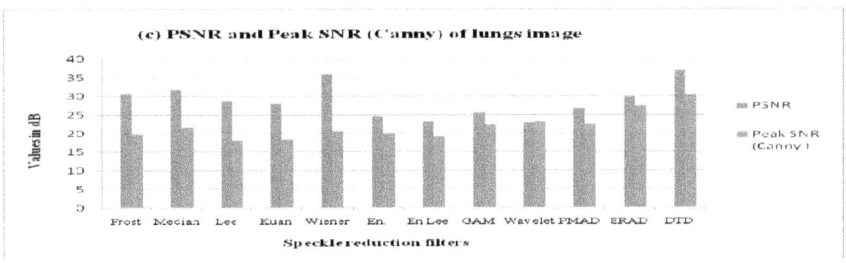
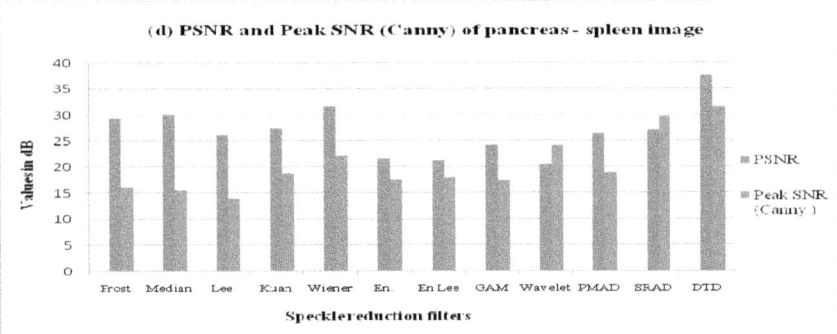

Fig A9 Histogram plot of the PSNR and Peak SNR (Canny) in the PCMAT system

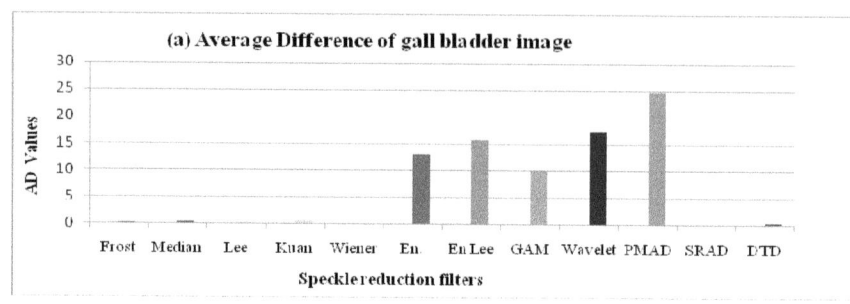

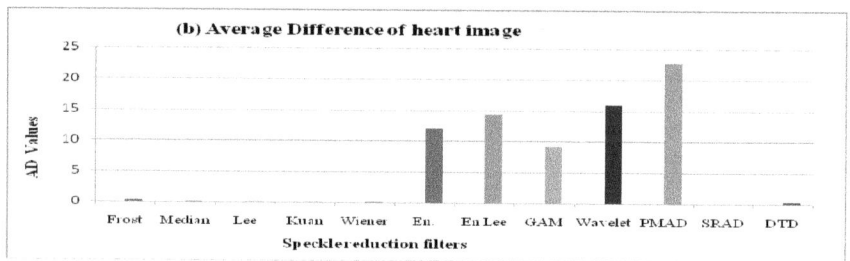

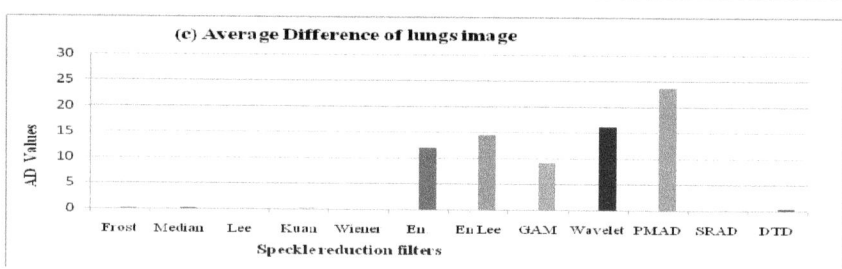

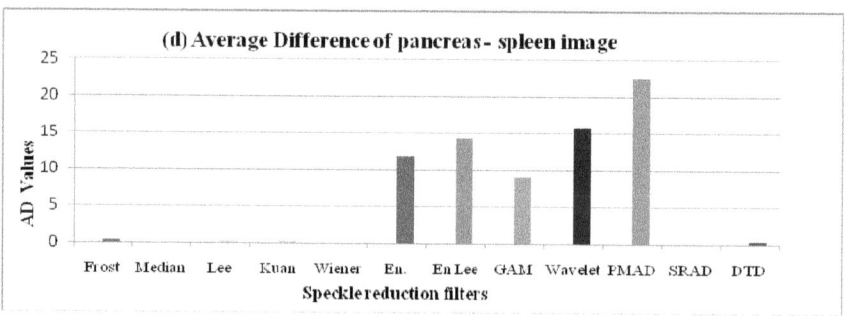

Fig A10 Histogram plot of the Average Difference (AD) in the PCMAT system

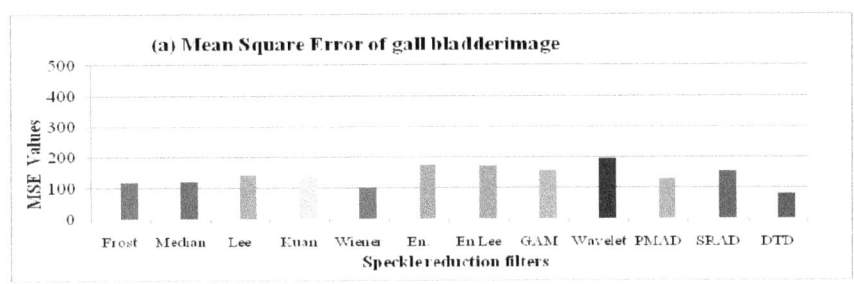
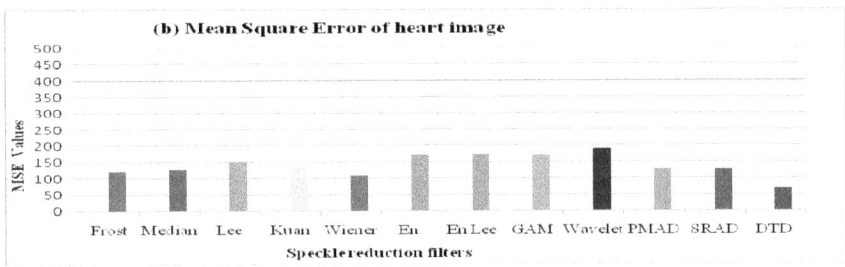
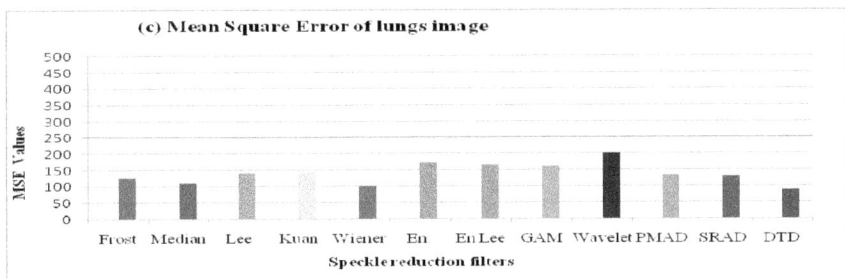
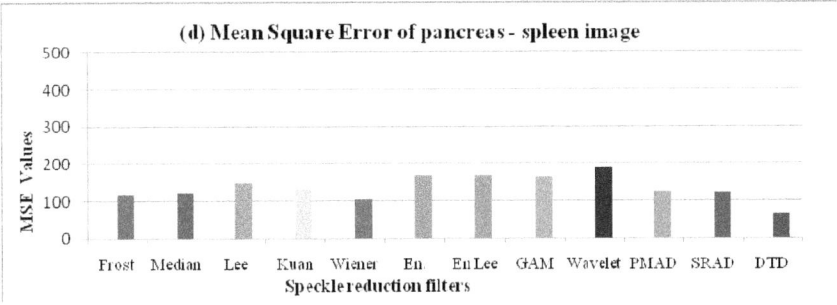

Fig A11 Histogram plot of the Mean Square Error (MSE) in the PCMAT system

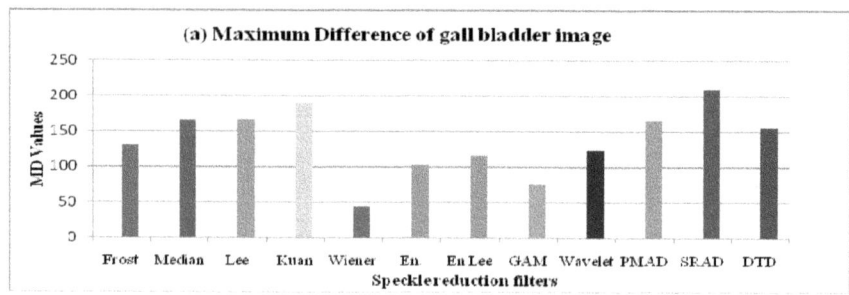
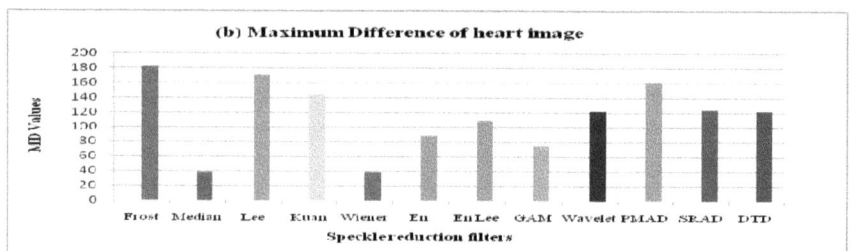
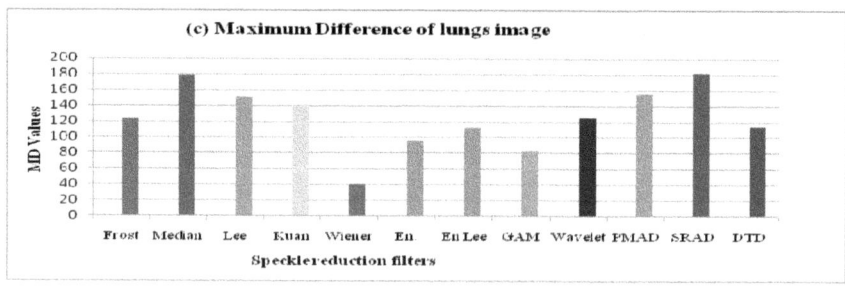
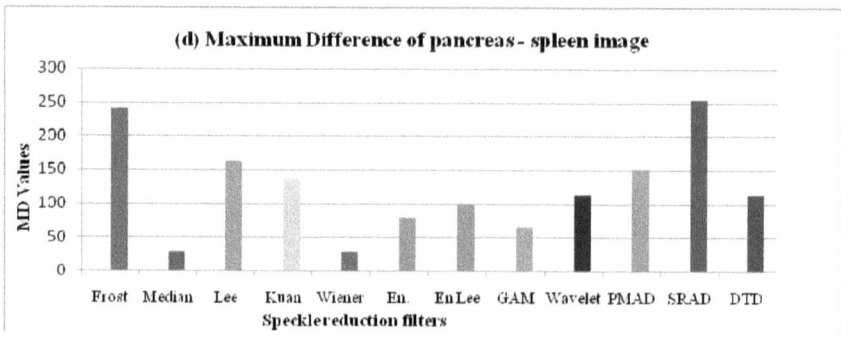

Fig A12 Histogram plot of the Maximum Difference (MD) in the PCMAT system

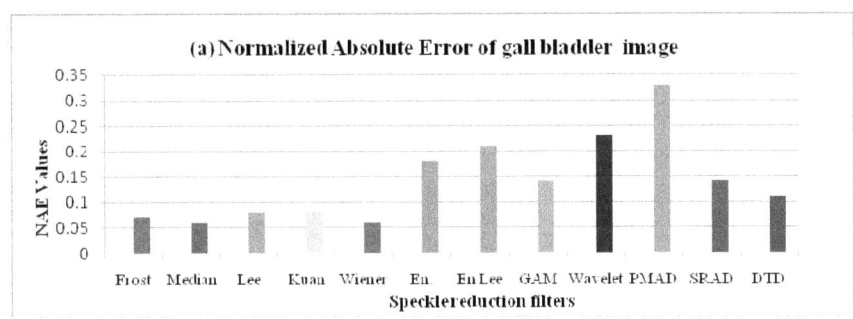
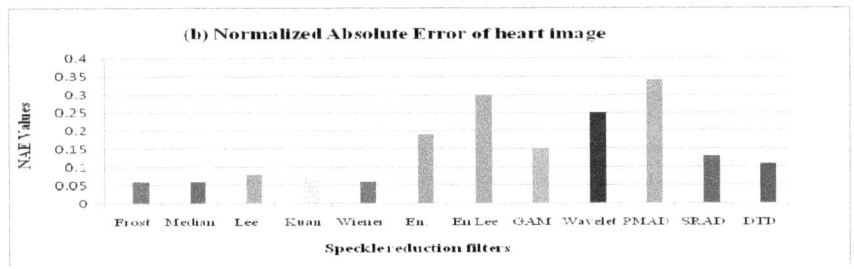
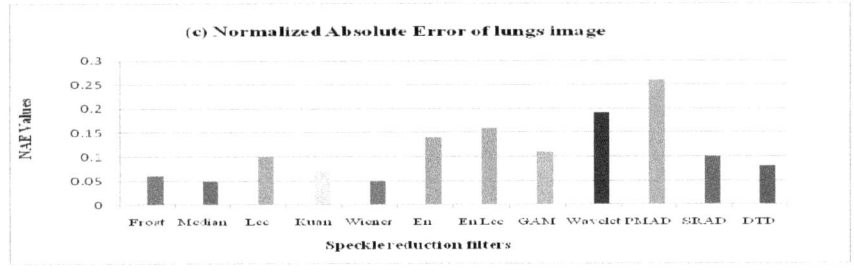
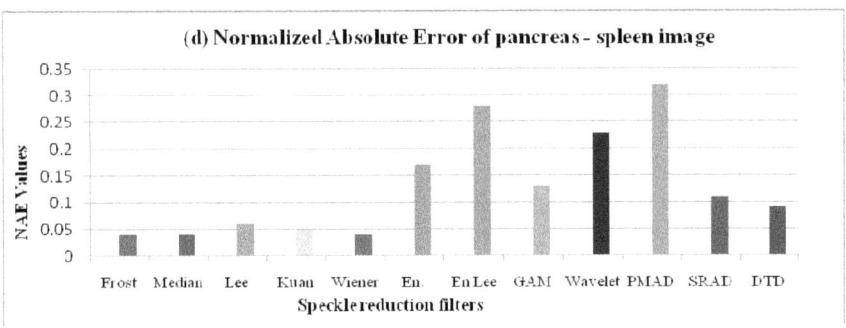

Fig A13 Histogram plot of the Normalized Absolute Error (NAE) in the PCMAT system

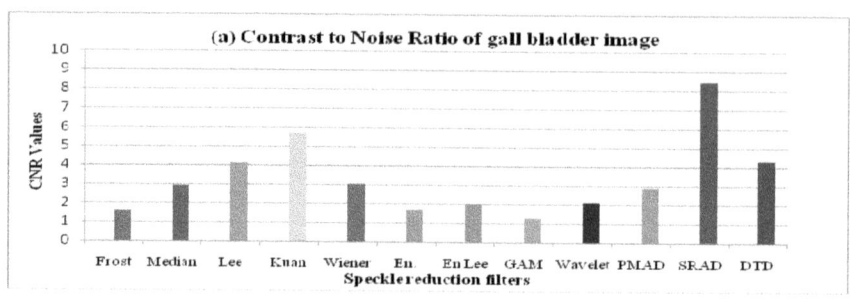
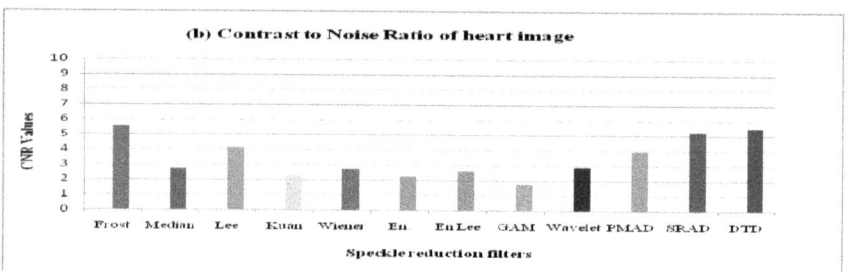
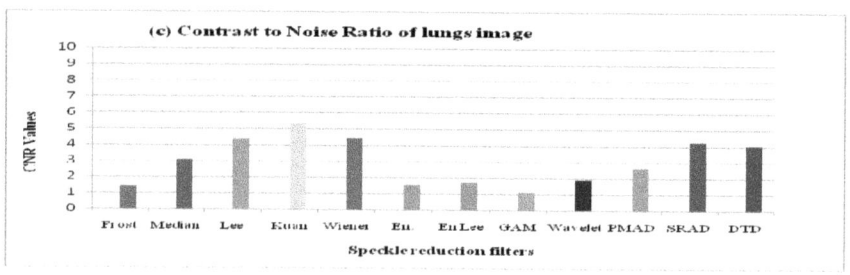
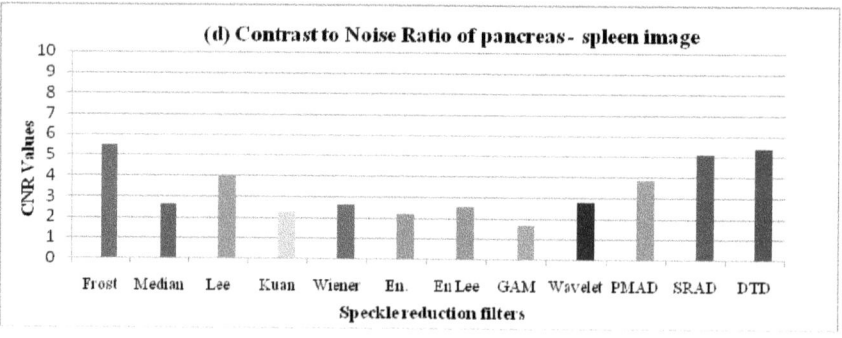

Fig A14 Histogram plot of the Contrast to Noise Ratio (CNR) in the PCMAT system

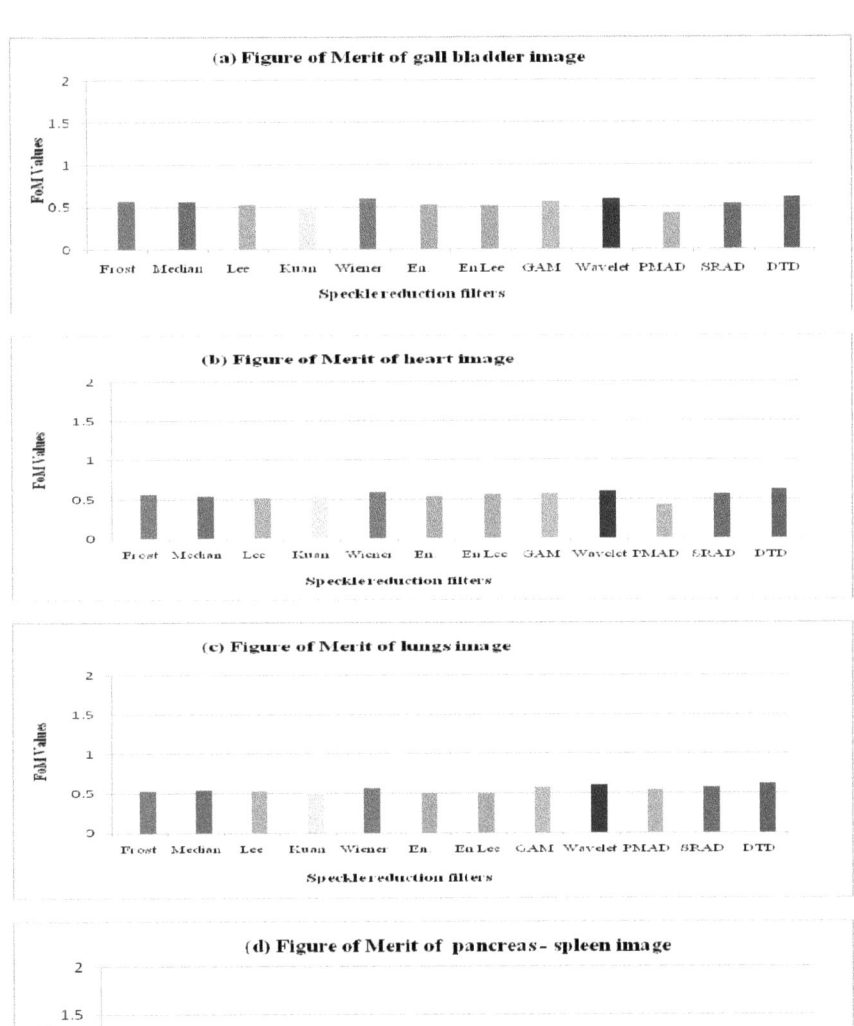

Fig A15 Histogram plot of the Figure of Merit (FoM) in the PCMAT system

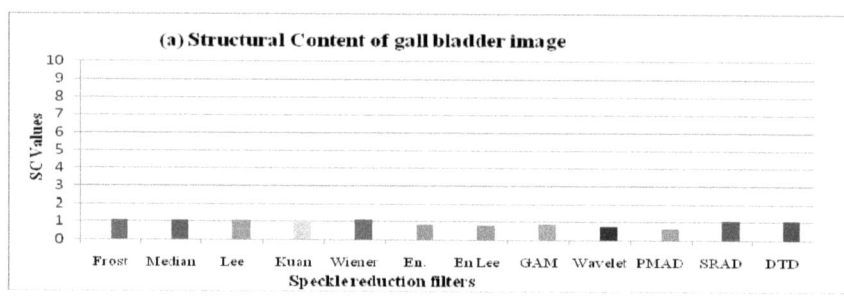
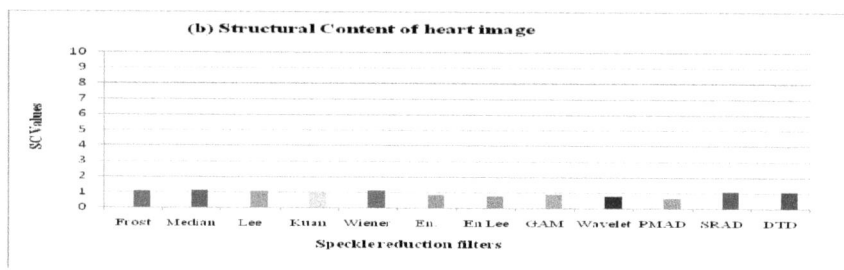
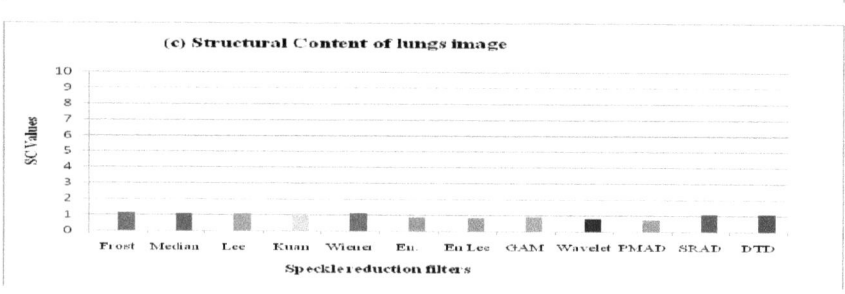
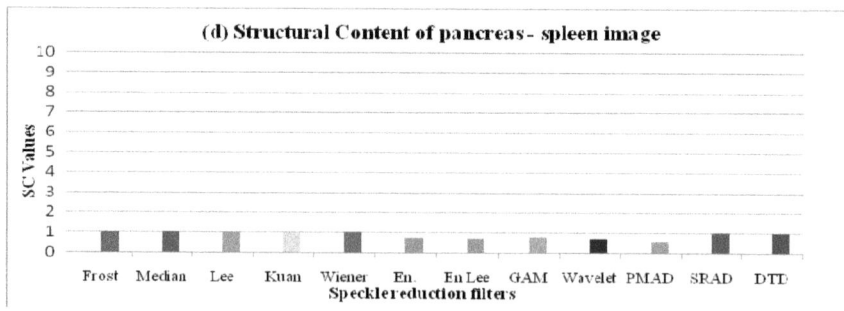

FigA16 Histogram plot of the Structural Content (SC) in the PCMAT system

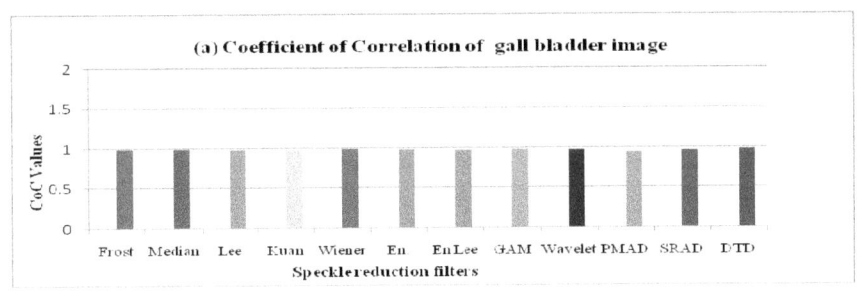
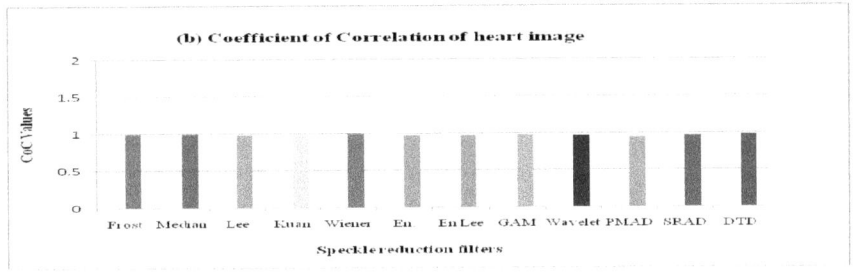
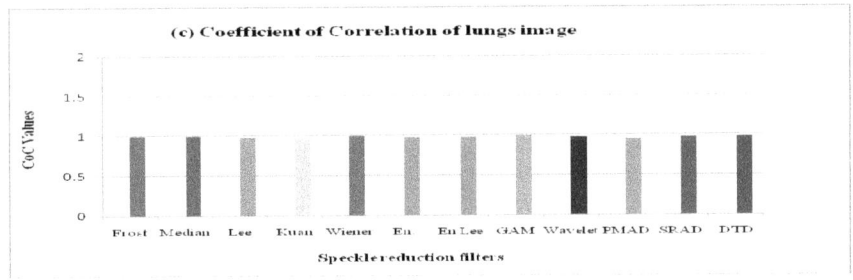
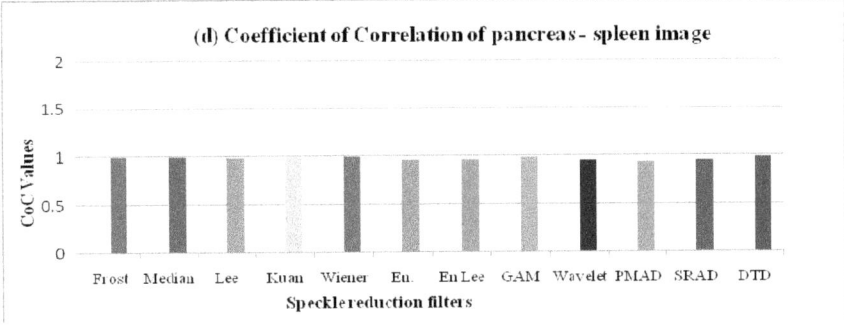

Fig A17 Histogram plot of the Coefficient of Correlation (CoC) in the PCMAT system

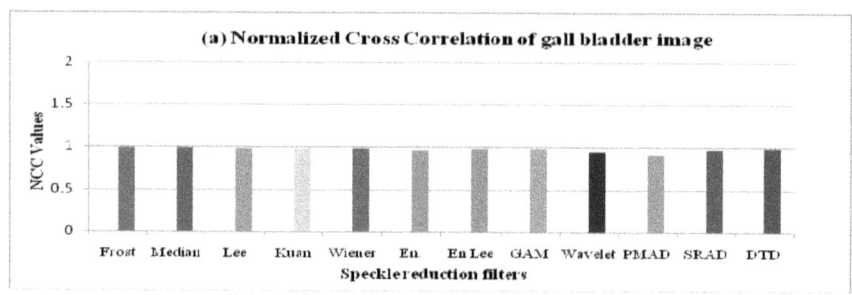
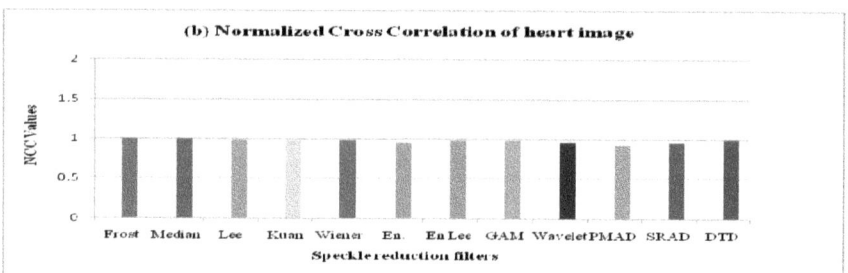
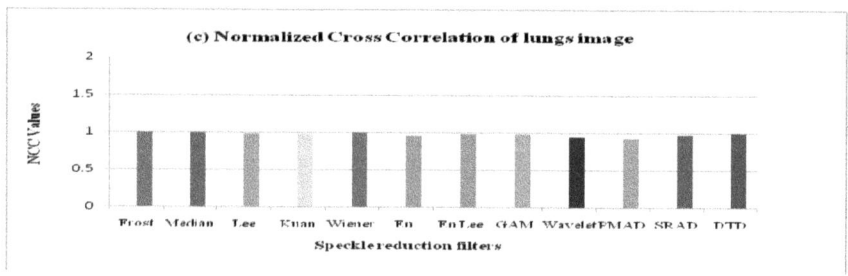
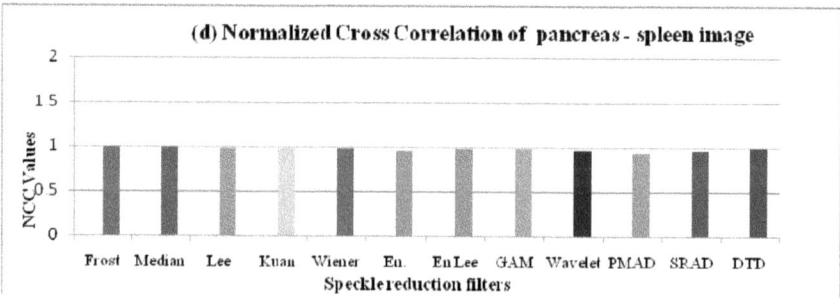

Fig A18 Histogram plot of the Normalized Cross Correlation (NCC) in the PCMAT system

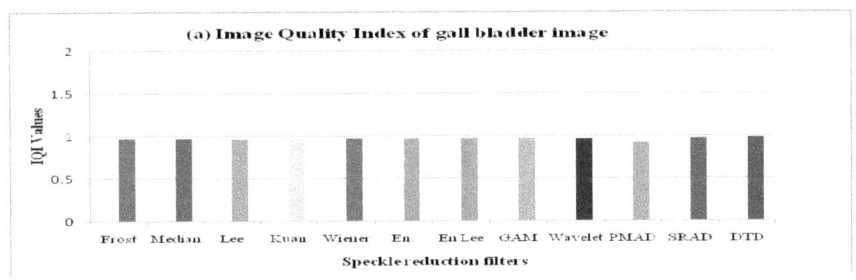
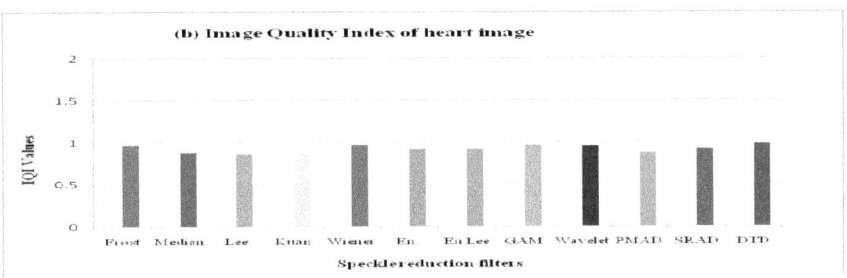
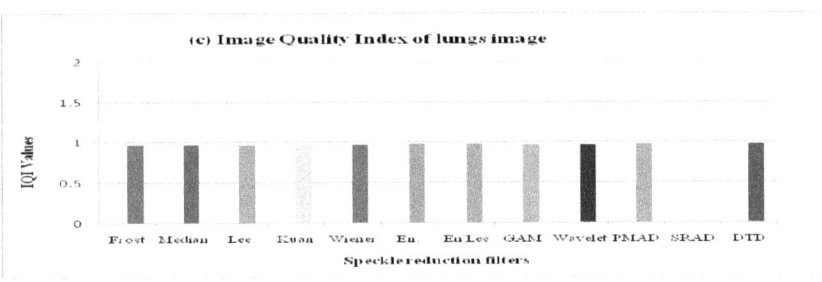
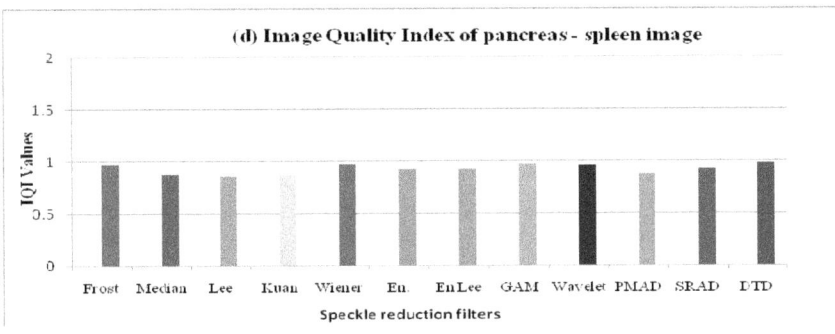

Fig A19 Histogram plot of the Image Quality Index (IQI) in the PCMAT system

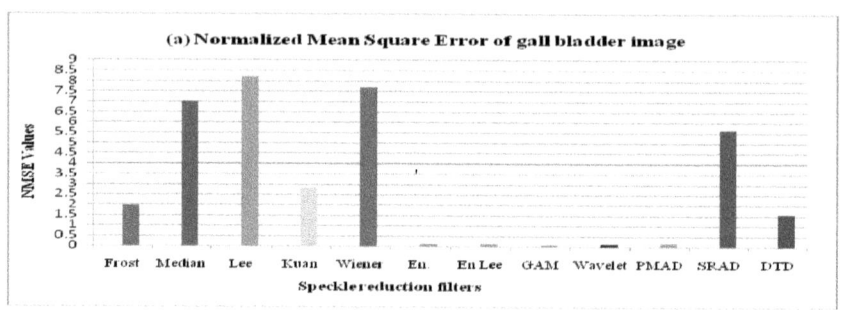
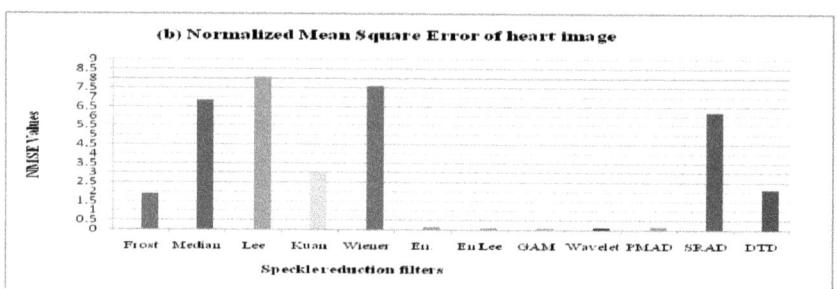
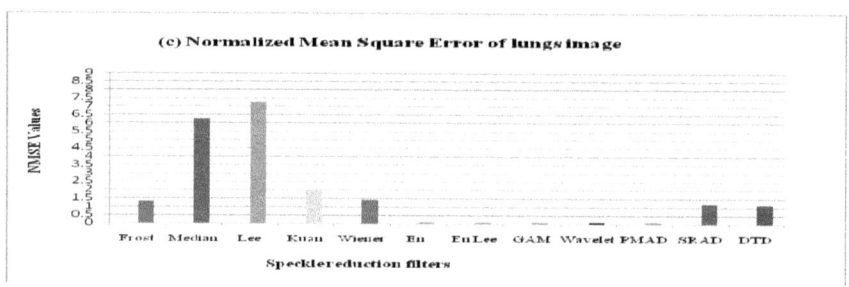
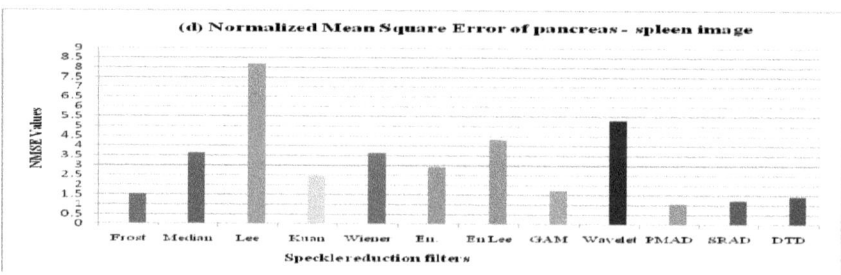

Fig A20 Histogram plot of the Normalized Mean Square Error (NMSE) in the PCMAT system

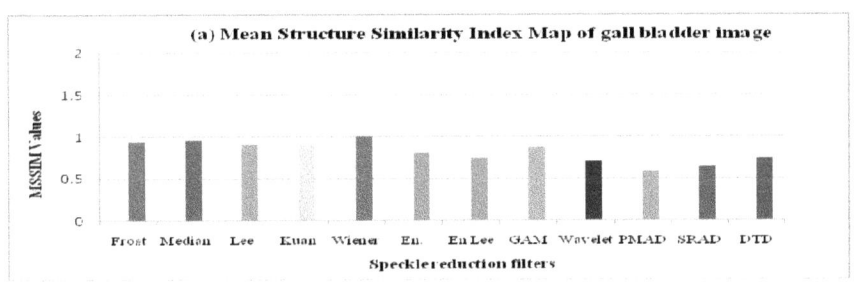
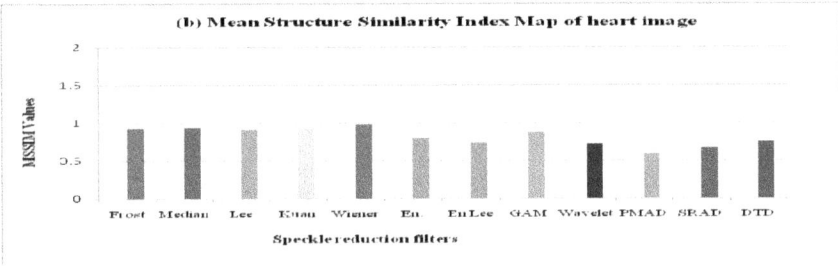
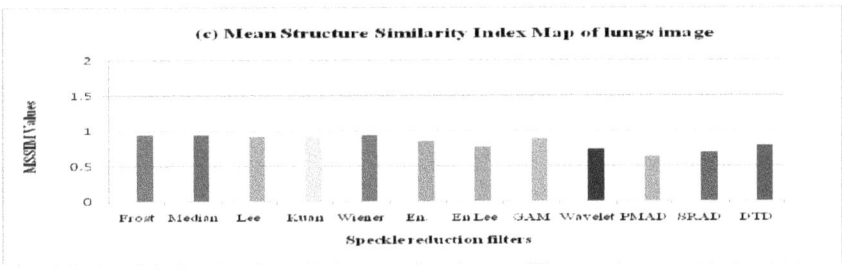
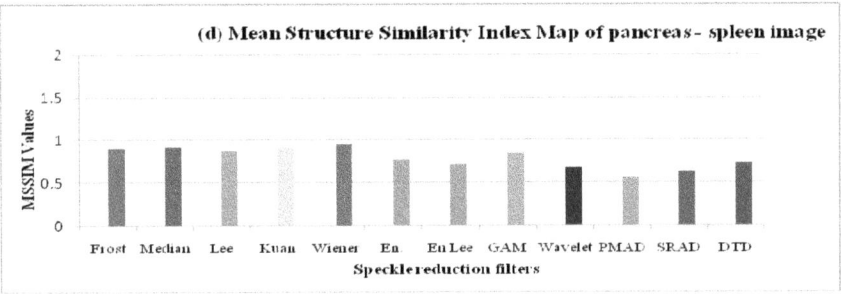

Fig A21 Histogram plot of the Mean Structure Similarity Index Map (MSSIM) in the PCMAT system

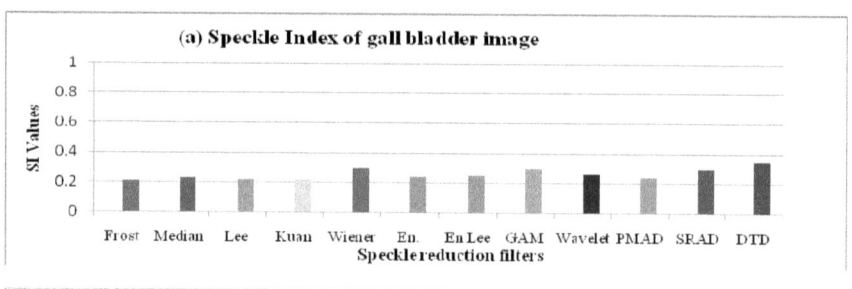
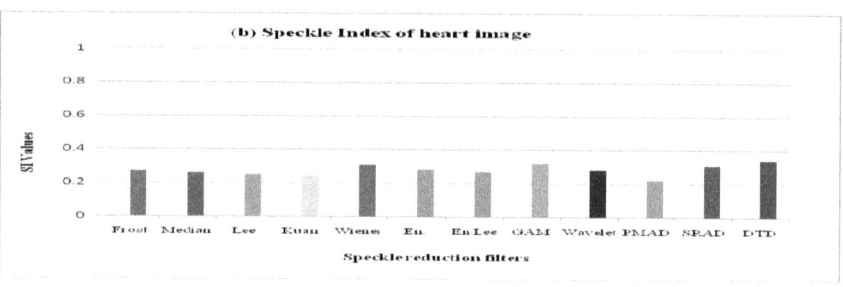
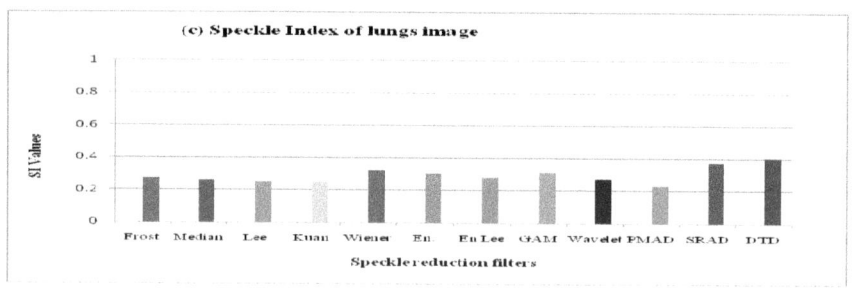
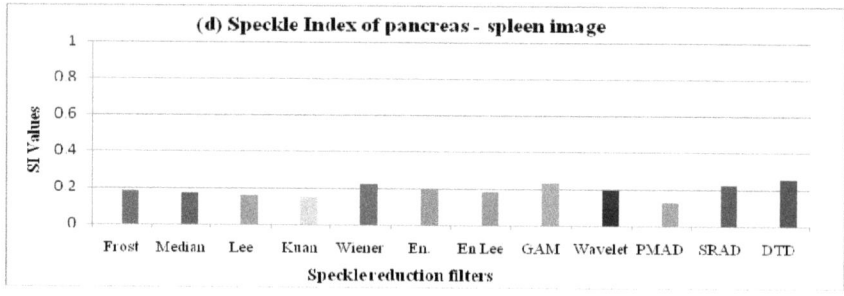

Fig A22 Histogram plot of the Speckle Index (SI) in the PCMAT system

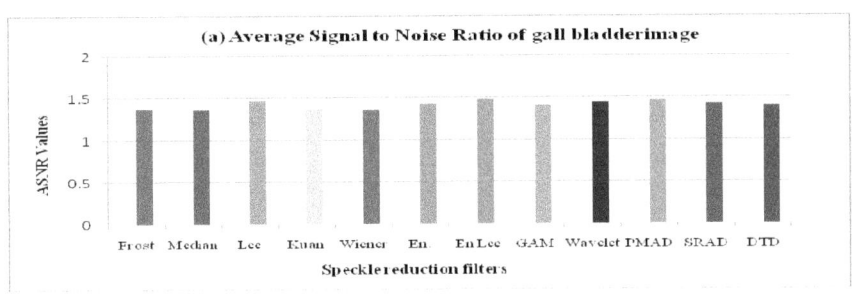
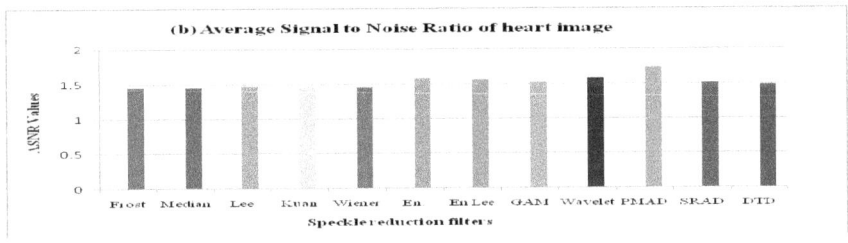
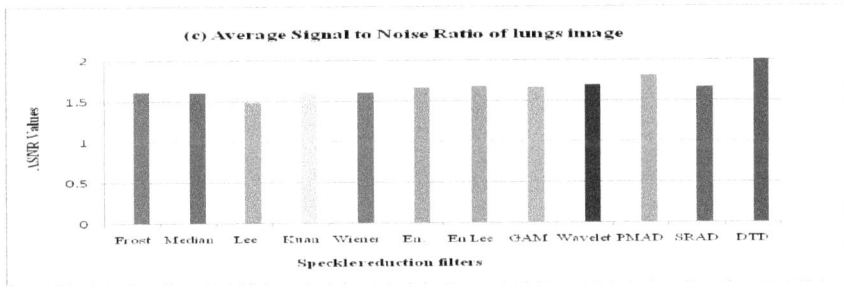
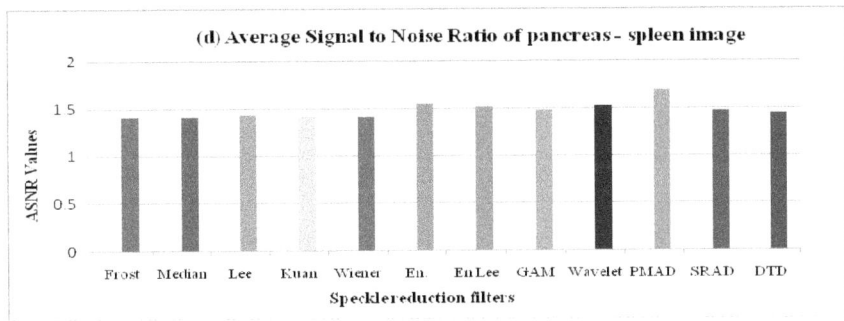

Fig A23 Histogram plot of the Average Signal to Noise Ratio (ASNR) in the PCMAT system

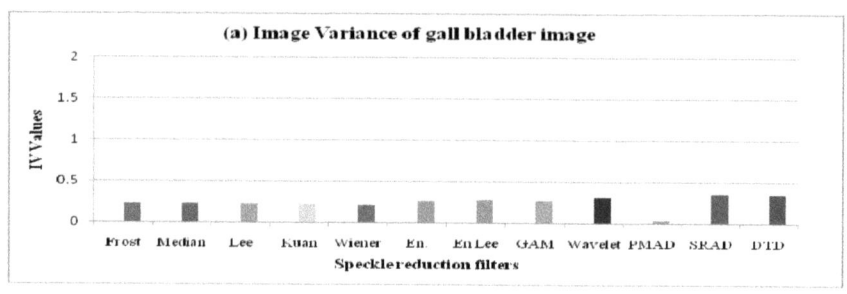
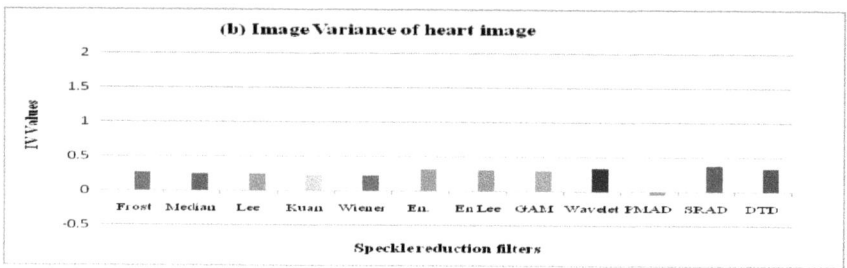
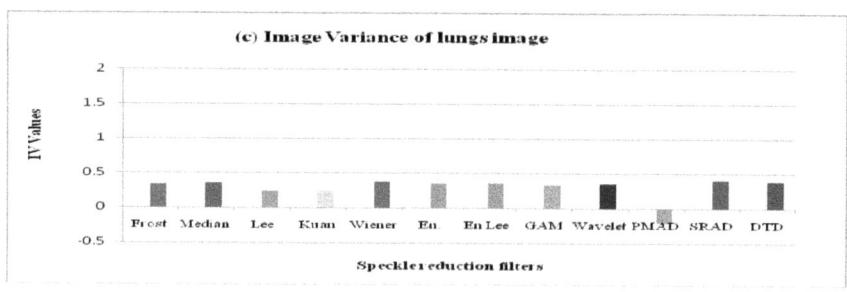
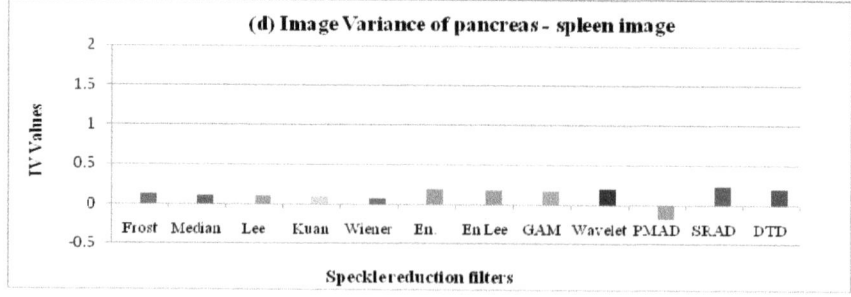

Fig A24 Histogram plot of the Image Variance (IV) in the PCMAT system

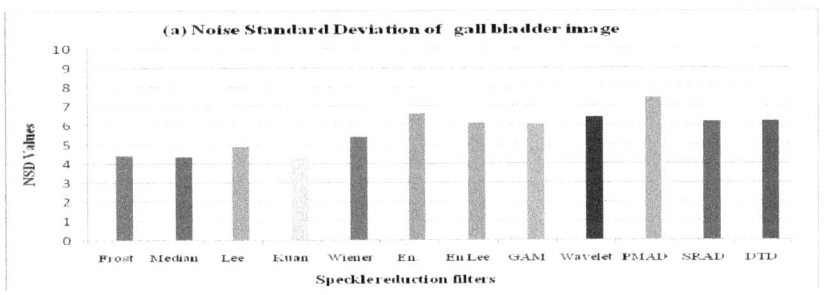
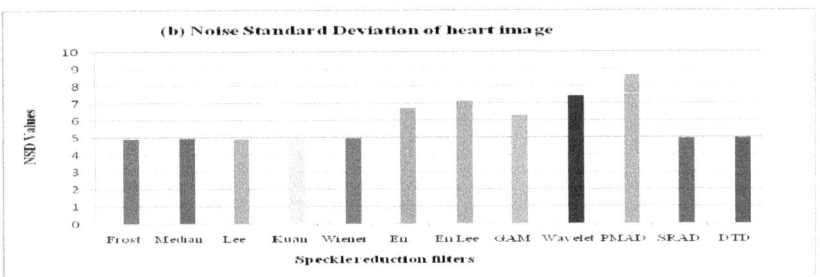
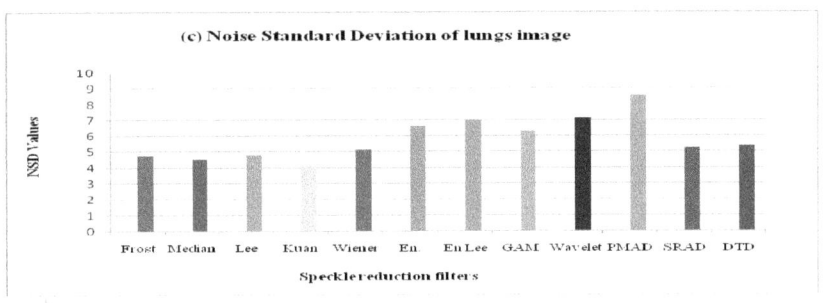
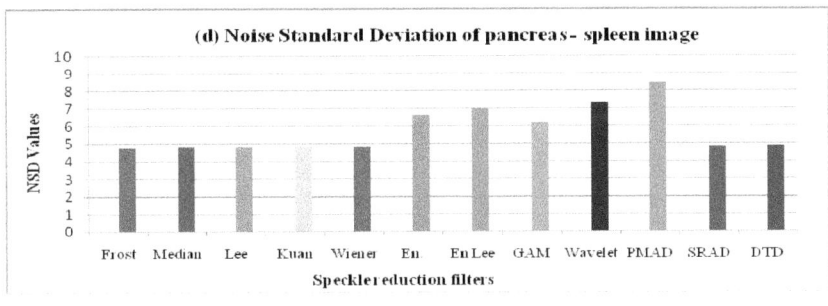

Fig A25 Histogram plot of the Noise Standard Deviation (NSD) in the PCMAT system

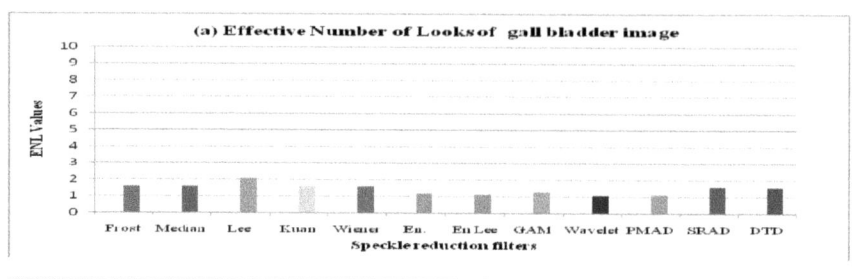
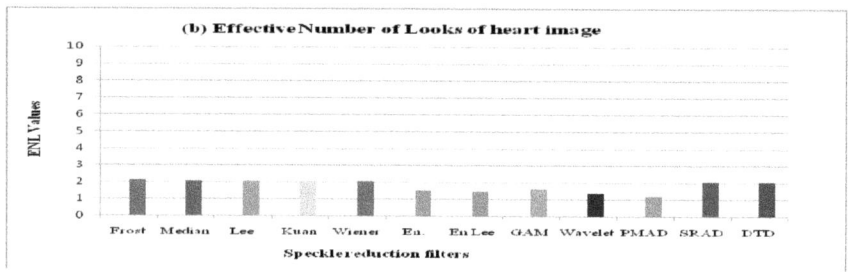
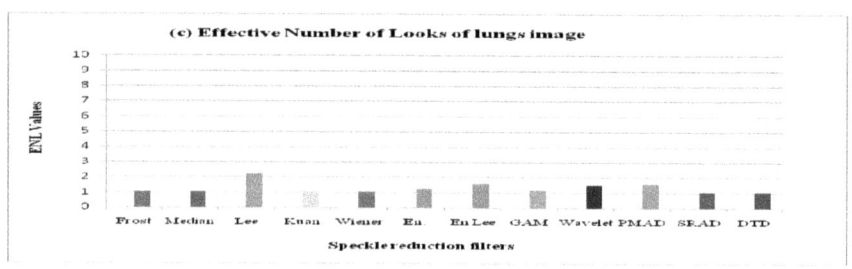
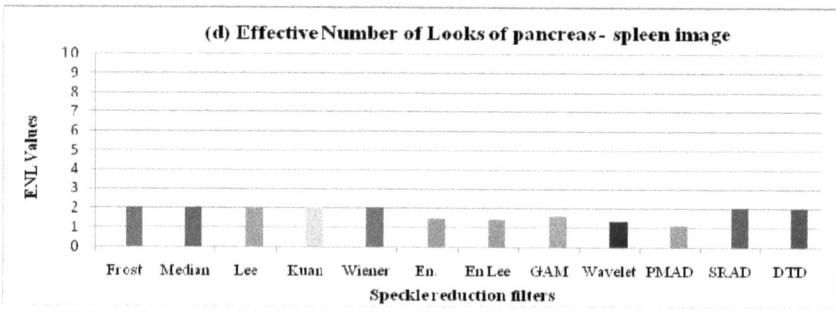

Fig A26 Histogram plot of the Effective Number of Looks (ENL) in the PCMAT system

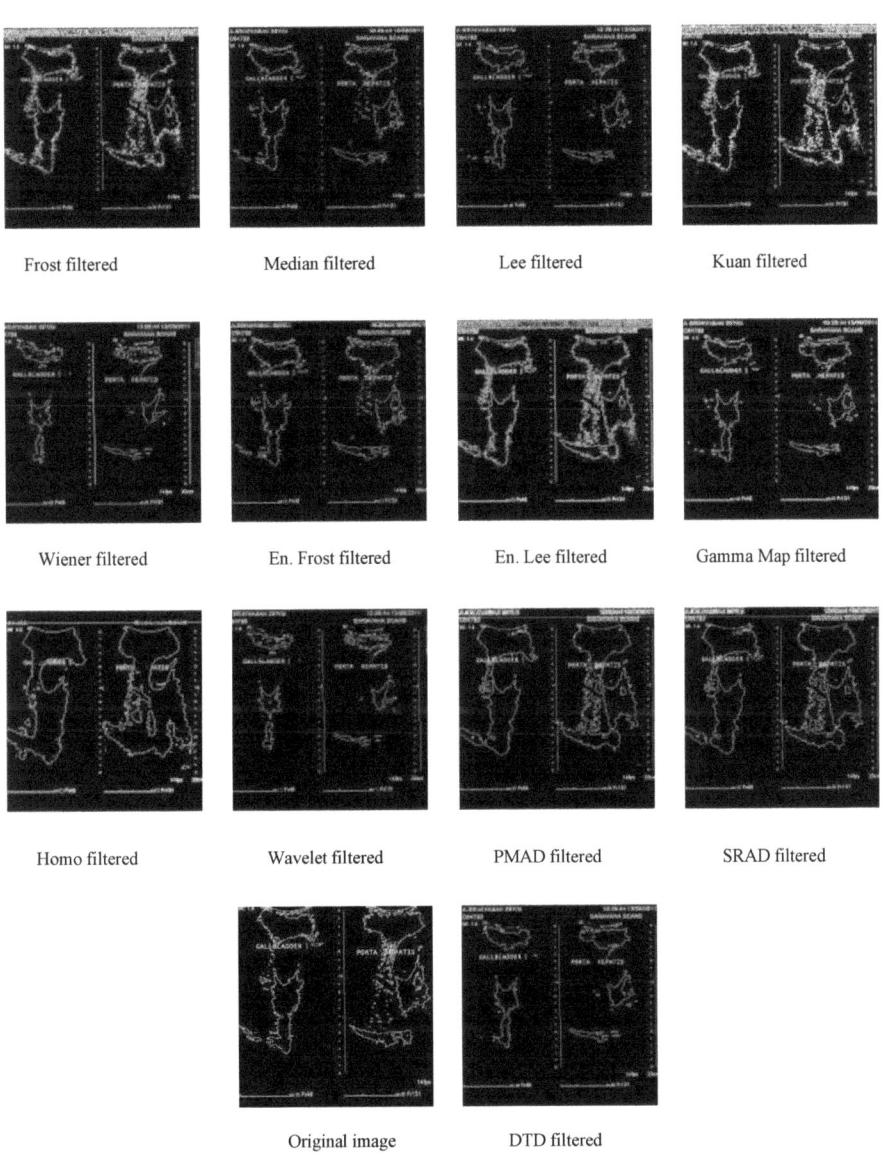

Fig B2 Canny edge detected images of gall bladder in the PCDSK system

Table B1 Calculated performance metrics of the despeckling filters applied on the gall bladder image in the PCDSK system

Group	Metrics	Frost	Median	Lee	Kuan	Homo morphic	Wiener	En. Frost	En Lee	GAM	Wavelet	PMAD	SRAD	DTD
Quality metrics	PSNR in dB	32.70	31.22	29.66	28.50	11.55	35.88	32.93	30.52	27.39	34.66	29.69	36.69	39.51
	PSNR (Canny) in dB	21.33	22.41	19.74	21.79	10.59	25.19	22.13	23.41	22.34	27.10	23.05	25.06	29.43
	AD	0.29	0.39	0.31	0.69	198.53	0.26	23.19	29.84	14.59	21.68	32.67	0.90	3.11
	MSE	115.04	120.98	140.95	136.68	7660.22	100.54	107.97	166.78	155.00	196.45	127.48	95.73	74.41
	MD	138.70	173.64	175.54	194.52	203.71	55.49	119.57	127.21	86.82	133.68	176.64	195.79	165.57
	NAE	0.06	0.03	0.04	0.07	1.77	0.03	0.15	0.18	0.11	0.20	0.30	0.11	0.08
	CNR	2.55	3.92	4.24	5.72	3.15	4.03	2.70	3.48	2.29	3.24	3.79	9.42	5.30
	FoM	0.62	0.59	0.52	0.56	0.24	0.68	0.53	0.57	0.59	0.62	0.43	0.59	0.72
Similarity metrics	SC	1.23	1.23	1.24	1.24	3881.58	1.29	0.99	0.95	1.04	0.93	0.84	1.26	1.24
	CoC	0.97	0.97	0.97	0.96	0.64	0.98	0.97	0.96	0.97	0.97	0.95	0.97	0.97
	NCC	0.98	0.99	0.98	0.98	0.02	0.98	0.96	0.98	0.98	0.94	0.91	0.97	0.99
	IQI	0.96	0.97	0.96	0.97	0.17	0.97	0.97	0.97	0.97	0.96	0.92	0.97	0.98
	GAE	0.00	0.00	0.00	0.00	0.00	0.00	0.00	0.00	0.00	0.00	0.00	0.00	0.00
	NMSE	2.09	7.13	8.34	2.95	1.16	7.82	0.23	0.23	0.22	0.24	0.29	5.78	1.68
	MSSIM	0.84	0.90	0.74	0.73	0.09	0.98	0.65	0.59	0.69	0.44	0.40	0.43	0.60
Speckle metrics	SI	0.29	0.27	0.25	0.18	0.22	0.23	0.29	0.39	0.41	0.26	0.29	0.46	0.36
	ASNR	1.48	1.47	1.57	1.47	1.16	1.46	1.53	1.59	1.51	1.55	1.57	1.53	1.50
	IV	0.29	0.28	0.30	0.28	253.35	0.27	0.32	0.34	0.33	0.37	0.10	0.40	0.42
	NSD	6.54	6.49	5.04	6.46	2.72	6.52	8.77	9.26	8.19	9.59	1.33	6.53	6.57
	ENL	1.69	1.73	2.02	1.71	1.11	1.70	1.28	1.22	1.37	1.18	1.22	1.69	1.68
	Execution time in sec	7.12	2.64	12.81	13.66	17.65	3.36	4.33	5.46	4.35	1.34	5.27	3.41	29.32

187

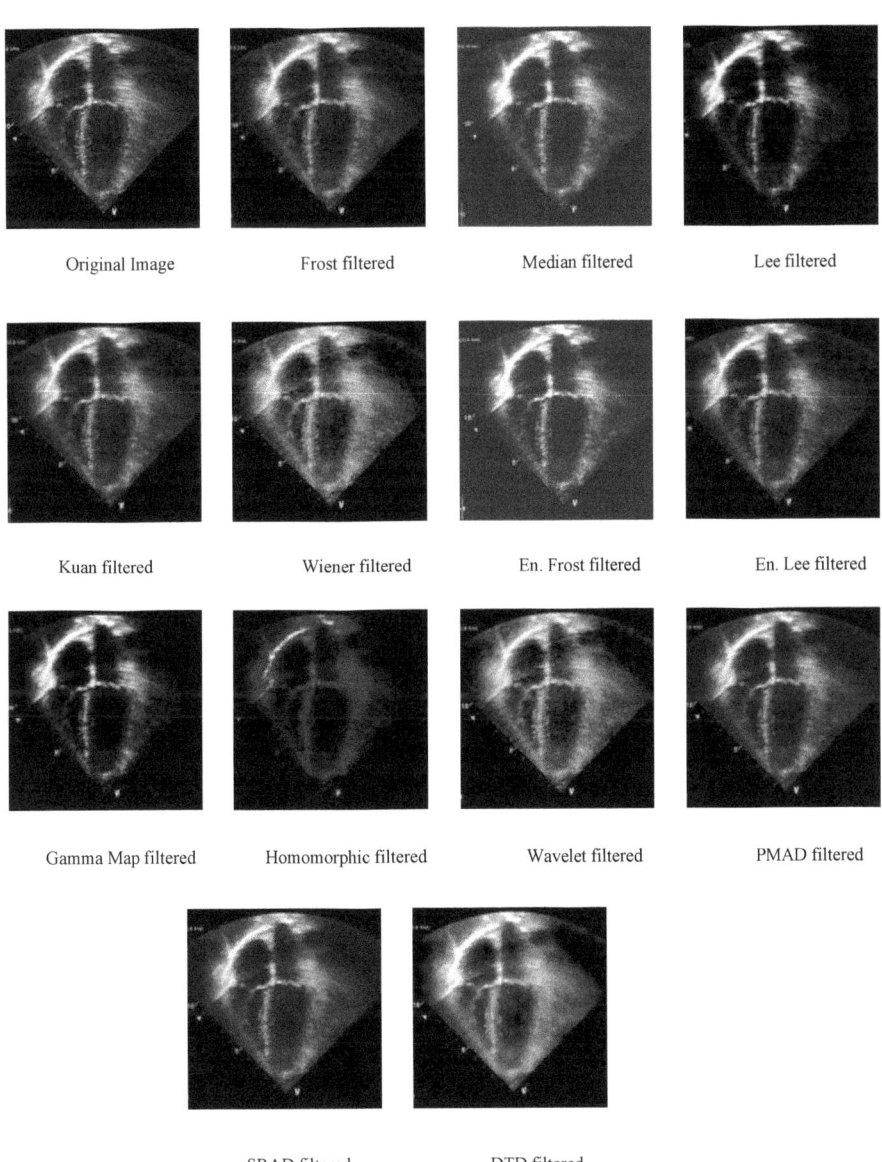

Fig B3 Original and despeckled images of heart in the PCDSK system

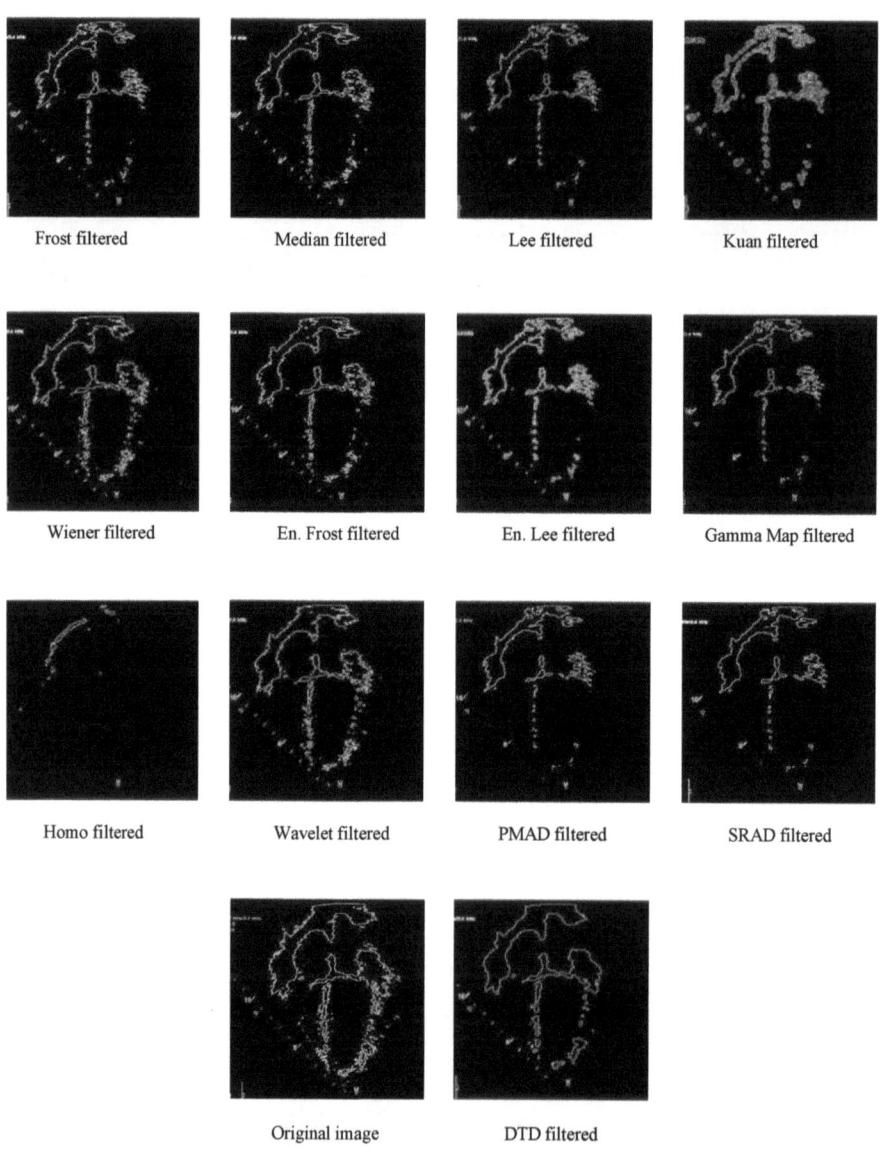

Fig B4 Canny edge detected images of heart in the PCDSK system

Table B2 Calculated performance metrics of the despeckling filters applied on the heart image in the PCDSK system

Group	Metrics	Frost	Median	Lee	Kuan	Homo morphic	Wiener	En. Frost	En Lee	GAM	Wavelet	PMAD	SRAD	DTD
Quality metrics	PSNR in dB	32.70	33.22	29.41	30.79	2.55	34.91	24.81	24.41	26.53	23.70	29.78	30.45	39.22
	PSNR (Canny)in dB	20.70	20.33	18.39	22.95	9.26	26.04	22.65	23.43	22.04	28.32	23.41	34.37	36.16
	AD	0.47	0.24	0.46	0.32	72.55	0.26	12.06	14.54	9.29	16.08	22.24	0.23	0.50
	MSE	120.36	123.77	150.25	134.96	8976.21	106.91	170.68	171.81	165.64	189.91	126.97	124.00	65.66
	MD	110.63	48.92	171.54	155.81	192.69	48.55	98.59	119.53	84.79	132.48	171.60	176.67	132.48
	NAE	0.03	0.03	0.05	0.04	0.96	0.03	0.16	0.27	0.12	0.22	0.31	0.10	0.08
	CNR	6.63	3.80	5.20	3.40	3.84	3.80	3.31	3.72	2.84	3.96	5.02	6.29	6.56
	FoM	0.61	0.64	0.58	0.61	0.20	0.76	0.55	0.56	0.65	0.66	0.45	0.56	0.68
Similarity metrics	SC	1.23	1.26	1.24	1.23	29.44	1.27	0.98	0.94	1.03	0.95	0.83	1.25	1.23
	CoC	0.98	0.98	0.98	0.96	0.47	0.98	0.97	0.96	0.97	0.97	0.95	0.97	0.99
	NCC	0.97	0.98	0.98	0.98	0.04	0.98	0.96	0.98	0.98	0.94	0.91	0.97	0.98
	IQI	0.97	0.98	0.96	0.97	0.32	0.97	0.97	0.97	0.98	0.96	0.92	0.97	0.98
	GAE	0.00	0.00	0.00	0.00	0.00	0.00	0.00	0.00	0.00	0.00	0.00	0.00	0.00
	NMSE	1.73	3.85	8.38	2.67	9.75	3.83	3.16	4.53	1.93	5.51	1.27	1.45	1.64
	MSSIM	0.83	0.87	0.75	0.69	0.05	0.97	0.64	0.63	0.72	0.48	0.33	0.48	0.63
Speckle metrics	SI	0.35	0.34	0.33	0.32	0.20	0.39	0.36	0.35	0.40	0.36	0.30	0.39	0.42
	ASNR	1.55	1.55	1.57	1.56	1.31	1.55	1.68	1.66	1.62	1.67	1.83	1.61	1.58
	IV	0.32	0.30	0.30	0.29	238.22	0.28	0.38	0.37	0.36	0.39	0.02	0.43	0.39
	NSD	5.03	5.07	5.04	5.08	2.69	5.07	6.86	7.28	6.42	7.54	8.77	5.07	5.10
	ENL	2.19	2.17	2.18	2.16	2.16	2.17	1.61	1.57	1.72	1.48	1.28	2.17	2.15
	Execution time in sec	8.19	2.18	11.57	4.13	17.63	2.13	4.14	5.73	2.39	2.27	4.63	3.27	24.53

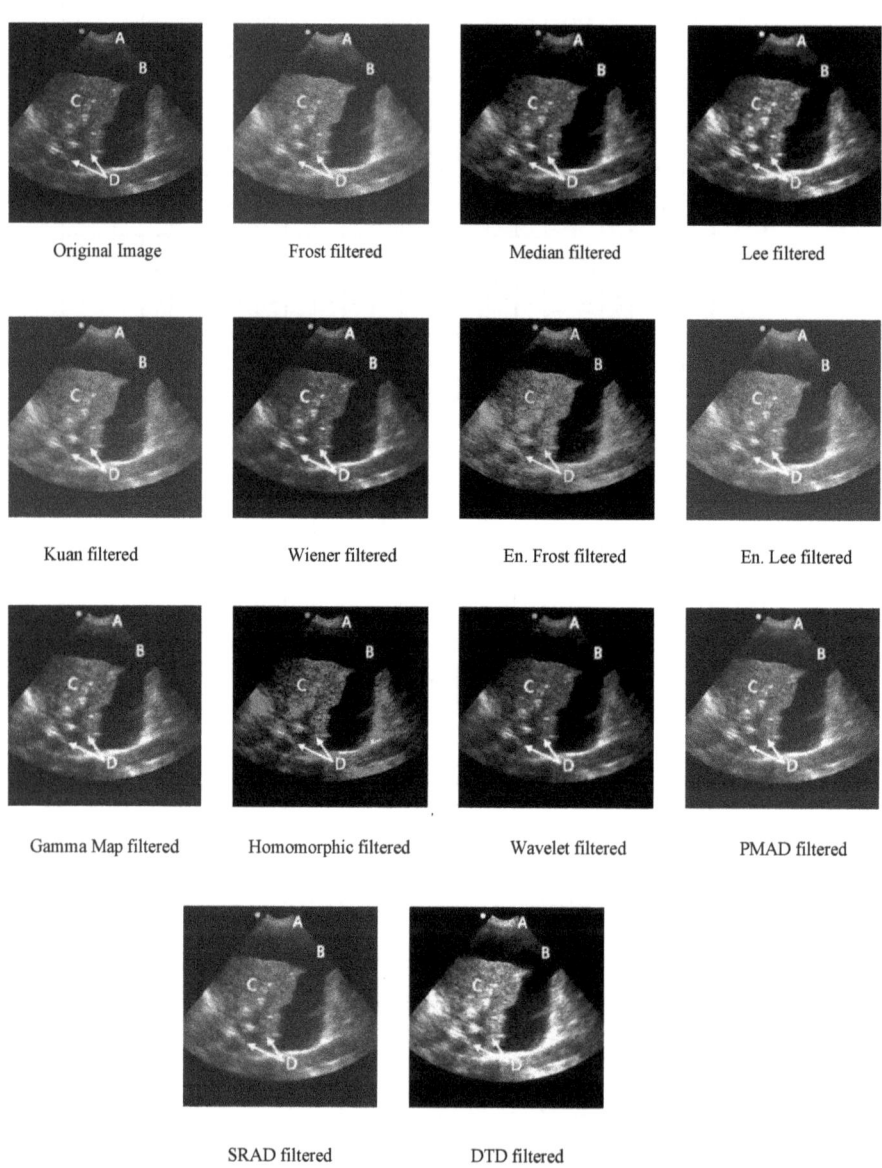

Fig B5 Original and despeckled images of lungs in the PCDSK system

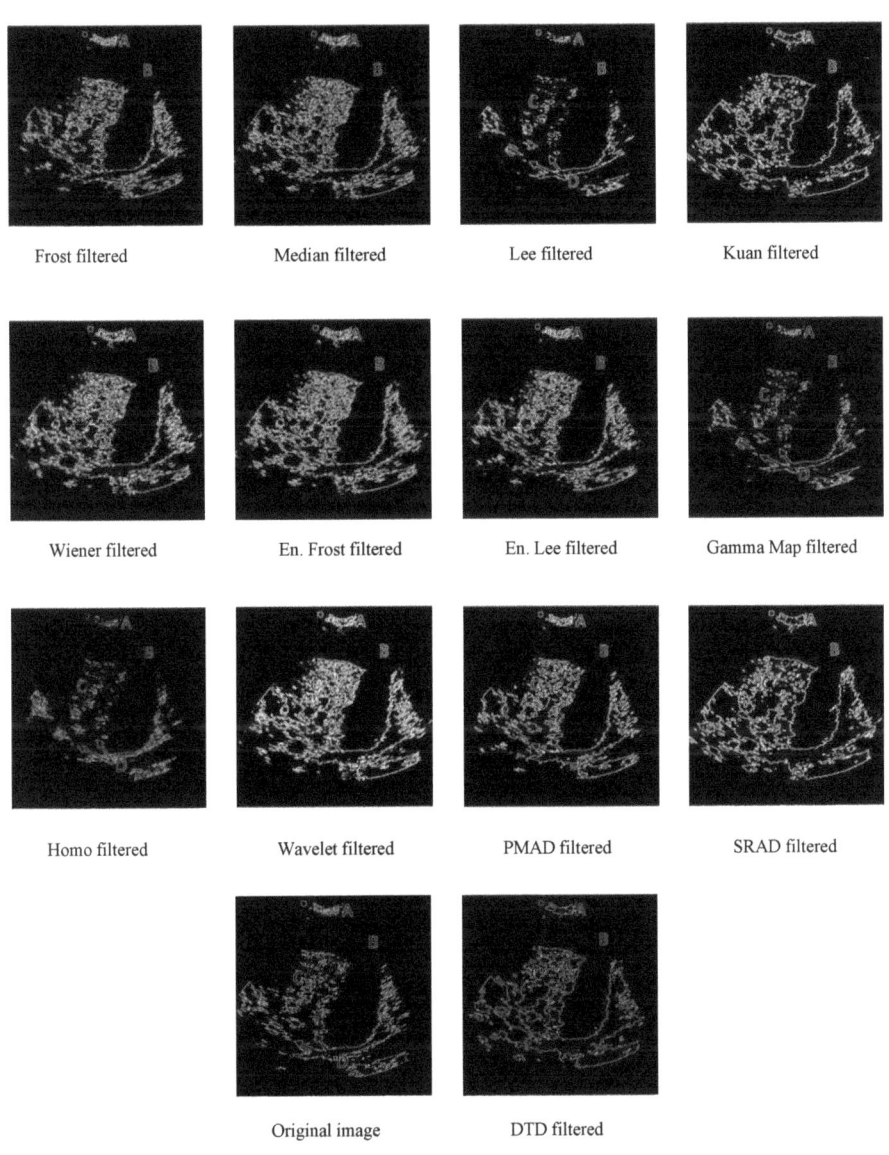

Fig B6 Canny edge detected images of lungs in the PCDSK system

Table B3 Calculated performance metrics of the despeckling filters applied on the lungs image in the PCDSK system

Group	Metrics	Frost	Median	Lee	Kuan	Homo morphic	Wiener	En. Frost	En Lee	GAM	Wavelet	PMAD	SRAD	DTD
Quality metrics	PSNR in dB	32.65	33.81	30.73	30.27	12.56	37.27	26.63	24.16	27.58	24.76	28.55	31.5	38.76
	PSNR (Canny)in dB	23.36	25.12	21.61	21.88	9.86	24.21	23.65	22.77	25.89	26.72	26.06	30.86	33.77
	AD	0.42	0.45	0.36	0.62	196.52	0.26	11.13	13.83	9.31	16.44	22.94	0.32	3.6
	MSE	127.84	113.54	144.38	144.98	7253.05	103.74	175.65	168.36	163.77	201.58	135.36	132.4	91.69
	MD	133.78	188.68	161.6	211.44	226.71	51.52	106.88	122.59	93.67	136.14	166.84	182.65	124.72
	NAE	0.03	0.04	0.07	0.04	0.97	0.02	0.11	0.13	0.08	0.16	0.23	0.07	0.05
	CNR	2.48	4.93	5.39	6.41	3.55	5.59	2.6	2.78	2.16	2.96	3.68	7.31	5.19
	FoM	0.59	0.6	0.59	0.57	0.25	0.62	0.56	0.55	0.63	0.66	0.6	0.63	0.68
Similarity metrics	SC	1.29	1.23	1.24	1.23	5240.37	1.27	1.03	1	1.07	0.98	0.9	1.24	1.23
	CoC	0.96	0.97	0.96	0.95	0.32	0.98	0.97	0.96	0.97	0.97	0.95	0.96	0.98
	NCC	0.98	0.98	0.98	0.98	0.03	0.98	0.96	0.98	0.96	0.96	0.94	0.97	0.98
	IQI	0.98	0.98	0.96	0.97	0.26	0.97	0.97	0.97	0.98	0.96	0.92	0.97	0.98
	GAE	0.00	0.00	0.00	0.00	0.00	0.00	0.00	0.00	0.00	0.00	0.00	0.00	0.00
	NMSE	1.4	6.35	7.49	2.12	9.9	1.49	0.21	0.22	0.2	0.22	0.25	1.31	1.25
	MSSIM	0.9	0.88	0.73	0.69	0.036	0.93	0.66	0.63	0.7	0.49	0.35	0.44	0.67
	SI	0.35	0.34	0.33	0.33	0.26	0.4	0.38	0.36	0.39	0.35	0.31	0.45	0.48
Speckle metrics	ASNR	1.71	1.7	1.58	1.7	1.26	1.7	1.76	1.78	1.76	1.79	1.91	1.76	159.14
	IV	0.54	0.56	0.45	0.45	179.59	0.58	0.56	0.57	0.54	0.56	0	0.61	0.59
	NSD	10	9.93	4.76	9.89	2.88	9.97	1.47	1.53	1.41	1.57	1.78	9.97	10.06
	ENL	1.14	1.14	2.29	1.15	13.86	1.14	2.17	2.79	2.61	2.57	2.68	1.14	1.14
	Execution time in sec	9.17	3.66	12.34	13.62	17.36	3.87	3.65	4.27	2.31	2.26	3.17	3.94	24.42

193

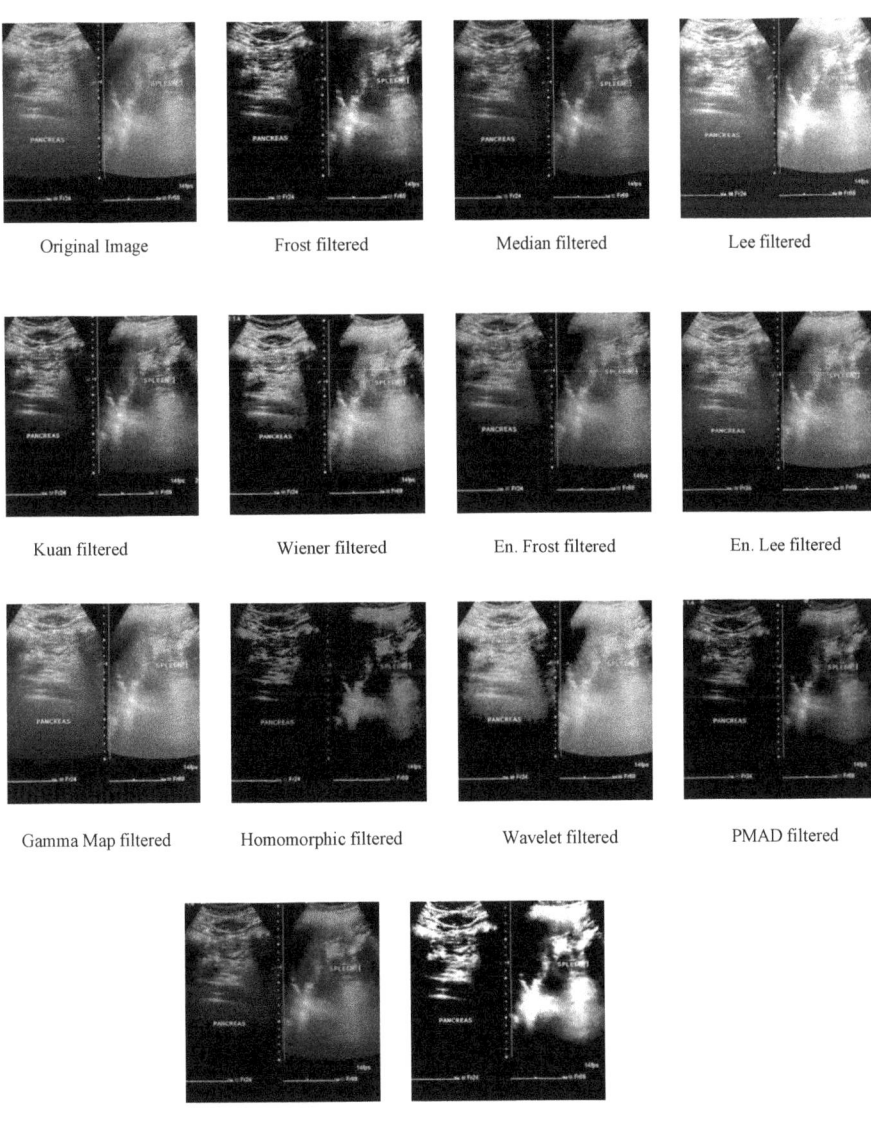

Fig B7 Original and despeckled images of pancreas - spleen in the PCDSK system

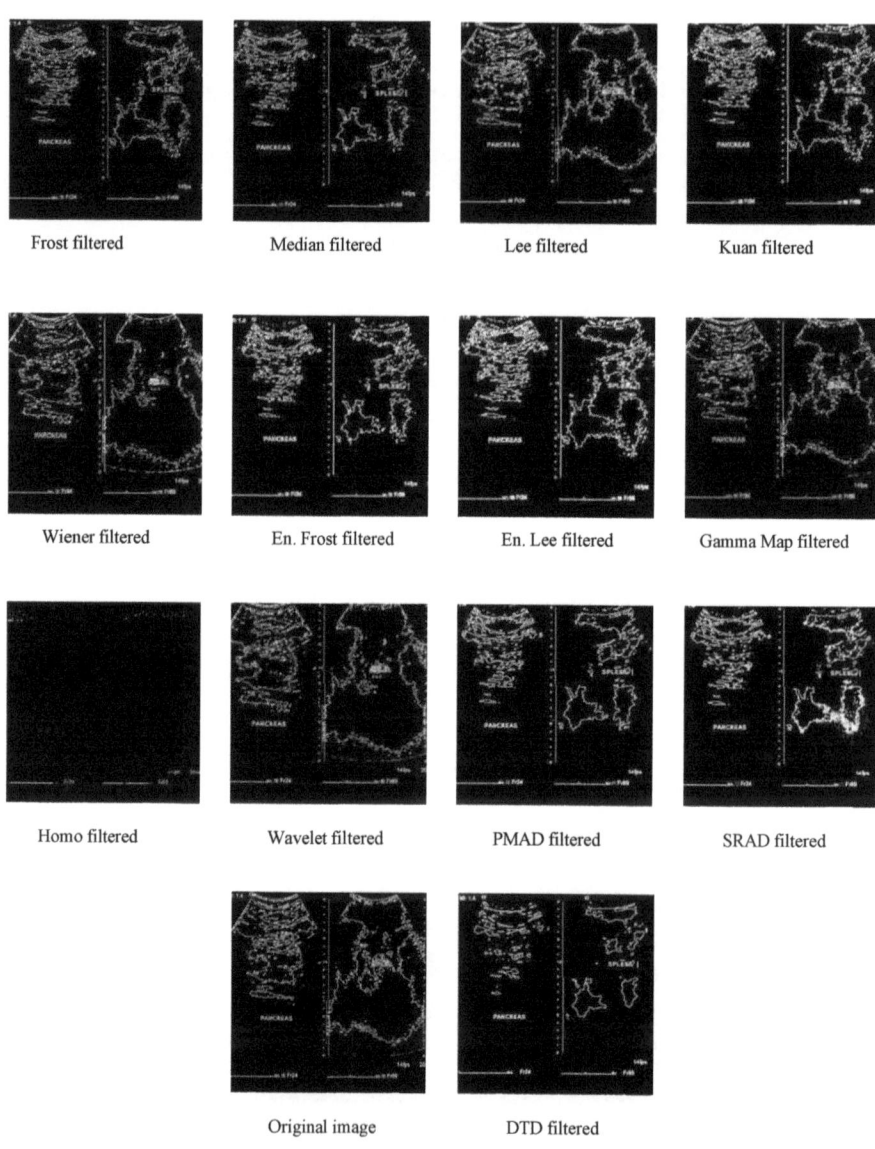

Fig B8 Canny edge detected images of pancreas - spleen in the PCDSK system

Table B4 Calculated performance metrics of the despeckling filters applied on the pancreas - spleen image in the PCDSK system

Group	Metrics	Frost	Median	Lee	Kuan	Homo morphic	Wiener	En. Frost	En Lee	GAM	Wavelet	PMAD	SRAD	DTD
Quality metrics	PSNR in dB	33.86	34.38	30.57	31.95	3.71	36.07	25.97	25.57	27.69	24.86	30.94	31.61	40.38
	PSNR (Canny)in dB	20.51	20.14	18.20	22.76	9.07	25.85	22.46	23.24	21.85	28.13	23.22	34.18	35.97
	AD	0.43	0.20	0.42	0.28	72.51	0.22	12.02	14.50	9.25	16.04	22.20	0.19	0.46
	MSE	118.97	122.38	148.86	133.57	8974.82	105.52	169.29	170.42	164.25	188.52	125.58	122.61	64.27
	MD	161.41	49.70	182.32	156.59	193.47	49.33	99.37	120.31	85.57	133.26	172.38	175.45	133.26
	NAE	0.04	0.04	0.06	0.05	0.97	0.04	0.17	0.28	0.13	0.23	0.32	0.11	0.09
	CNR	6.64	3.81	5.21	3.41	3.85	3.81	3.32	3.73	2.85	3.97	5.03	6.30	6.57
	FoM	0.66	0.69	0.63	0.66	0.25	0.81	0.60	0.61	0.70	0.71	0.50	0.61	0.73
Similarity metrics	SC	1.24	1.27	1.25	1.24	29.45	1.28	0.99	0.95	1.04	0.96	0.84	1.26	1.24
	CoC	0.98	0.98	0.98	0.96	0.47	0.98	0.97	0.96	0.97	0.97	0.95	0.97	0.99
	NCC	0.97	0.98	0.98	0.98	0.04	0.98	0.96	0.98	0.98	0.94	0.91	0.97	0.98
	IQI	0.97	0.98	0.96	0.97	0.32	0.97	0.97	0.97	0.98	0.96	0.92	0.97	0.98
	GAE	0.00	0.00	0.00	0.00	0.00	0.00	0.00	0.00	0.00	0.00	0.00	0.00	0.00
	NMSE	1.70	3.82	8.35	2.64	9.72	3.80	3.13	4.50	1.90	5.48	1.24	1.42	1.61
	MSSIM	0.84	0.88	0.76	0.70	0.06	0.98	0.65	0.64	0.73	0.49	0.34	0.49	0.64
	SI	0.37	0.36	0.35	0.34	0.22	0.41	0.38	0.37	0.42	0.38	0.32	0.41	0.44
Speckle metrics	ASNR	1.58	1.58	1.60	1.59	1.34	1.58	1.71	1.69	1.65	1.70	1.86	1.64	1.61
	IV	0.41	0.39	0.39	0.38	238.31	0.37	0.47	0.46	0.45	0.48	0.11	0.52	0.48
	NSD	5.11	5.15	5.12	5.16	2.77	5.15	6.94	7.36	6.50	7.62	8.85	5.15	5.18
	ENL	2.21	2.19	2.20	2.18	14.18	2.19	1.63	1.59	1.74	1.50	1.30	2.19	2.17
	Execution time in sec	10.42	2.41	12.18	13.36	17.92	3.36	4.37	5.96	2.62	2.07	3.25	3.73	29.76

Table B5 Comparison of execution time of algorithms tested on the four images in the PCMAT and PCDSK systems

Images	System	Frost	Median	Lee	Kuan	Homo morphic	Wiener	En. Frost	En Lee	GAM	Wavelet	PMAD	SRAD	DTD
Gall-Bladder	PCMAT	17.82	4.57	23.78	26.12	5.16	4.52	18.52	25.89	20.45	2.59	8.74	7.16	38.56
	PCDSK	7.12	2.64	12.81	13.66	17.65	3.36	4.33	5.46	4.35	1.34	5.27	3.41	29.32
Heart	PCMAT	18.57	4.52	23.35	26.14	4.74	3.89	19.12	25.08	21.19	3.52	9.57	8.78	37.41
	PCDSK	8.19	2.18	11.57	4.13	17.63	2.13	4.14	5.73	2.39	2.27	4.63	3.27	24.53
Lungs	PCMAT	16.83	4.19	22.32	24.17	4.11	4.28	17.89	23.14	19.08	3.52	7.42	6.43	37.08
	PCDSK	9.17	3.66	12.34	13.62	17.36	3.87	3.65	4.27	2.31	2.26	3.17	3.94	24.42
Pancreas-Spleen	PCMAT	18.23	4.17	23.78	26.52	4.81	3.89	18.13	24.89	20.73	3.74	8.92	7.56	38.17
	PCDSK	10.42	2.41	12.18	13.36	17.92	3.36	4.37	5.96	2.62	2.07	3.25	3.73	29.76
Average execution time (sec)	PCMAT	17.862	4.362	23.307	25.737	4.705	4.145	18.415	24.75	20.362	3.342	8.662	7.482	37.805
	PCDSK	8.725	2.722	12.225	11.192	17.64	3.18	4.122	5.355	2.917	1.985	4.08	3.587	27.007
Difference in Average execution time in sec		9.137	1.64	11.082	14.545	-12.935	0.965	14.293	19.395	17.445	1.357	4.582	3.895	10.798

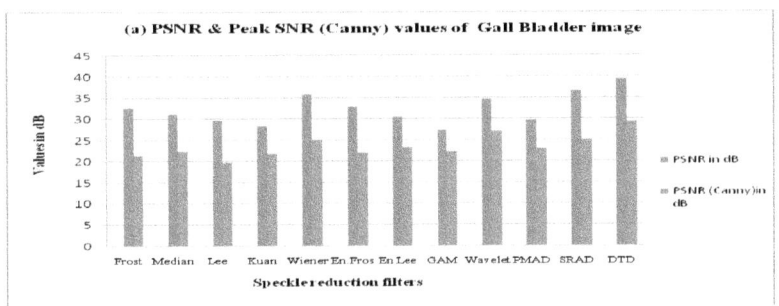
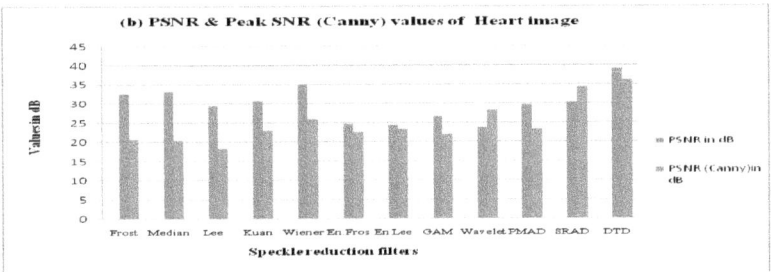
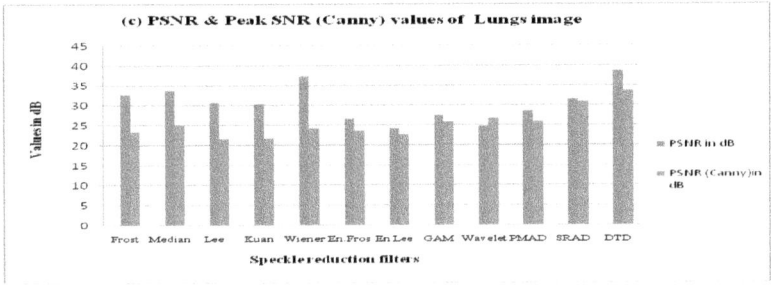
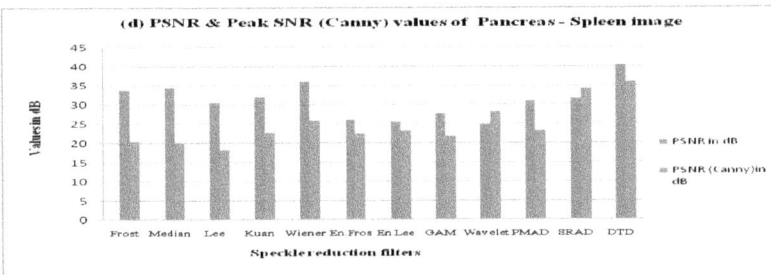

Fig B9 Histogram plot of the PSNR and Peak SNR (Canny) in the PCDSK system

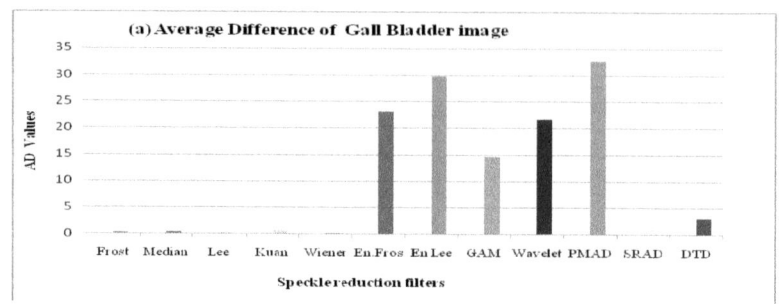
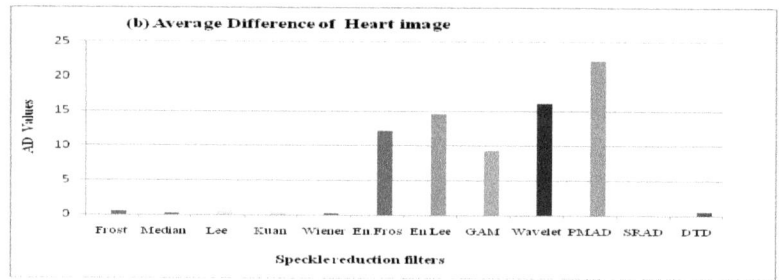
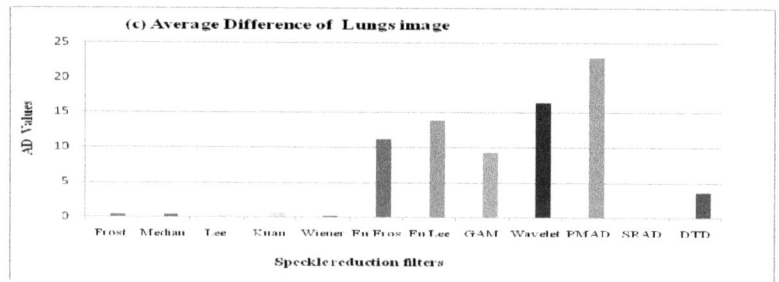
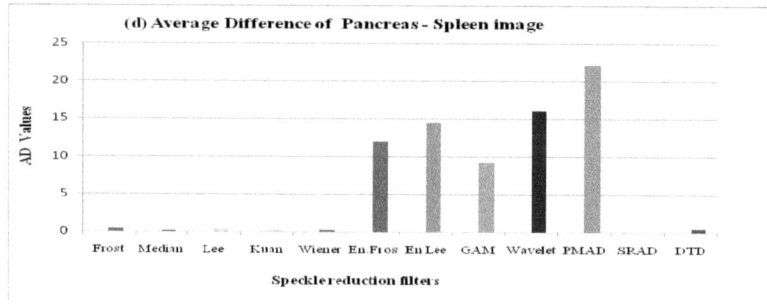

Fig B10 Histogram plot of the Average Difference (AD) in the PCDSK system

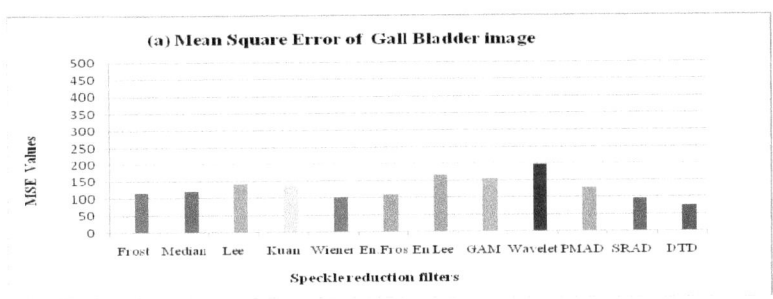

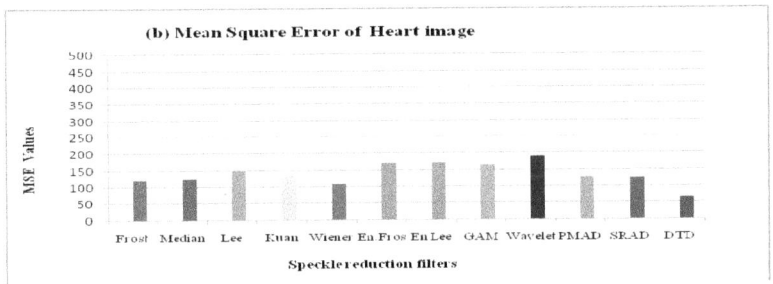

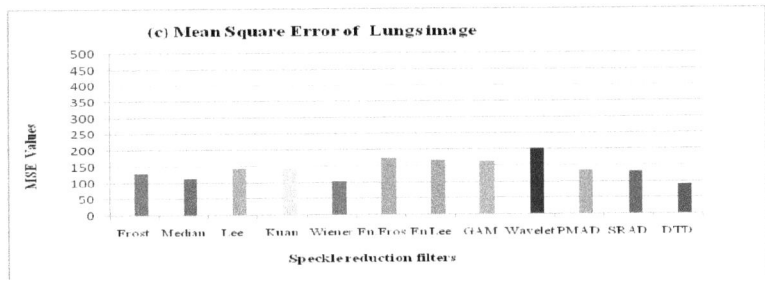

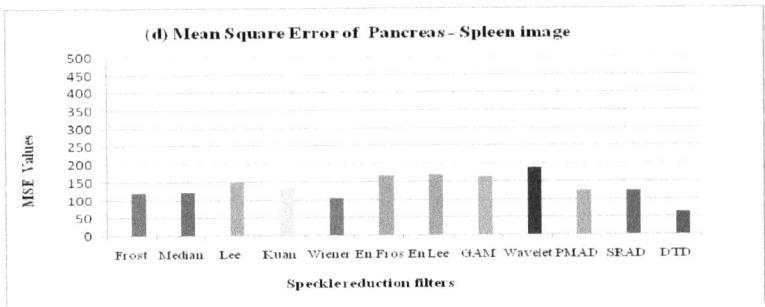

Fig B11 Histogram plot of the Mean Square Error (MSE) in the PCDSK system

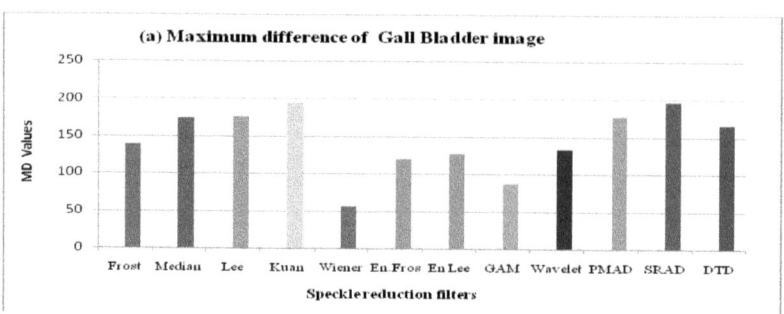
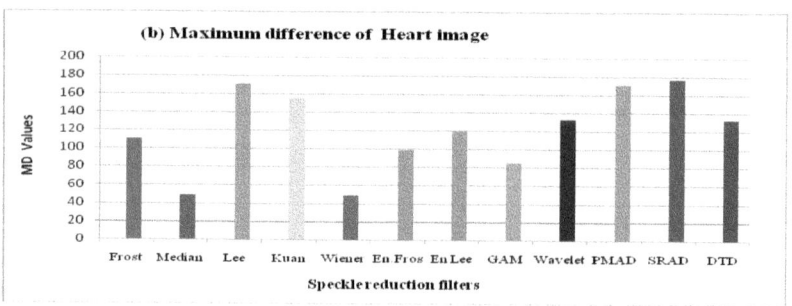
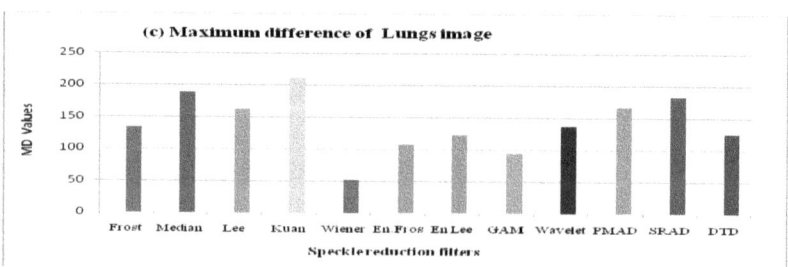
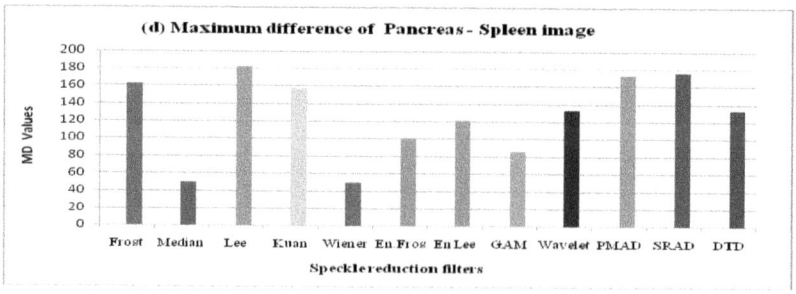

Fig B12 Histogram plot of the Maximum Difference (MD) in the PCDSK system

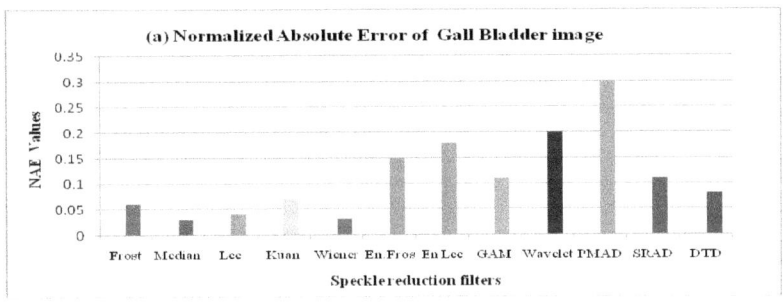
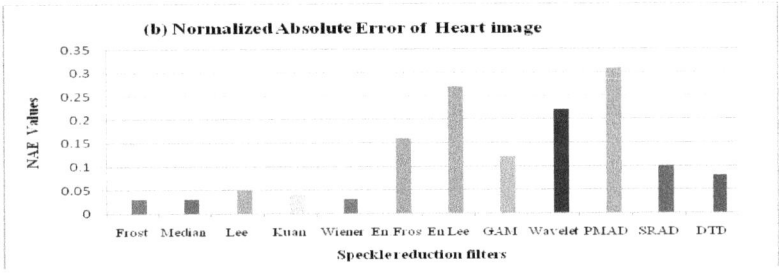
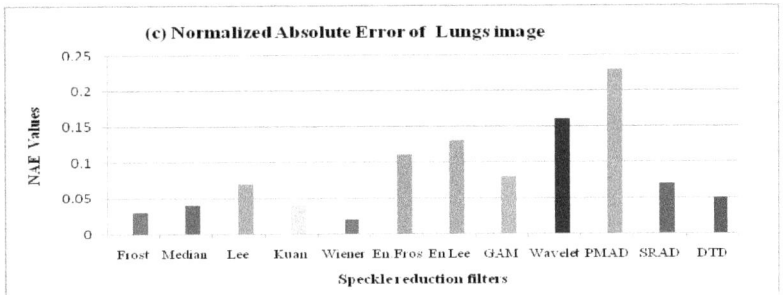
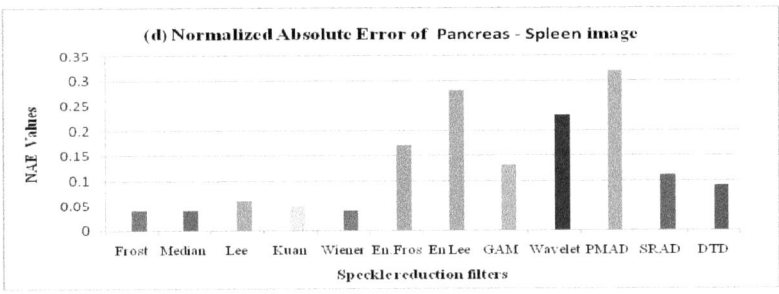

Fig B13 Histogram plot of the Normalized Absolute Error (NAE) in the PCDSK system

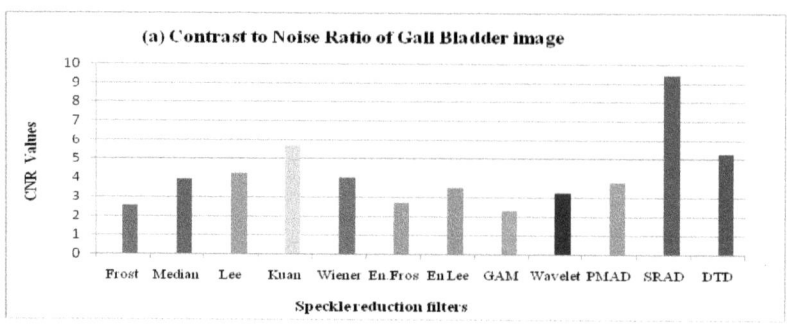
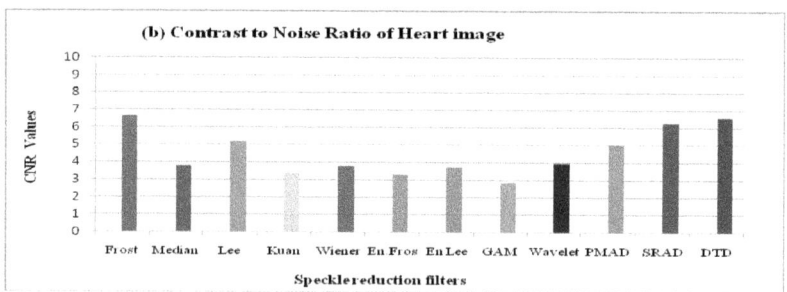
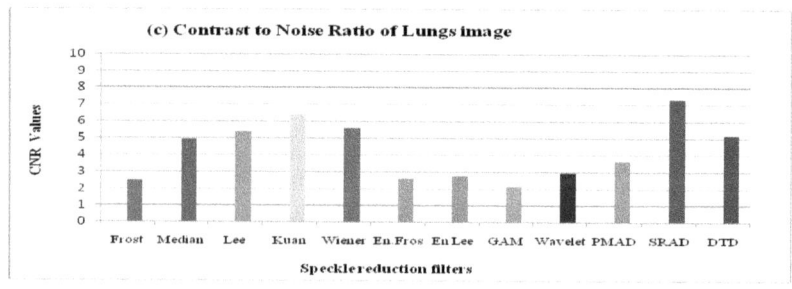
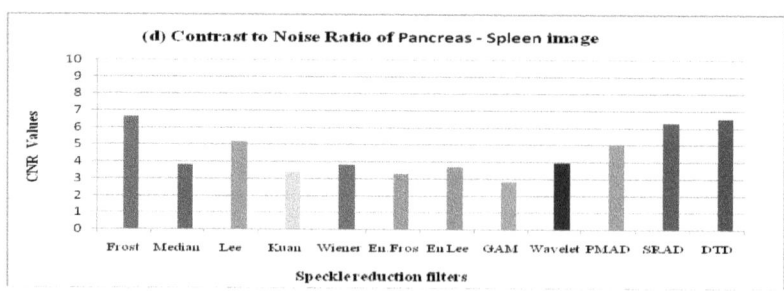

Fig B14 Histogram plot of the Contrast to Noise Ratio (CNR) in the PCDSK system

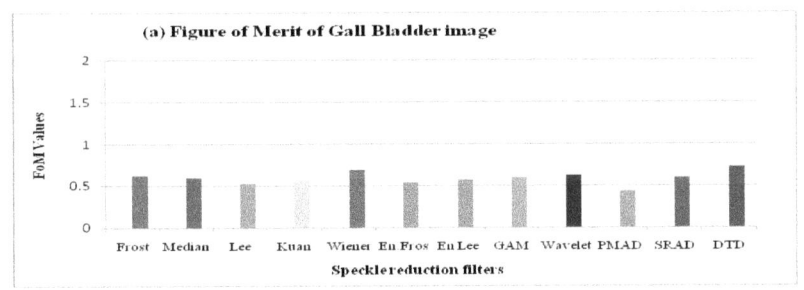
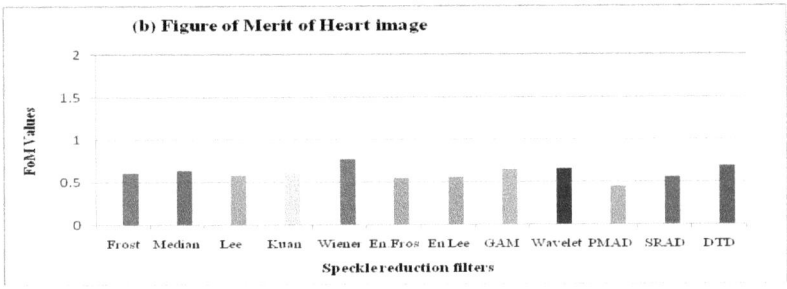
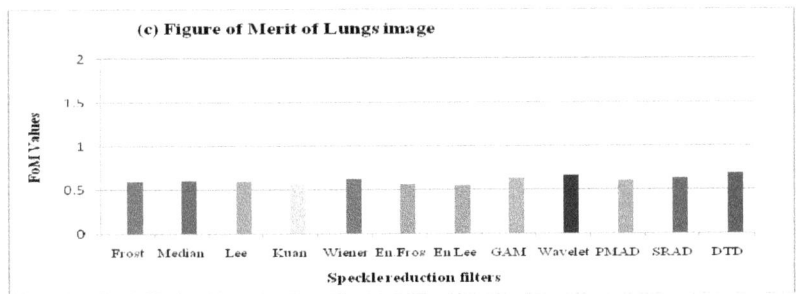
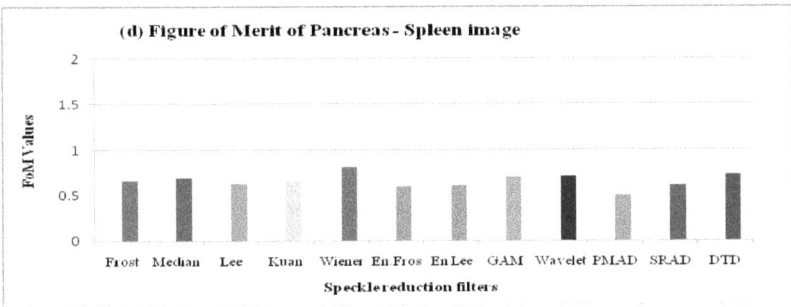

Fig B15 Histogram plot of the Figure of Merit (FoM) in the PCDSK system

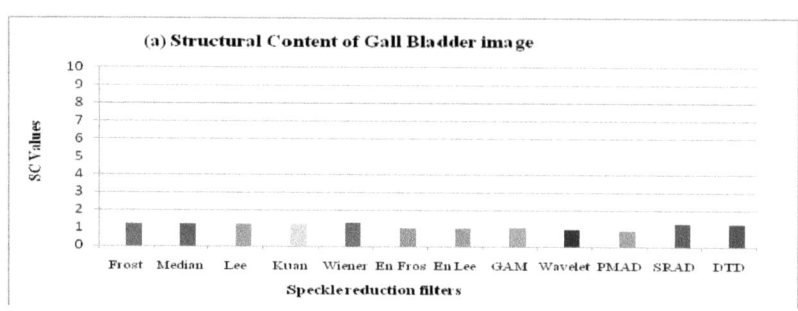
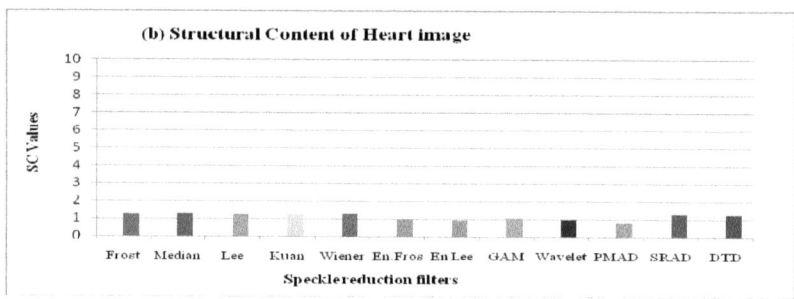
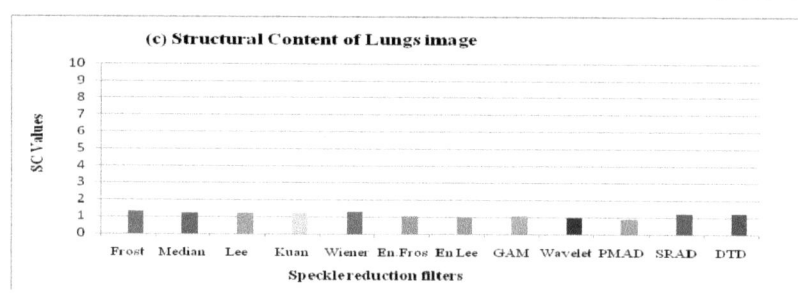
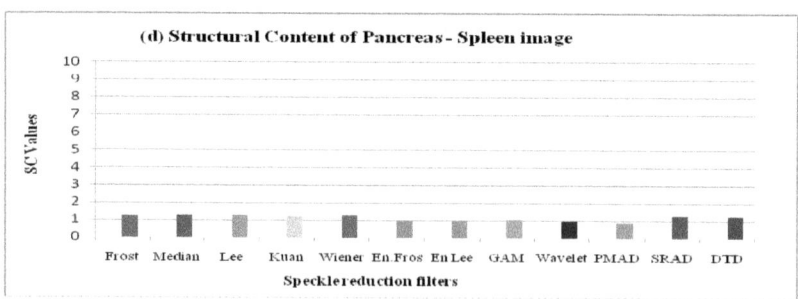

Fig B16 Histogram plot of the Structural Content (SC) in the PCDSK system

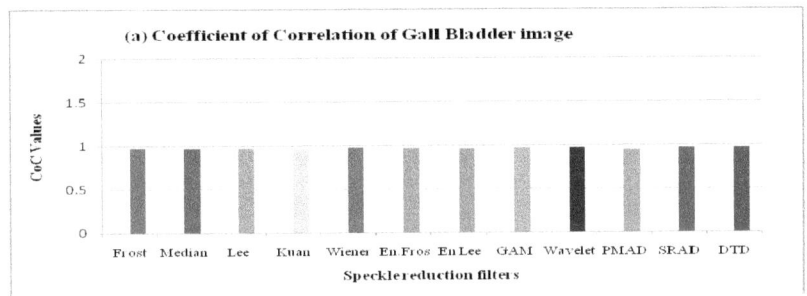
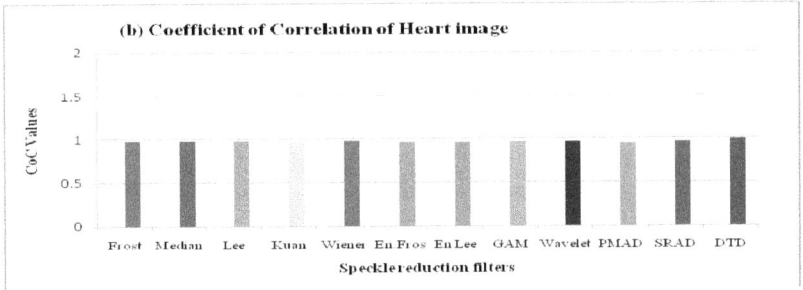
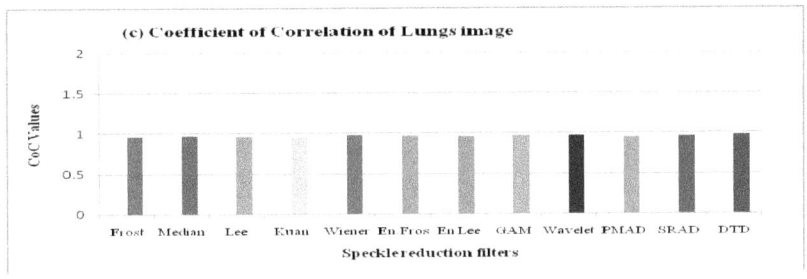
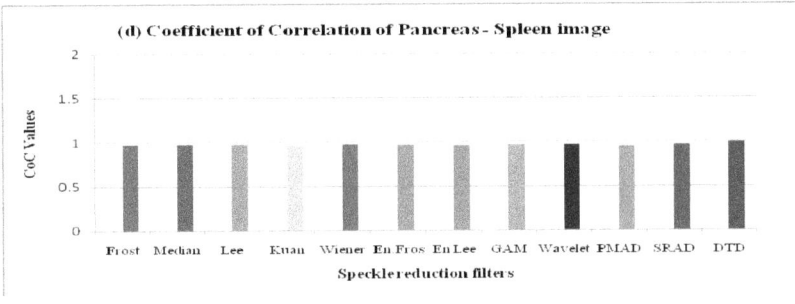

Fig B17 Histogram plot of the Coefficient of Correlation (CoC) in the PCDSK system

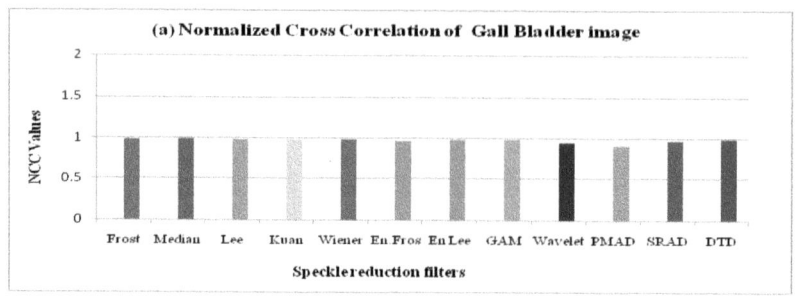
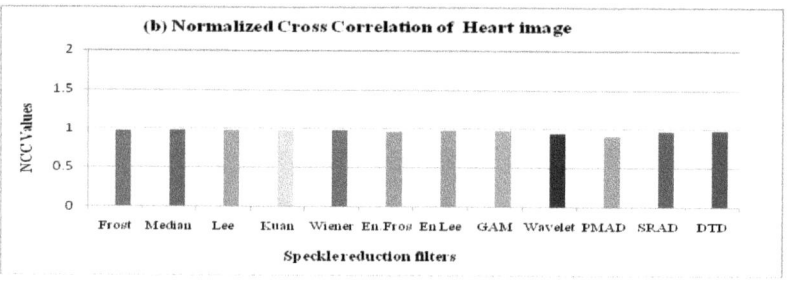
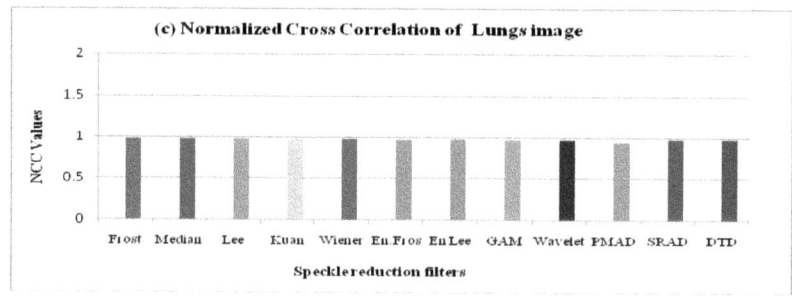
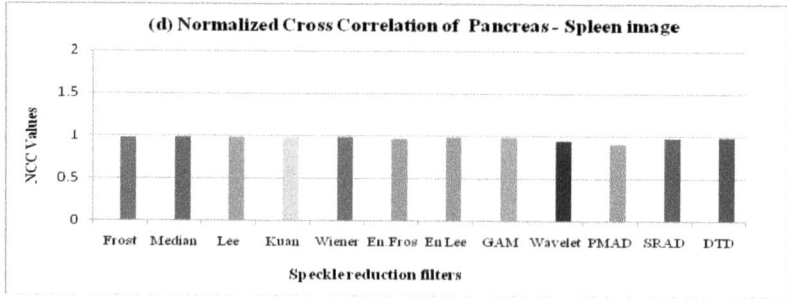

Fig B18 Histogram plot of the Normalized Cross Correlation (NCC) in the PCDSK system

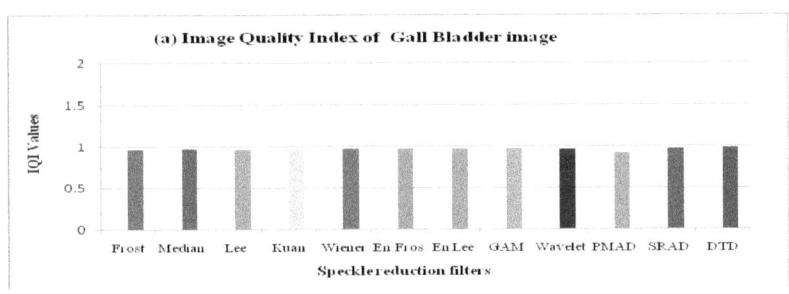
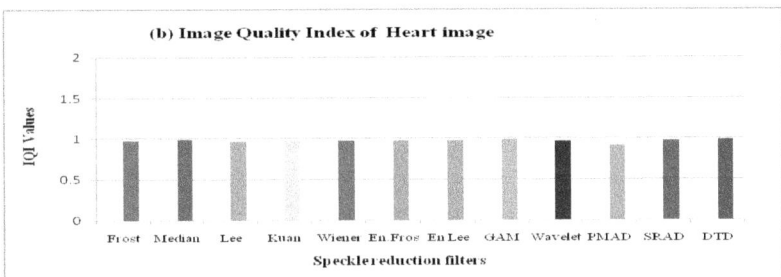
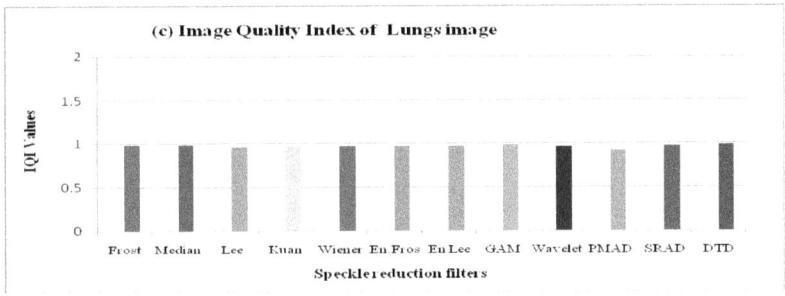
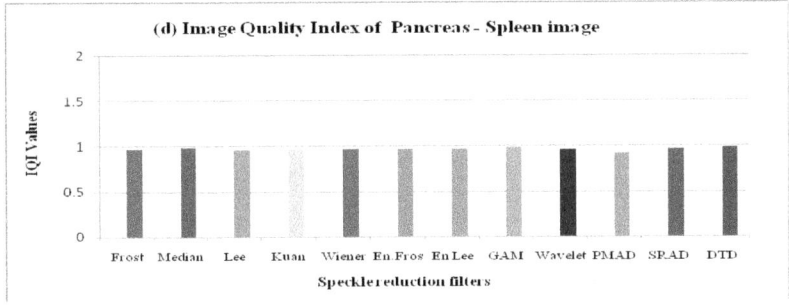

Fig B19 Histogram plot of the Image Quality Index (IQI) in the PCDSK system

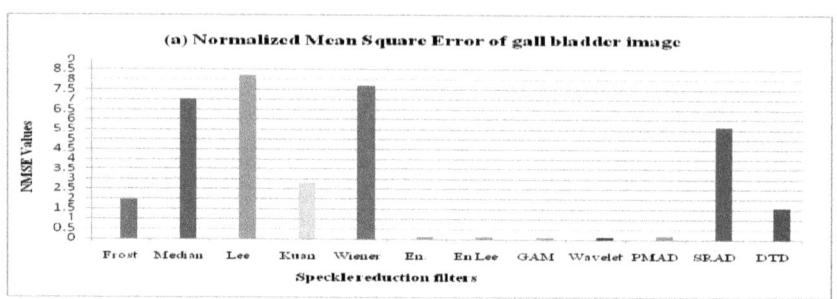
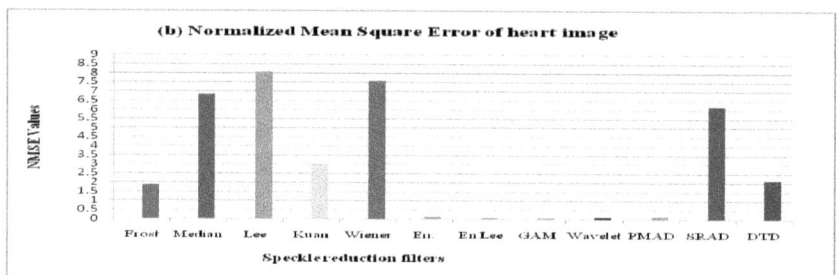
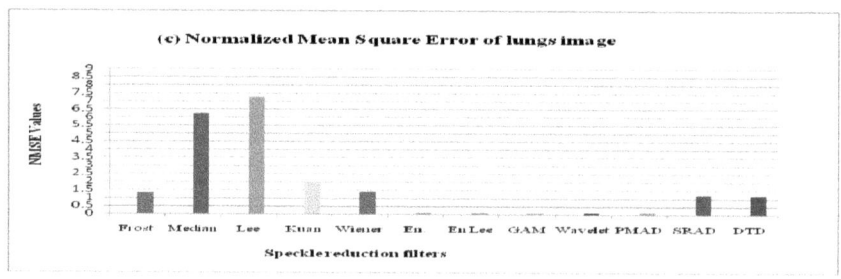
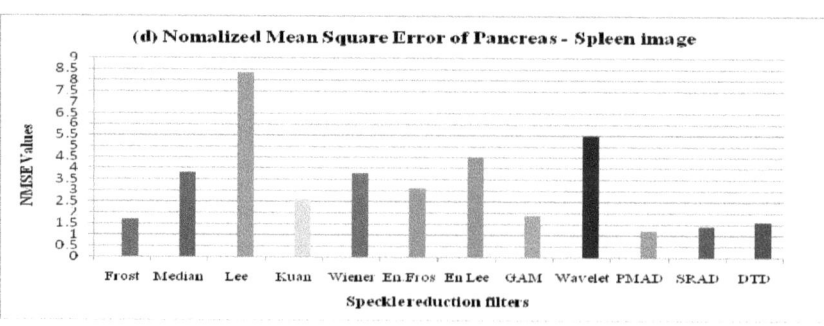

Fig B20 Histogram plot of the Normalized Mean Square Error (NMSE) in the PCDSK system

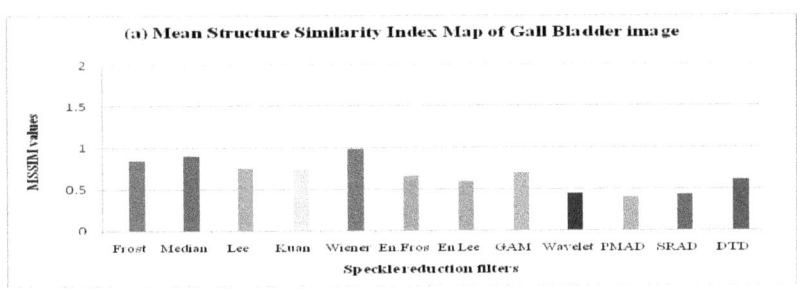
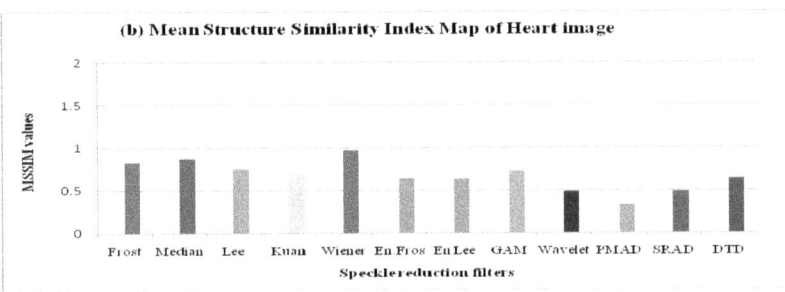
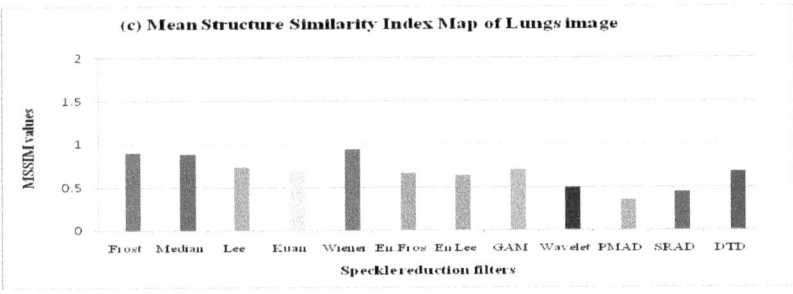
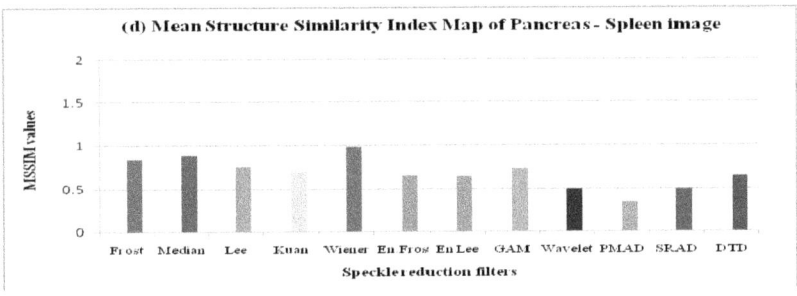

Fig B21 Histogram plot of the Mean Structure Similarity Index Map (MSSIM) in the PCDSK system

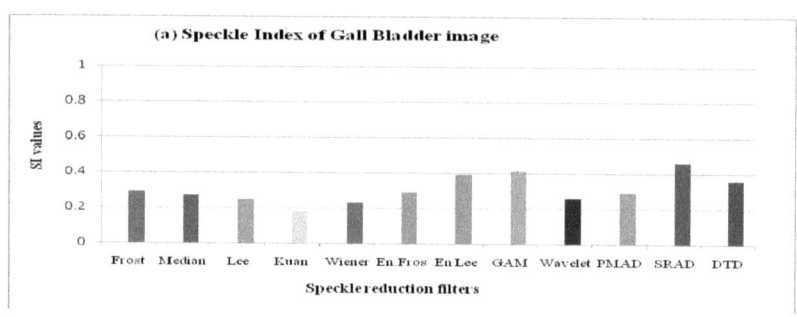
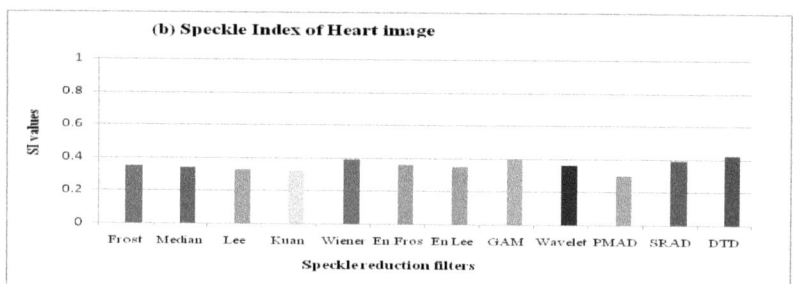
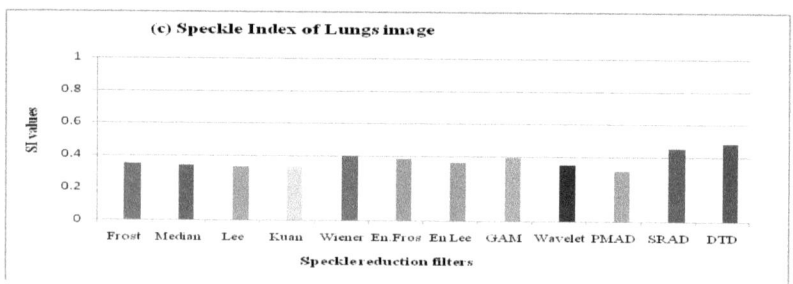
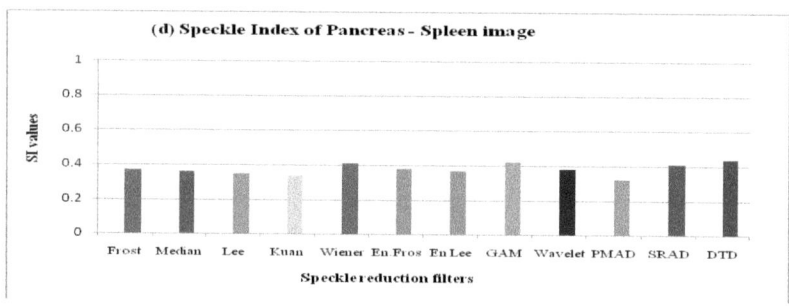

Fig B22 Histogram plot of the Speckle Index (SI) in the PCDSK system

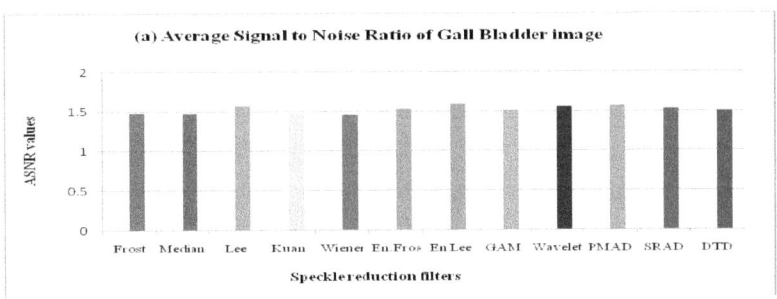
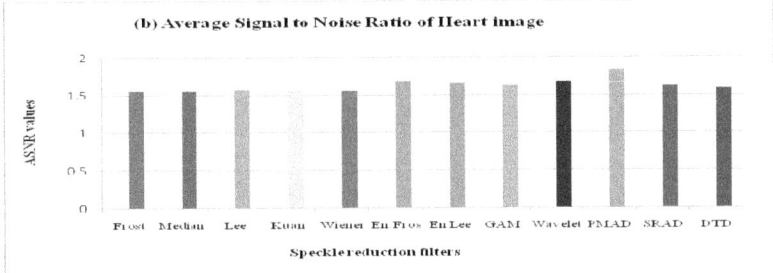
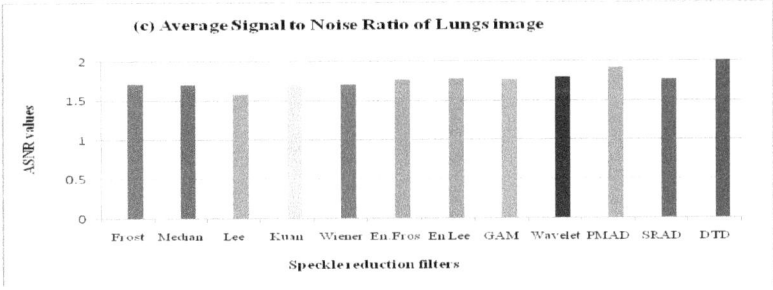
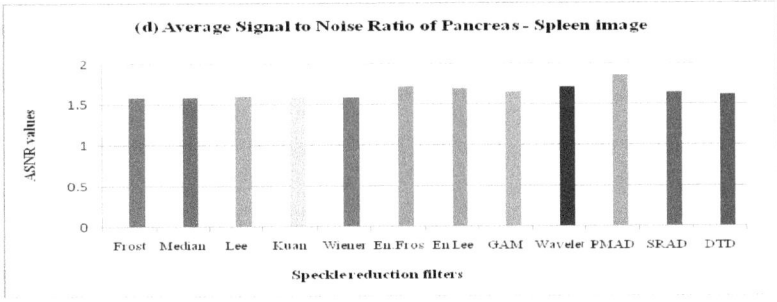

Fig B23 Histogram plot of the Average Signal to Noise Ratio (ASNR) in the PCDSK system

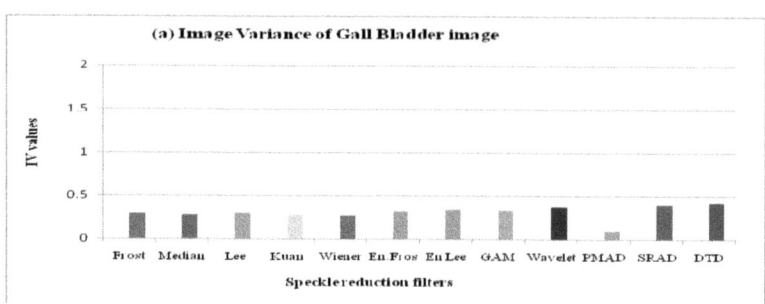
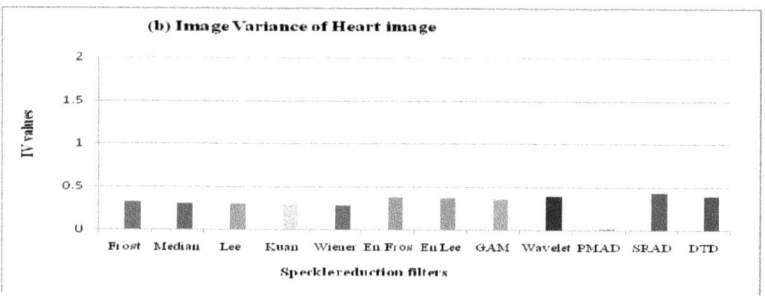
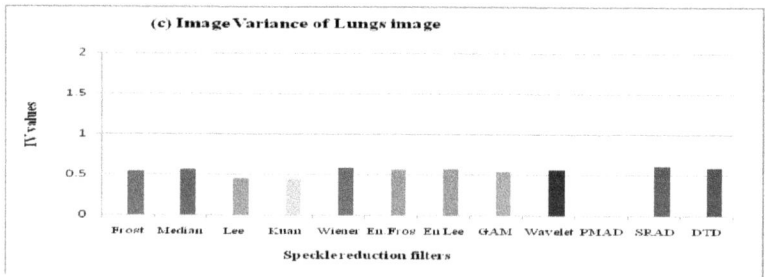
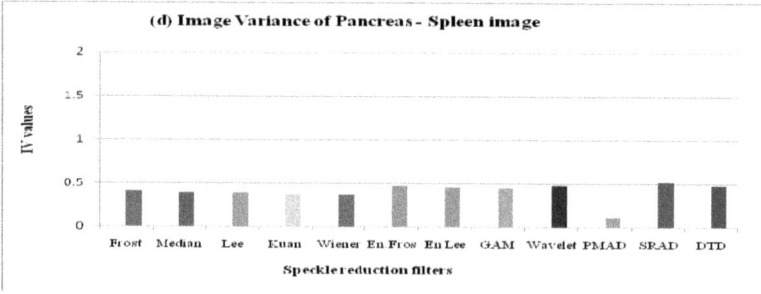

Fig B24 Histogram plot of the Image Variance (IV) in the PCDSK system

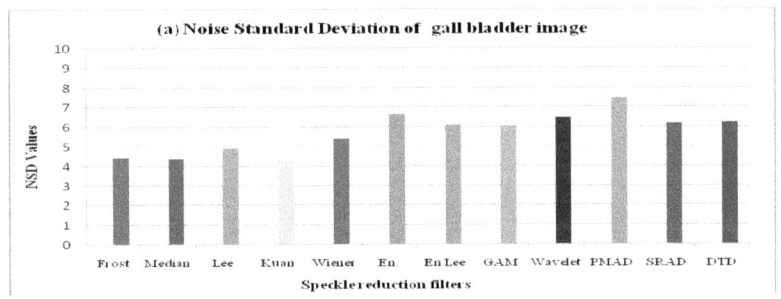
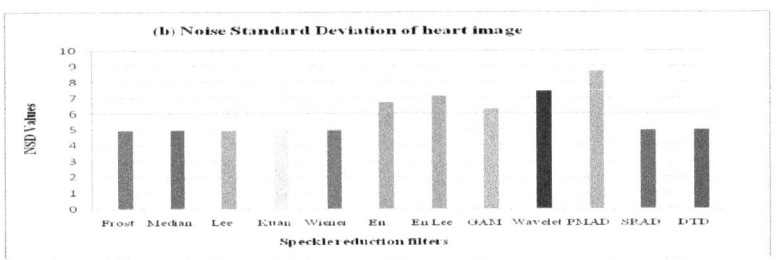
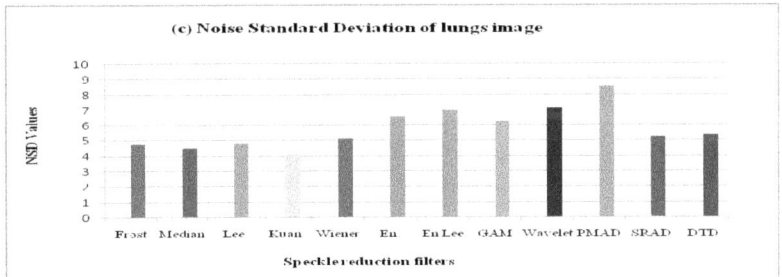
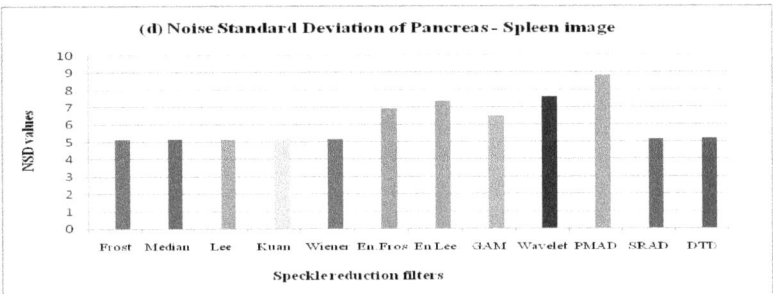

Fig B25 Histogram plot of the Noise Standard Deviation (NSD) in the PCDSK system

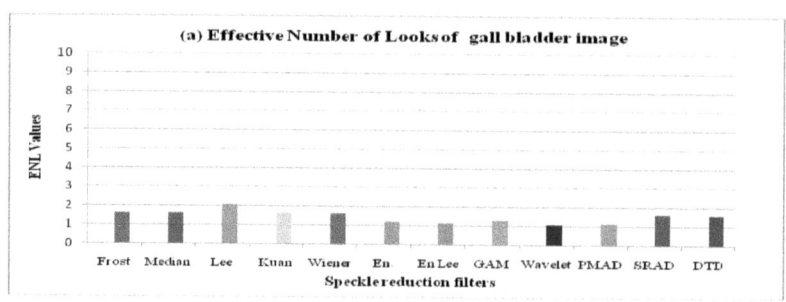
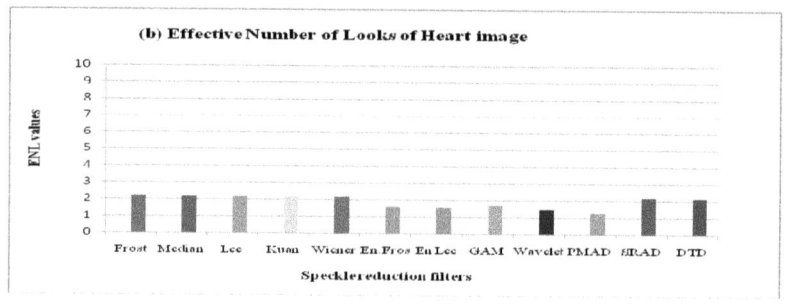
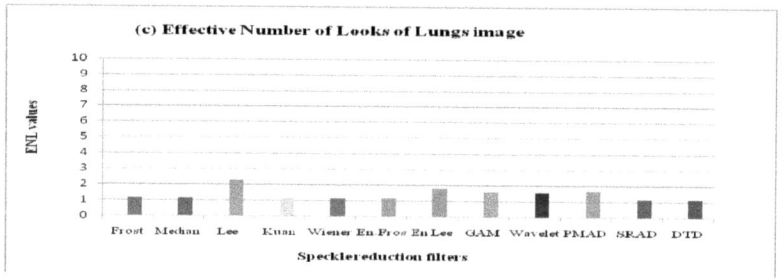
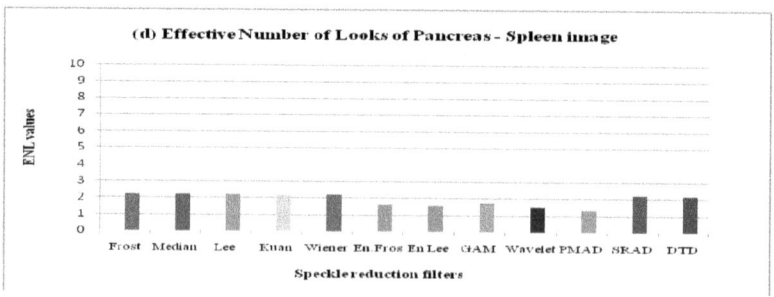

Fig B26 Histogram plot of the Effective Number of Looks in the PCDSK system

www.ingramcontent.com/pod-product-compliance
Ingram Content Group UK Ltd.
Pitfield, Milton Keynes, MK11 3LW, UK
UKHW022228230426
12048UKWH00016BA/1131